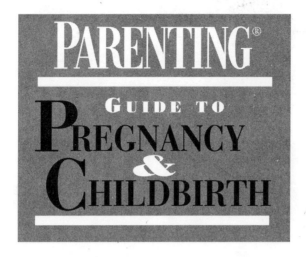

PARENTING®

GUIDE TO
PREGNANCY
&
CHILDBIRTH

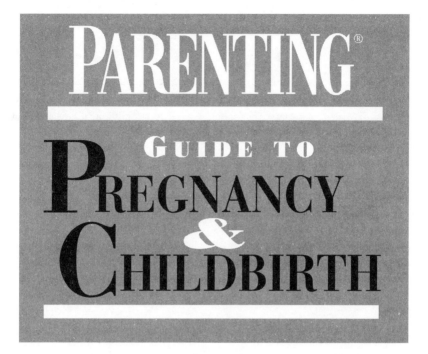

PARENTING®

GUIDE TO
PREGNANCY & CHILDBIRTH

Paula Spencer
with the Editors of PARENTING Magazine

BALLANTINE BOOKS
NEW YORK

A Ballantine Book
Published by The Ballantine Publishing Group

Copyright © 1998 by PARENTING Magazine

All rights reserved under International and Pan-American Copyright Conventions. Published in the United States by The Ballantine Publishing Group, a division of Random House, Inc., New York, and simultaneously in Canada by Random House of Canada Limited, Toronto.

http://www.randomhouse.com

Library of Congress Cataloging-in-Publication Data
Spencer, Paula.
   Parenting guide to pregnancy and childbirth / Paula Spencer with the editors of Parenting magazine. — 1st ed.
      p.   cm.
   Includes index.
   ISBN 0-345-41179-X (pbk.)
   1. Pregnancy.   2. Childbirth.   I. Parenting (San Francisco, Calif.)   II. Title.
RG525.S648 1998
618.2—dc21   97-35736
                                                                              CIP
Text design by Michaelis/Carpelis Design Assoc., Inc.
Cover design by Dreu Pennington-McNeil
Cover photo by David Roth; stylist, Karen Kozlowski; hair and makeup, Annaliese

Manufactured in the United States of America

First Edition: March 1998

10 9 8 7 6 5 4 3 2 1

CONTENTS

Foreword   xi

Acknowledgments   xiii

Medical Advisory Board   xv

Introduction   xvii

If You're Not Yet Pregnant . . .   2

CHAPTER 1: YOUR FIRST TRIMESTER (Conception to Twelve Weeks)   5

Week-by-Week Highlights   6

What's Going on in Your Body   8
Am I pregnant? • Confirming a pregnancy • When is your due date?
• Calculate your due date • Common aches and pains • Avoiding
infections • Checklist: What to watch out for • Checklist: When to call
the doctor • *Mother to Mother:* "How I quit smoking"

What's Going on in Your Head   28
Conflicting thoughts • More ways to feel good • Good Advice: Spreading
the news • *Mother to Mother:* "I worried about a prior miscarriage" • *Mother to
Mother:* "Going it alone"

Checkups and Tests   35
Choosing a caregiver • The first exam • First-trimester tests • Cautions on
prenatal testing • Genetic counseling • Checklist: Questions to ask at your first
visit • Good Advice: Getting the most out of checkups • CVS or amnio?

What Should I Eat?   48
Why this trimester is unique • Healthy practices to start now • How much weight gain? • If you're overweight at the start • Try these recipes! • Checklist: Best/worst foods for the first trimester • Filling in the "problem four" • Good Advice: How to drink more water • *Mother to Mother:* "Eating vegetarian" • *Mother to Mother:* "I was overweight at the start"

Fit for Pregnancy   63
Why be in shape? • Rating the workouts • Expect differences • How much is enough? • Good habits to start now • Prenatal exercise class • Checklist: Who should exercise caution?

The Pregnant Look   69
Early changes • No-waistline dressing tricks • Good Advice: Buying comfortable lingerie

What About Sex?   74
Libido lost and found • Staying close • Checklist: When to abstain

Special Situations   76
Who's high-risk? • Multiple pregnancy • First-trimester bleeding • Early miscarriage • Ectopic pregnancy • Checklist: Could I be expecting multiples? • *Mother to Mother:* "It's twins!"

Work Worries   87
Telling your colleagues • Planning your leave • Avoiding hazards on the job • Staying productive • Good Advice: Negotiating a better leave • Checklist: Insurance questions

Other Big Deals   94
Dealing with the "pregnancy police" • Traveling • Choosing baby names • *Mother to Mother:* "Mum's the word"

CHAPTER 2: YOUR SECOND TRIMESTER (Thirteen to Twenty-eight Weeks)   99

Week-by-Week Highlights   99

What's Going on in Your Body   102
Common aches and pains • The kick-off kick • Dental care • Sleeping smart

What's Going on in Your Head   109
Smooth sailing • Body image • Test anxiety • *Mother to Mother:* "Being pregnant made me finally like my body" • Good Advice: On advice givers

Checkups and Tests 113
Second-trimester exams • *Mother to Mother:* "We had a prenatal test scare"

What Should I Eat? 118
Nutrition basics now • Are nutrition shortcuts okay? • Try these recipes!
• Smart swaps • Good Advice: Sneaking in nutrients

Fit for Pregnancy 128
Exercising caution • Relaxation • The tip-top ten • Good Advice:
Remember to Kegel

The Pregnant Look 133
Maternity clothes: A buyer's and borrower's guide • Good Advice:
A professional look

What About Sex? 138
What's normal now? • Dad's views • *Mother to Mother:*
"Pregnant sex was great"

Special Situations 142
Gestational diabetes • Preterm labor • Late bleeding • Bedrest
• *Mother to Mother:* "Sentenced to bedrest"

Work Worries 147
Planning childcare • Which type of childcare? • Checklist: Smart snacks
to stash at your desk

Other Big Deals 150
Finding out: Boy or girl? • Choosing a childbirth class • Taking other
classes • Going out and about • Readying the nursery

CHAPTER 3: YOUR THIRD TRIMESTER (Twenty-nine to Forty Weeks) 159

Week-by-Week Highlights 159

What's Going on in Your Body 162
Preparing for the big day • How does your baby lie? • Common aches
and pains • Checklist: When to call your doctor • *Mother to Mother:*
"False alarm!"

What's Going on in Your Head 168
The fog • Nesting • Fears of the unknown • Pregnant dreams
• Good Advice: Pamper yourself in the homestretch • *Father to Father:*
"*We're* pregnant"

Checkups and Tests   175
Last-trimester visits • Planning for birth • Checklist: Your birth plan

What Should I Eat?   180
Do a diet check • Try these recipes!

Fit for Pregnancy   185
Posture basics

The Pregnant Look   187
Skin changes • Good Advice: When you're sick of maternity clothes

What About Sex?   190
Homestretch intimacy

Special Situations   190
Preeclampsia • Placenta problems • The overdue baby • *Mother to Mother:*
"My baby was born early" • *Mother to Mother:* "My 10-month pregnancy"

Work Worries   196
Preparing your exit • Seeking work-family balance

Other Big Deals   199
Decisions, decisions • Checklist: Before you deliver • Checklist: Best shower
gifts to ask for • Checklist: What to pack for delivery

CHAPTER 4: YOUR BABY'S BIRTH (Labor and Delivery)   215

The Right Attitude   217
Common worries about labor • Easing fears • The fashion factor

Is This It?   221
Signs of labor • At the hospital • True labor or false labor?
• Checklist: Alert your doctor if . . .

Childbirth Basics   230
Every labor's different • Stage one: Dilatation • Stage two: Pushing and
birth • Stage three: After the birth • Complications • *Mother to Mother:*
"My speedy labor" • *Mother to Mother:* "My labor lasted forever"
• *Mother to Mother:* "My home birth" • *Father to Father:*
"A dad's view of labor"

All About Pain   249
What does labor feel like? • Nonmedical pain management • Medical pain
management • Should you have an epidural? • Checklist: Ways coaches can

help • *Mother to Mother:* "My drug-free delivery" • *Mother to Mother:*
"My epidural" • *Mother to Mother:* "I felt all my labor in my back"

Special Situations   268
Cesarean birth • Vaginal birth after Cesarean (VBAC) • Multiple births
• *Mother to Mother:* "My two C-sections" • *Mother to Mother:* "My VBAC"

Right After Delivery   275
What happens to your baby • What happens to you • Baby's first test
• Good Advice: Newborn security • Checklist: Are you ready to go home?
• Checklist: Handy items to bring home

CHAPTER 5: YOUR "FOURTH TRIMESTER" (Recovery and Newborn Care) 287

What's Going on in Your Body   287
The biology of recovery • Cesarean recovery • Good Advice: Best rest ideas
• Checklist: When to call the doctor

What's Going on in Your Head   294
First feelings • The baby blues • Sanity savers • Checklist:
Have you been good to yourself today? • *Mother to Mother:* "I had
postpartum depression" • *Mother to Mother:* "Our road to sibling
revelry"

Checkups and Tests   302
The postpartum exam

Feeding Your Baby   303
Breastfeeding basics • Overcoming common setbacks • Expressing
breast milk • Checklist: For successful breastfeeding • Bottle-feeding
basics • Burping basics • Checklist: Is your baby eating enough?
• *Mother to Mother:* "I had trouble nursing at first" • Good Advice:
Public nursing

What Should I Eat?   322
Losing weight • Nutrition now • Try these recipes!

Fit for Motherhood   329
First exercises • Working up to workouts • A postpartum abdominal
workout • *Mother to Mother:* "How I got back in shape"

What About Sex?   335
When to resume? • But do I have to? • Making sex better • Birth control
after baby • *Mother to Mother:* "Give it time"

Newborn-Care Basics 342

Sleeping • Crying and colic • Swaddling • Dressing • Diapering • Cord and circumcision care • Bathing • Outings and visitors • Jaundice • Checkups • Not quite picture-perfect? • Checklist: When to call your pediatrician • Good Advice: Soothing baby's cries • *Mother to Mother:* "Easing early jitters"

Illustration Credits 363

Index 365

FOREWORD

From PARENTING's Editor

As the mother of two, I remember full well the joys of carrying a baby for nine months. But I also recall being filled with uncertainty during that time. Like Paula Spencer, the author of this guide, I read just about everything I could get my hands on.

But finding the explanations, reassurance, and advice I craved wasn't easy. Books about pregnancy abound, yet no single volume spoke to all my concerns. Some charted an expectant mom's physical journey but skipped her mental one. Others were full of cheery encouragement, but short on the sometimes annoying, sometimes worrisome, realities of pregnancy.

I realized what I wanted was a complete sourcebook, one that delivered answers to everything from the mystery of fetal development and mom-to-be's moods to the stages of labor and delivery. And I wanted one that presented the information in a way that was quick and easy to access. I wanted to be able to sort through a book on pregnancy in much the same way I could read a magazine article on the topic—much as we present information in Parenting magazine.

I wasn't alone. My frustrations reflected those of other staffers on our magazine as well as those of many of our readers. And so, you're holding a book that addresses a mother-to-be's concerns from the angle that Parenting knows best: what real women really want to know. Alongside the health facts, it covers the little concerns and big plans that make up the sum total of being pregnant. It prepares you for all you need to know during the miraculous nine months from conception to birth, and for the months that follow.

I know you'll find this book comprehensive, friendly, and easy to use—and that it will become your essential Guide to Pregnancy and Childbirth.

Janet Chan
Editor in Chief
PARENTING

ACKNOWLEDGMENTS

*J*ust as a mother requires the assistance of a whole team—partner, doctor, nurses, childbirth educator, et al.—to bring her baby into the world, so it was with the creation of this book. I am indebted to PARENTING's editor for franchise development, Bruce Raskin, for the opportunity to write it and for his line-by-line input and encouragement throughout its gestation.

I'd also like to thank the following individuals: For interviewing all the mothers whose profiles appear here, Heidi Kotansky. For their research assistance, Carrie Spector, Valerie Fahey, Kristen Philipkoski, and Laura Linden. For research and for writing most of the photo captions, Dawn Margolis. For providing the book's recipes, Kathy Gunst, author of *The PARENTING Cookbook*. For art and photo editing, Lisa Hilgers. For shooting many of the photos, David Roth. For her wonderful illustrations, Narda Lebo. For photo styling, Karen Kozlowski. For editorial assistance, Renee Swanson. I'm also indebted to Anne Krueger, Melanie Haiken, and Patti Anderson. And for providing detailed feedback on the manuscript, my thanks to the entire medical advisory board. For an additional medical eye, Ronald J. Reiss, M.D., F.A.C.O.G.

The book's ultimate midwife was Elisa Wares, senior editor at Ballantine Books.

I'm also grateful to all the parents and experts whom I've interviewed on these subjects over the years. Thanks, too, to the professionals who helped me transform all this academic information into personal experience during my own pregnancies and deliveries: Dr. Ken Taylor, Dr. Kathleen Edmunds, Dr. Donald Larmee, Sharon Fogarty, Cat Clayton, Rhonda Moretto, Susan Rutherford, and Jane Duarte.

Finally, deserving special credit are those to whom I dedicate this book: George, my husband and partner in parenthood and in life, and the fruits of our labors—Henry Hartsfield, Eleanor Louie, and Margaret Meriwether.

P.S.

The Medical Advisory Board for *Parenting Guide to Pregnancy and Childbirth*

Paula Spencer and the editors of PARENTING wish to thank the UCLA Center for Healthy Children, Families, and Communities and its affiliated faculty for carefully reviewing the manuscript of this book.

INTRODUCTION

When I'm reading up on a life-changing event—especially one, like pregnancy, that will change my body, my mind, my relationship, and nearly every other aspect of my life—I like to hear the unvarnished truth about it from an insider, from someone who's been there. Well, in the case of this book, I haven't just "been there," I was in the middle of being there as I wrote. In a stranger-than-fiction twist of fate, one Monday morning, the editors of PARENTING asked me if I would be interested in writing a book about pregnancy. On Tuesday, I realized that my period was late. A home-pregnancy test issued a bright blue line of confirmation. You can bet that my interest in writing such a book spiked higher than my hCG levels. (That's human chorionic gonadotrophin, a hormone that skyrockets in your system to say, "Yup, you're growing a baby.") What's more, my deadline for finishing the book turned out to be . . . the day before my due date.

Coincidence? Or something that was meant to be? Soon I was off and writing about first-trimester bladder changes between trips to the bathroom—and without the benefit of my usual deadline fuel, coffee and M&Ms. (Alas, I'd lost all taste for them.) By the second trimester, it was easy to write about what it felt like to feel a baby move; all I had to do was pause at the keyboard and wait for a kick. I could also empathize with questions like "What should I do if the alpha-fetoprotein test looks suspicious?" and "How can I survive bedrest without going crazy?" And so it went for nine months. I delivered the manuscript 10 days early "just in case," then promptly delivered the baby early too. Finally, I revised the finished text while childbirth and the first weeks with a newborn were fresh in my mind—and by then, in another coincidence, my editor at Ballantine, Elisa Wares, was expecting as well.

The lucky timing of writing a pregnancy guide while I was pregnant enabled me to tune in to the minutiae of these special months in a much keener way than if I were strictly doing research and looking back on my previous four experiences. (I'd already had two children, ages 4 and 2, and two miscarriages.) This in-the-trenches perspective also reminded me what a topsy-turvy experience having a baby is. I love being pregnant. But that's not to say I loved every minute of every pregnancy. The high of hearing the fetal heartbeat was balanced by the low of having heartburn. I welcomed going to my doctor's appointments but dreaded giving blood for tests (and worrying about the potential results). Along with every fun decision about how to decorate the nursery seemed to lurk a cranky argument with my husband over what to name the baby. And let's not talk about varicose veins.

Being pregnant also allowed me to capture the endless questions, big and small, that shadow a woman like so many curious toddlers during this unique slice of life. Is it safe to eat this? Was that twitch normal? Is it really true (as my own mom cautioned) that reaching my arms over my head would cause the umbilical cord to knot?

The first time I was pregnant, for example, I was dogged by a secret terror that I'd be inept at motherhood. I was the one who'd always tiptoe backward out of the office when a young child came to visit the place I worked. I'd never baby-sat. I'd never even held an infant. To bolster my confidence, my husband and I took a newborn parenting course. It covered all the basics: breastfeeding, burping, bathing, and so on. Then came a chance for hands-on experience, diapering lifelike baby dolls. I cowered. I hung back and let my husband go first. When he insisted I try, I flushed. I fumbled. Yes, I even dropped the doll. Eight months pregnant, hurtling toward motherhood with no turning back, I cried all the way home. But then, just a few weeks later, this same apprehensive mama-to-be soldiered through 12 hours of labor and greeted a new day with a slippery, robust newborn in her arms. A baby! I did it! And now, several pregnancies later, here I am, writing a book about the subject. Believe me, if I can ease through pregnancy to parenthood—loving it—anyone can.

That's why, above all, this is a real person's guide to having a baby. Both practical and reassuring, it's fully appreciative of the fact that everyone—and every pregnancy—is different. It presents a total picture of pregnancy and childbirth, from the latest medical facts to enduring old wives' tales, from what's going on in your body to what's going on in your head and your heart and even your closet. You'll find explanations, advice, and ideas. But it skips the preachy lectures and scientific treatises that sound more pre-med than prenatal.

Such a guide is not, of course, created from one mom's experiences alone; I've woven together the perspectives of doctors, nurses, childbirth educators, scientists, and researchers. Importantly, you'll also read the advice of other expectant parents, who know that pregnancy is about more than measuring your fundus and consuming folic acid. (Though you can be sure those important details are here too!)

I tried to organize the book the way a pregnant woman thinks. (Again, gestating while I typed really helped.) Each 3-month trimester is handled separately and in depth, to reflect the unique differences between early, middle, and late pregnancy. Covered within each trimester are all of the main preoccupations of a pregnant woman's life: Physical changes, emotional changes, health-care visits, diet, exercise, sexuality, appearance, work, and "other big deals" (such as decorating a nursery and choosing a pediatrician). Labor and the first weeks with a newborn merit their own chapters.

This book is for women like you, who—like me—in the course of 9 amazing months will find themselves transformed, from big-bellied blank slates to experience-rich mothers. May it help make your long strange trip the best it can be, with the happiest ending.

Paula Spencer

P.S. In my case, that happy ending was an 8-pound, 9-ounce daughter named Margaret Meriwether Spencer.

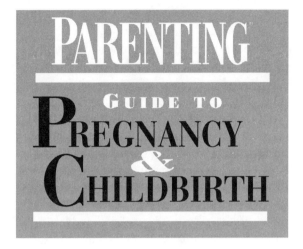

PARENTING

GUIDE TO

PREGNANCY
&
CHILDBIRTH

If You're Not Yet Pregnant . . .

Your timing's wonderful if you picked up this book because you're thinking about having a baby or have recently abandoned birth control to try to conceive. In recent years, doctors have learned plenty about what a woman can do even before she conceives to better her odds of an uncomplicated 9 months' gestation and the safe delivery of a healthy baby. Called *pre-pregnancy planning*, it involves making health, nutrition, and lifestyle adjustments based on the latest medical knowledge.

And you thought all the action started once your pregnancy test turned positive!

In fact, planning ahead for pregnancy is more commonsensical than complicated. No one can guarantee you a perfect baby, of course. But following the guidelines below can help ferret out many serious threats to a child's well-being. (Many of these topics are covered in depth later in the book.) Take advantage of the extra time you have now to make these smart, baby-healthy changes.

• **Get a preconceptional checkup.** Why see an obstetrician-gynecologist even before you've conceived? Because it can be the most important doctor visit of your pregnancy. He or she can give your overall health a green light or help you identify and clear up any problems that could interfere with fertility or a healthy pregnancy. If you haven't had or haven't been exposed to rubella (German measles), for example, an inoculation at least 3 to 6 months before you conceive can protect you against this common cause of birth defects. Diabetics can drastically reduce their risk of miscarriage or defects by controlling blood-sugar levels before they conceive. You'll also get advice on how to safely stop birth control, keep accurate menstrual records, time intercourse to conceive, and care for yourself in early pregnancy, such as by taking vitamin supplements. That's vital stuff, considering that the first prenatal appointment typically takes place after you've been pregnant for 2 months or more, once your baby's genetic map is already unfolding. If hereditary disorders run in your family, special tests and counseling can help, too. Be frank about your medical and lifestyle history.

This checkup also gives you the opportunity to evaluate your caregiver: Is he or she attentive and informative? Do you share philosophies about childbirth? If you have reservations, begin interviewing new doctors or midwives now.

• **Take care of dental work, mammograms, and other special health needs.** You won't want to get X-rayed, for example, while pregnant if you can avoid it.

• **Kick dangerous habits.** You probably already know that smoking, drinking, and taking illicit drugs don't mix with motherhood. Quitting can be tough—but *not* quitting once you're pregnant is worse. So give yourself a head start now to do it right.

• *Avoid hazardous substances.* Some potential dangers—passive smoke, pesticides—are obvious. Others may surprise you, including hot tubs, certain vitamin supplements, and cat litter. Kelp supplements, for example, are high in iodine and can cause fetal thyroid abnormalities. The oral acne drug Accutane increases the risk of miscarriage and birth defects and should be suspended at least 2 months before you try to conceive. Review your home and work routines. Check with your doctor about any nutrition supplements or medications you take. Note that some of these hazards affect the father's sperm, too. (See Checklist: "What to Watch Out For," page 20)

• *Stock up on nutrients—particularly folate.* A balanced diet helps improve your overall health and fertility. There are also specific foods to stock up on now, most notably those containing folate (folic acid), which has been linked to neural tube defects (such as spinal bifida) in the babies of women who didn't consume enough of it before pregnancy and during the first weeks after conception. Women planning to conceive should consume 800 micrograms of folate a day. If you've been on birth-control pills, are a vegetarian, or have certain health problems, your folate reserves may be especially depleted and a supplement may be prescribed. Vegetarians should review their entire diet with an expert.

• *Shape up while you can.* Start by getting as close to your optimal weight as possible. Overweight mothers tend to have more complications in pregnancy (such as gestational diabetes) and larger babies that result in harder deliveries—not to mention more trouble getting back in shape afterward. Underweight women may have difficulty conceiving or nourishing a fetus. What's more, if you're accustomed to regular exercise before you conceive, you're apt to feel better and weather the ordinary strains of pregnancy better than someone who's out of shape. It's dangerous to diet or to start any ambitious or new exercise program during pregnancy, so make the effort now.

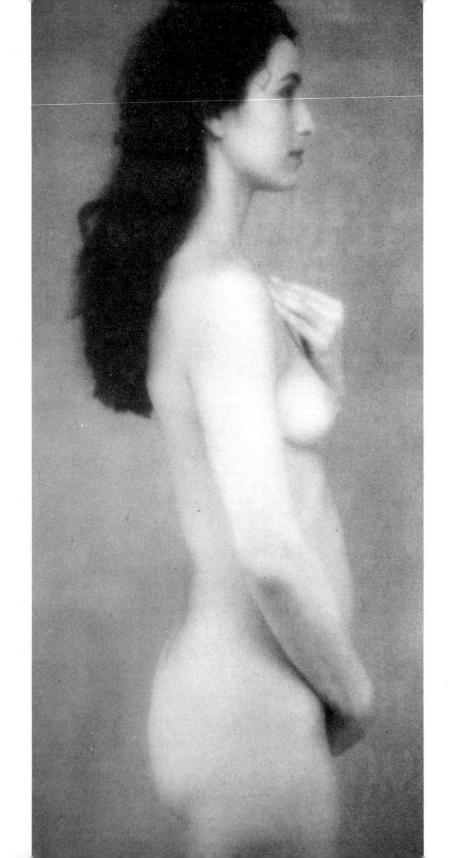

CHAPTER 1

YOUR FIRST TRIMESTER

CONCEPTION TO TWELVE WEEKS

So you're pregnant! *Now what?*

Whether this baby was painstakingly planned or a complete surprise, whether it's taken years to arrive or you conceived on your first try, the next 9 months will be unlike any you've ever experienced. Many of the changes will be thrilling. Others can be unnerving, even frightening. It's downright strange—and more than a little miraculous—to wake up every day wearing a new body that's slightly different from the one you went to sleep in.

At first, you may not notice the transformations taking place. In fact, you may feel impatient about the lag time, waiting for physical reactions to catch up with all the mental ones crowding your thoughts. Then, soon enough, you feel swamped by sensations ranging from fatigue to mood swings. You may feel inexplicably hesitant and private, or like shouting your news from the rooftop. You may be panic-stricken, scared, or elated by the prospect of what's ahead. Things may seem to be unfolding much too quickly, or frustratingly slowly. And if you feel all of those responses, well, that's normal, too.

In body, mind, and soul, the first trimester (weeks 0 to 12) is a time for the pregnancy to take hold.

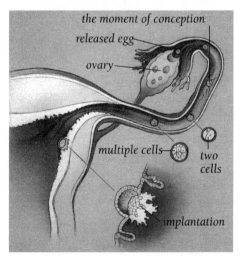

the moment of conception

released egg

ovary

multiple cells

two cells

implantation

After an egg is released from the ovaries, it moves into one of the fallopian tubes. If a single sperm manages to penetrate the egg's tough outer membrane, the cells will begin to multiply as they continue to travel toward the uterus.

Week-by-Week Highlights

How does your baby grow? How do *you* grow? What are the milestones of prenatal care? Here are some of the major first-trimester developments:

Week 1: This is the week of your menstrual period. The first day of significant bleeding is considered the official start date of the pregnancy (that's because it's an easier date to recognize and remember than conception).

Week 2: As it does each month in anticipation of new life, the uterus forms a lush, blood-rich lining of tissue. At the same time, the ovaries ripen eggs in fluid-filled sacs called follicles.

Week 3: Around mid-cycle (day 14 of the typical 28-day cycle), one of the eggs is swept into the fallopian tube. This is *ovulation*. If, in the next 24 hours, 1 of the 350 million sperm in the average ejaculate can trek all the way from the vagina through the uterus and to the fallopian tube to penetrate the egg, bingo—fertilization. (Sperm can live in the tube awaiting a mature egg for 1 to 4 days.) The fertilized egg, called a *zygote*, immediately closes its outer membrane to the other 300 or so sperm that have made it this far and begins dividing into identical cells as it floats down the fallopian tube to the uterus.

Week 4: The fluid-filled cluster of cells, still multiplying madly, is now called a *blastocyst*. It nests in the uterus, where it divides into two parts. The half attached to the uterine wall becomes the placenta, the blood-vessel–filled support system that nourishes the developing life, and the other half will become

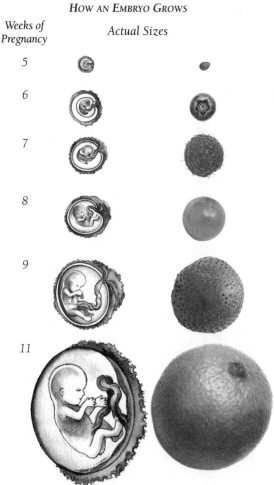

HOW AN EMBRYO GROWS

Weeks of Pregnancy   *Actual Sizes*

5

6

7

8

9

11

Why compare an embryo to an apple seed? To show its dramatic growth in just six weeks.

the baby. By the end of this week, you miss a period, though slight staining called *implantation bleeding* is possible.

Week 5: The ball of cells, about the size of an apple seed, has become an *embryo*. The placenta and umbilical cord, through which the baby will receive nourishment and oxygen, are on the job. Many women now first suspect pregnancy; a home pregnancy test can confirm it. Call your doctor to schedule an initial visit and discuss any medication you are currently taking, to be sure it is safe during pregnancy. Ask about taking a folate supplement even before your first checkup. Weeks 5 to 10 are critical to the baby's development. (See "Checklist: What to Watch Out For," page 20.)

Week 6: The embryo looks more like a tadpole than a human. Its heart, no bigger than a poppy seed, has begun to beat. Other major organs, including kidneys and liver, have begun to develop and the neural tube (which connects the brain and spinal cord) closes. The physical sensations of pregnancy—nausea, sore breasts, fatigue, frequent urination—kick in. The first prenatal checkup is usually scheduled between 6 and 10 weeks.

Week 7: The embryo is the size of a small raspberry. It has an oversized head in proportion to the body, dark spots where the eyes and nostrils are beginning to form, pits that mark the ears, and protruding buds that will become the arms and legs.

Week 8: Now grape size, the embryo has distinct fingers and toes, slightly webbed. Its skin is thin as parchment. Your expanding uterus is now the size of a peach.

 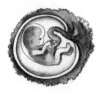 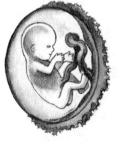

Month 1: By the end of the first month, the head and body are already taking shape, as well as the beginnings of arms and legs. On day 25, the heart begins to beat.

Size: 1/2 inch long
Weight: less than 1 ounce

Month 2: By month's end eyelids are in place, although they remain closed. Appendages, including fingers, toes, and ears also appear.

Size: 1 inch long
Weight: less than 1 ounce

Month 3: Fingers and toes are now developing rapidly. Hair may also be growing on the head. The kidneys begin to function, and by the end of this month the body is fully formed.

Size: 4 inches long
Weight: a little more than an ounce

Week 9: By now you'll be spilling out of your old bra and need better support. The strawberry-size being is now called a *fetus*. It is constantly moving, though you won't be able to feel the movements for some time.

Week 10: In both shape and size, the fetus looks a bit like a medium shrimp. Its genitals begin to form, though you can't yet tell the sex by looking at a sonogram. The prenatal test *chorionic villus sampling* (CVS) is usually performed around 10 to 12 weeks.

Week 11: Your uterus is the size of a grapefruit. The fetus, about 2 inches long and weighing less than half an ounce, is swallowing and kicking. Its vital organs are fully developed. Each day more minute details fill in, such as fingernails and hair. Beginning about now, its rapid "whooshing" heartbeat can be heard through a *Doppler*, a hand-held sound-wave stethoscope.

Week 12: For you, nausea begins to wane and energy picks up. The uterus moves up to front-and-center of your abdomen, from its usual spot on the pelvic floor, which relieves pressure on the bladder. Now about 2½ inches long, the fetus is fully formed—from toothbuds to toenails. Its primary task during the next 6 months will be to grow larger and stronger until it can survive on its own. With the most critical development past, the odds of miscarriage drop considerably after 12 weeks.

What's Going on in Your Body

Am I Pregnant?

A few clairvoyant women claim to know they're pregnant almost from the moment of conception, while others can go weeks without suspecting a thing. Those who know early may be unusually tuned in to their body's signals, such as exactly when they ovulate. That's pretty rare, though. Sometimes a pregnancy sneaks by unnoticed for a while. That can occur, for example, if persistent bleeding misleads a woman into thinking she's had a period when she hasn't. Likewise, an irregular cycle, severe stress, or breastfeeding (if she's recently had a baby) may cause her to ovulate without knowing exactly when.

The majority of women, however, rely on a few basic clues to determine a pregnancy fairly early in the first trimester. The first sign is usually a missed period. Sometimes you may notice a slight staining around the time you would normally get a period; this is called *implantation bleeding*, caused by a sloughing off of uterine cells when the fertilized blastocyst (which will become the baby) first burrows into the womb. During those first few uncertain days, however, you might feel as though your period will start any day. You may have tender breasts or mild cramps. More than one woman has been fooled into thinking she's coming down with the flu or worse.

Within a week of the fertilized egg's implantation in the uterus, your breasts seem to take on a life of their own: sensitive to the touch, even painful, and slightly swollen. You may not want your partner to come near them. It may hurt to lie on your stomach. You'll probably crave sleep—to the point where the mere act of picking up the TV remote seems too strenuous—and you nod off at the slightest opportunity. You may begin to use the bathroom more often (even every hour). Telltale nausea strikes by the fifth or sixth week. Thought to be caused by the firestorm of hormones that pregnancy ignites, nausea can range from a vague, fleeting queasiness to day-long vomiting. (See "Common Aches and Pains: Pregnancy sickness," page 13.) Smells that you once found delicious—bacon frying, garlic, your favorite shampoo—may suddenly make your stomach churn. Newly sensitive taste buds accompany this newly sensitive nose; familiar flavors may seem metallic or simply unappealing. A yen for those female staples, coffee and chocolate, is often the first to go.

Since every woman bears her pregnancy differently, you may be affected mildly or severely by any of these symptoms. If you're lucky, you may even escape a few of them.

If you think you're pregnant and are still taking birth-control pills, take a home pregnancy test or see your doctor right away. If a home test is positive, discontinue the pills without waiting for a doctor's confirmation that you're expecting; if it turns out you have not actually conceived, you can always finish out the cycle on another contraceptive method. It's unlikely that taking the pill for a week or two of pregnancy will damage the developing embryo, however.

Confirming a Pregnancy

Most women nowadays put a few of these omens together and rush out for a home pregnancy test; these tests are sold over the counter in pharmacies and grocery stores. Home tests have improved dramatically since their arrival in the late 1970s, and if performed properly, they're now nearly 99 percent accurate. Home tests are also private, cheap ($10 to $20), easy to use, and quick, reporting results in minutes. The simplest brands require you to urinate onto a special stick; chemicals interact with your urine to screen for the presence of a hormone called *human chorionic gonadotrophin* (hCG), which is produced by the placenta and doubles every 2 to 3 days, beginning within a week of conception. A color change in a special window on the stick represents the result. Another type of home test involves two steps: first urinating in a cup, then adding a few drops to a well or test tube containing an hCG-detecting chemical.

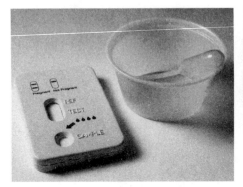

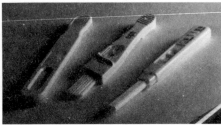

Done properly, home pregnancy tests are 99 percent accurate. Several different types are available over-the-counter.

For best test results, always read the package insert and follow instructions exactly. Common mistakes include placing the wrong end of a stick in the urine or allowing the windows that show the test results to get splashed. Wait until the day your period is due for accurate results (though many leading brands are now so sensitive they can detect hCG even sooner). Most tests promise an accurate result at any time of day, but if you're testing on or before the day your period was due, your first urine of the morning will have the greatest concentration of hCG. Read the results right away because if you wait 10 or 20 minutes more than instructed, a negative result can turn positive, even though you are not pregnant.

It's smart to buy the tests economically packaged in twos, since you'll want to retest a few days later. If you've tested yourself too early or have irregular cycles, or if your pregnancy is ectopic (a rare event in which the fertilized egg has implanted itself outside of the uterus), you could get a false-negative reading—meaning you really are pregnant even though the test indicated you're not. It's also wise to reconfirm if you tested positive, though false-negatives are more common than false-positives. Fertility drugs containing hCG can give a false-positive, as can certain medications (such as some for urinary-tract infections and depression); check with your doctor if you're taking anything. Antibiotics should have no impact. Test results can also be skewed for women over age 40 because of hormonal changes that begin to occur in the premenopause years.

Call your doctor as soon as you suspect a pregnancy. He or she can make a definite verification. An internal exam, for example, will reveal if your cervix is tightly closed and a distinct purply-blue, the result of increased blood supply to the area if you're pregnant. Since hCG is present in both your urine and your blood, a serum pregnancy test (by drawing blood) can also detect the hormone. An ultrasound shows the baby and its beating heart as early as 6 to 9 weeks. By 10 to 12 weeks (but sometimes as early as 7 weeks), the heartbeat can be heard with a Doppler, or sound-wave stethoscope.

When Is Your Due Date?

The average pregnancy lasts 280 days, a period equal to 9 months that are each about 4½ weeks long. Ninety-five percent of all babies are born within 2 weeks of this norm. To figure out how far along you are, most doctors count from the first day of your last menstrual period (LMP). In a typical 28-day cycle, conception takes place around the 14th day of the pregnancy, not the first day. By 40 weeks (full-term), you will actually have been pregnant for 38 weeks.

The usual formula is to take your LMP date, add 3 months, and then subtract 7 days. To calculate your due date, use the chart on page 12.

Note: Some doctors date pregnancy from the time of conception, which means that when you are "13 weeks pregnant" your fetus is 13 weeks old. This is called *fertilization age.* Be sure you know which system of measuring your doctor is using. In this book, we use the more common *gestational age,* or *menstrual age,* which counts the first day of your menstrual period as the first day of your pregnancy. Thus, "13 weeks pregnant" means you have actually been pregnant for 11 weeks.

Though it's the date you'll memorize—and pin all your plans on—don't forget that a due date is merely an *estimation.* It tells you little more than that you'll probably have your baby within 2 weeks on either side of that target. If you can't remember when your period began, if you tend to have longer or shorter cycles than average, or if your cycles are irregular, it can be hard to specify just when you ovulated and conceived. Even if you're ordinarily very regular, your dates might be off if you recently quit the pill, which can distort menstrual cycles for up to 3 months afterward. Nor can you predict your precise due date, even if you're sure of the moment of conception, because the number of days a baby spends in the womb varies, influenced by many factors.

Doctors rely on a due date to help monitor your pregnancy. Each visit, the doctor will check the growth of your uterus (and maybe once or twice, through ultrasound, the growth of your baby) against the typical growth for someone at your stage of pregnancy. The reliability of some prenatal tests also depends on knowing how far along you are. If anything seems amiss, the doctor will want to know why: you may be carrying more than one fetus, for example. Your doctor may revise your date based on information from tests or ultrasound exams. In the first trimester, when the fetus grows at predictable rates, an ultrasound can pinpoint how far along you are to within a couple of days; after that, growth rates vary and ultrasound is less reliable as a tool to determine dates.

Calculate Your Due Date

To determine your due date (also known as *estimated date of delivery*, EDD, or *estimated date of confinement*, EDC), find the first day of your last menstrual period on the following chart. The date in the colored box below is your due date—9 months and 7 days after your last menstrual period. Only about 1 in 20 babies is born promptly on its due date; the majority come within the 2 weeks before or the 2 weeks after.

JANUARY	1 2 3 4 5 6 7 8 9 10 11 12 13 14 15 16 17 18 19 20 21 22 23 24 25 26 27 28 29 30 31
OCTOBER	8 9 10 11 12 13 14 15 16 17 18 19 20 21 22 23 24 25 26 27 28 29 30 31 1 2 3 4 5 6 7
FEBRUARY	1 2 3 4 5 6 7 8 9 10 11 12 13 14 15 16 17 18 19 20 21 22 23 24 25 26 27 28
NOVEMBER	8 9 10 11 12 13 14 15 16 17 18 19 20 21 22 23 24 25 26 27 28 29 30 1 2 3 4 5
MARCH	1 2 3 4 5 6 7 8 9 10 11 12 13 14 15 16 17 18 19 20 21 22 23 24 25 26 27 28 29 30 31
DECEMBER	6 7 8 9 10 11 12 13 14 15 16 17 18 19 20 21 22 23 24 25 26 27 28 29 30 31 1 2 3 4 5
APRIL	1 2 3 4 5 6 7 8 9 10 11 12 13 14 15 16 17 18 19 20 21 22 23 24 25 26 27 28 29 30
JANUARY	6 7 8 9 10 11 12 13 14 15 16 17 18 19 20 21 22 23 24 25 26 27 28 29 30 31 1 2 3 4
MAY	1 2 3 4 5 6 7 8 9 10 11 12 13 14 15 16 17 18 19 20 21 22 23 24 25 26 27 28 29 30 31
FEBRUARY	5 6 7 8 9 10 11 12 13 14 15 16 17 18 19 20 21 22 23 24 25 26 27 28 1 2 3 4 5 6 7
JUNE	1 2 3 4 5 6 7 8 9 10 11 12 13 14 15 16 17 18 19 20 21 22 23 24 25 26 27 28 29 30
MARCH	8 9 10 11 12 13 14 15 16 17 18 19 20 21 22 23 24 25 26 27 28 29 30 31 1 2 3 4 5 6
JULY	1 2 3 4 5 6 7 8 9 10 11 12 13 14 15 16 17 18 19 20 21 22 23 24 25 26 27 28 29 30 31
APRIL	7 8 9 10 11 12 13 14 15 16 17 18 19 20 21 22 23 24 25 26 27 28 29 30 1 2 3 4 5 6 7
AUGUST	1 2 3 4 5 6 7 8 9 10 11 12 13 14 15 16 17 18 19 20 21 22 23 24 25 26 27 28 29 30 31
MAY	8 9 10 11 12 13 14 15 16 17 18 19 20 21 22 23 24 25 26 27 28 29 30 31 1 2 3 4 5 6 7
SEPTEMBER	1 2 3 4 5 6 7 8 9 10 11 12 13 14 15 16 17 18 19 20 21 22 23 24 25 26 27 28 29 30
JUNE	8 9 10 11 12 13 14 15 16 17 18 19 20 21 22 23 24 25 26 27 28 29 30 1 2 3 4 5 6 7
OCTOBER	1 2 3 4 5 6 7 8 9 10 11 12 13 14 15 16 17 18 19 20 21 22 23 24 25 26 27 28 29 30 31
JULY	8 9 10 11 12 13 14 15 16 17 18 19 20 21 22 23 24 25 26 27 28 29 30 31 1 2 3 4 5 6 7
NOVEMBER	1 2 3 4 5 6 7 8 9 10 11 12 13 14 15 16 17 18 19 20 21 22 23 24 25 26 27 28 29 30
AUGUST	8 9 10 11 12 13 14 15 16 17 18 19 20 21 22 23 24 25 26 27 28 29 30 31 1 2 3 4 5 6
DECEMBER	1 2 3 4 5 6 7 8 9 10 11 12 13 14 15 16 17 18 19 20 21 22 23 24 25 26 27 28 29 30 31
SEPTEMBER	7 8 9 10 11 12 13 14 15 16 17 18 19 20 21 22 23 24 25 26 27 28 29 30 1 2 3 4 5 6 7

Common Aches and Pains

Expect some physical reactions to kick in as your body begins to accommodate the new life that's rapidly taking shape within you. More than one newly pregnant woman has remarked, "It's as if my body is running on autopilot, with someone else telling me when to eat and when to sleep." In the first trimester, the most common side effects include the following.

• *Pregnancy sickness (nausea).* The familiar term "morning sickness" is losing favor because, as any sufferer knows, nausea and vomiting have no time limits. (The name stems from the fact that, for many women, symptoms are worst upon waking.) No two cases are alike. Some women feel little worse than a come-and-go upset stomach and never throw up, while others are left sprinting to the toilet all day long. Still others wish they could retch but can't. If you're lucky, you may be able to identify which smells or tastes set you off, and avoid them. But you may also get ill without a clear-cut trigger. The precise cause of this common malady, which affects most pregnant women to some degree, remains one of the great medical mysteries.

The leading suspects are rising levels of the hormones hCG and possibly estrogen and progesterone. The presence of hCG, for example, runs suspiciously parallel to the usual pattern of nausea: its production steadily rises just after the fertilized egg implants in the womb and begins to ebb around week 12, then remains low from the fourth month through to delivery. (Rarely, a few unlucky women stay nauseous for the duration.) Some speculate that this pattern of nausea may have an evolutionary root: because it occurs exactly during the key weeks of the embryo's growth, a sensitivity to odors, tastes, and certain food associations may serve as natural protection from poisons that might otherwise get ingested by the mother during that critical phase.

Nausea tends to be worsened by a woman's eating habits—more specifically, by her *not* eating. Many expectant mothers unwittingly fall into a vicious cycle of cutting back on how often or how much they eat because they feel nauseous, which then perpetuates or even worsens the sickness.

What *doesn't* cause pregnancy sickness is emotional stress, though stress can exacerbate its severity; being in poor physical shape; difficulty adjusting mentally to motherhood; or an unvoiced displeasure with being pregnant.

The best coping advice is to find ways to take control of this potentially overwhelming condition. Graze on small amounts of foods you can tolerate throughout the day to ward off the extreme nausea that an empty stomach can bring on. It's less important that you eat plentifully, or even especially nutritiously, during the first trimester, than it is to keep something in your stomach to stay as healthy as possible, while avoiding substances that could endanger the developing embryo. The fetus requires very few nutrients at first. Follow your instincts. If the smell of dog food turns your stomach, get someone else to feed the dog. If sitting in a dim room or sleeping alone seems to help, do so. If you can tolerate only bland pasta, stick with noodles. Don't worry if you wind up losing a little weight in the first 2 or 3 months; total weight gain is rarely more than a few pounds in the first trimester, regardless of one's degree of pregnancy sickness.

Comfort yourself, too, with the knowledge that smell and taste aversions may be actually protecting your developing baby. Your sense of smell, for example, sharpens in the first trimester, helping steer you from spoiled dairy products or smoky rooms. (It returns to normal in mid-pregnancy before worsening by the ninth month.) What's more, feeling nauseous should actually reassure you that the pregnancy is proceeding normally. Your baby, by the way, doesn't notice a thing.

More pregnancy-sickness tips:

- Quit eating three big preplanned meals in favor of day-long mini-meals; even snacking as often as once an hour can make a big difference. Bland snacks that work well for some women include rice cakes, pretzels, cold cereal (such as Cheerios or Rice Chex), and saltine crackers.
- To circumvent morning nausea, don't go hungry at night. Have half a sandwich and a glass of milk before you retire, or make middle-of-the-night refrigerator raids for light snacks.
- Drink lots of fluids to avoid dehydration. Cold juice, milk, or lemonade may appeal more than warm or hot beverages.
- Don't forget other sources of liquids: popsicles (look for brands made of 100 percent juice), frozen juice or sorbet, Jell-O, frozen grapes or melon balls, bouillon.
- When you're not chewing food, try hard candy or peppermints to prevent irritating stomach acids from building up (as they do on an empty stomach).
- Nibble crackers, cereal, or cheese before you get out of bed and wait 15 to 20 minutes before standing up.
- Try the fresh lemon cure: sniff a wedge or suck one, either plain or sprinkled with salt.
- Keep a window open or a fan running at night, since stale air can worsen nausea.
- Quit cooking. Order take-out or hand the spatula and apron to your partner. (Restaurants, with their many odors, may not appeal.)
- Switch to unscented soaps, detergents, and lotions.
- Skip perfume.
- Beware herbal medicines (such as gingerroot) purported to quell nausea;

they may work, but they are potentially toxic and unstudied in terms of birth defects.
- Try an acupressure wristband designed for seasickness, available at boating stores or pharmacies.
- Sleep!

Never take motion-sickness pills or any other medications for nausea without your doctor's okay. Get medical help if you can't keep anything down for several days or if you lose weight rapidly. This can lead to a severe dehydration known as *hyperemesis gravidarum*, which sometimes requires hospitalization. A combination of antinausea drugs and intravenous fluids may be needed to combat the dehydration and restore your body's chemical balance. These are safe for the fetus, who will also be monitored carefully.

- *Fatigue.* The phrase "comalike sleep" will take on new meaning. This unbelievable tiredness is your body's way of hanging out a sign: HARD AT WORK! All body systems are taxed trying to accommodate the new, rapidly multiplying cells within you, which themselves demand a great deal of energy to grow the fetal organs and the placenta. What's more, the ovaries' production of the hormones estrogen and progesterone speeds up in the early weeks to help sustain the pregnancy. Progesterone has a sedative effect, while estrogen can interfere with deep, non-REM sleep, causing you to toss and turn more.

This initial tumult eases up around the fourth month, when hormone levels stabilize and the fetus's organs have formed, giving most pregnant women a renewed sense of energy. Meanwhile, *make rest a priority*. Short naps (under 90 minutes) actually work better to boost energy without disrupting nighttime sleep. Even putting your feet up in a quiet room can be restorative. Beware of sugar and caffeine; they can give you a rush of energy, followed by a low period that makes you feel even worse. If you have older children, rely on videotapes and reading books together; let Dad or baby-sitters take them outside for an hour or so while you relax.

When bedtime finally arrives, you'll be ready. In fact, you may need several more hours of sleep per night than usual. But if restlessness or nausea interferes, try the following before bed to improve the quality of sleep:

- Fit in some exercise during the day (even a brisk 20-minute walk).
- Avoid caffeine and drink milk instead, warm if you can tolerate it.
- Try a bubble bath—by candlelight.
- Make your bedroom as dark and quiet as possible (no TV, no radio).

Fatigue can also be a warning sign of anemia. Typically caused by an iron deficiency, this is a common condition during pregnancy because the blood supply is so taxed. Women who have severe pregnancy sickness or whose children are closely spaced tend to be especially susceptible. A blood test can confirm iron-deficiency anemia, which is usually easily resolved with an iron supplement pill.

• **Frequent urination.** The expanding uterus sits right on your bladder in early pregnancy, squeezing out its usual storage space for urine. The kidneys also begin working overtime to flush out waste products from the blood at a faster-than-normal pace. What you feel is an almost constant urge to use the bathroom, day and night. Even in the middle of a deep sleep, dreams about oceans or toilets nag you awake: *Oh yeah, gotta go again.* This sensation usually eases by the end of the first trimester, when the uterus rises up in your abdomen and away from the bladder. Because of the increased volume of fluids in your system, however, you may find frequent urination a fact of pregnant life.

In the meantime, go with the flow (so to speak). Don't try to cut back on your liquids. In fact, you may even notice that you are thirstier than usual; this early-warning sign of dehydration is your body's way of reminding you that it needs plenty of water to perform all the amazing tricks taking place inside. Nor should you try to hold it in, which may lead to a urinary tract infection (UTI, or *cystitis*). Alert your doctor if you experience these signs of UTI: feeling like you need to urinate but producing little urine; painful or burning urination; blood in the urine; fever.

• **Increased vaginal discharge.** A clear-to-yellowish, faintly odorous secretion (*leukorrhea*) increases in production during pregnancy. It's similar in its mucus texture and quantity to what's released just prior to ovulation. Produced by the cervix, vaginal discharge is probably a defense mechanism against infection.

To feel fresher, keep the vaginal area as clean and dry as possible. Wear light absorbent pads (not tampons and not the other, newer products designed to absorb menstrual flow internally, such as the disposable or reusable cup). Change your underwear as needed throughout the day (100 percent cotton is most comfortable and absorbent). Don't douche. Alert your doctor if the color or odor changes significantly or is accompanied by any pink, red, or brown staining or bleeding, or if urination becomes painful. These are signs of a vaginal infection. Also inform your doctor if the discharge becomes watery, which is a warning sign of cervical incompetence, in which the cervix begins to dilate very prematurely, threatening the pregnancy.

• **Dizziness.** Changes in blood pressure that occur during pregnancy can make you feel lightheaded if you stand up quickly. If you do feel faint, sit down slowly, breathe deeply, and avoid making any sudden movements. Or lie down with your feet elevated, if you can. Actual fainting is pretty uncommon.

• *Headaches.* Hormonal changes, hunger, or feeling overheated can bring on headaches; try fresh air, temple massage, or rest before resorting to medication. Acetaminophen (Tylenol) is considered safe for occasional use. Aspirin is not, unless specifically prescribed by a doctor, because it thins the blood, which can have consequences for mother and baby. Nor is ibuprofen (Advil, Nuprin) recommended, as it can thin the blood and may cause heart disease in the baby. The best bet is to check with your doctor first. Always report persistent headaches, which, when accompanied by swelling of the face or hands, may indicate high blood pressure.

Three-quarters of women who suffer from migraines find that their headaches disappear during pregnancy, particularly after the first trimester. Estrogen is thought to have a protective effect, and the tendency for pregnant women to abstain from caffeine and take other steps to improve their general health may also help.

• *Nasal congestion.* Hormonal changes can cause a long-lasting stuffy nose. This irritation, combined with your blooming blood supply, sometimes leads to nosebleeds. Though most common in winter, the condition can last throughout pregnancy. Rely on nonmedication relief, such as a humidifier to moisten air, and a dab of petroleum jelly inside each nostril. (Avoid nasal sprays and antihistamines.)

• *Bloating and gassiness.* Your insides are working overtime, and the hormones that support pregnancy, especially progesterone, also can slow some of your other organs' routine tasks. The results are unflattering but unavoidable: abdominal pain, flatulence, burping, and a heavy feeling about your middle can all be traced to sluggish intestines. Indigestion and heartburn, as well as constipation, may also result. (See chapter 2, "Common Aches and Pains," pages 102–106.)

You can't make these sensations go away, though you may reduce their severity by avoiding gas-producing foods. These include cabbage; some beans; foods high in fat (lamb, pork, hotdogs); greasy foods (french fries, chips, fried pies); and carbonated beverages. Choose whole grains over refined grains, since the latter retain more fluid and take longer to digest (on top of being less nutritious). Try eating a half-cup of yogurt as an appetizer before meals. The beneficial bacteria in yogurt can improve digestion and reduce or eliminate heartburn, bloating, and gassiness. Another unexpected preventive is exercise; a brisk 20-minute walk can improve digestion, thus reducing gassiness.

How to relieve indigestion? It's safe to take products such as Rolaids or Tums, which have the added benefit of being calcium rich. Most antacids containing aluminum and magnesium (Maalox, Mylanta) also seem to pose no risk to the fetus. Check labels to be sure the products don't contain aspirin (as does Alka-Seltzer). Caveat: don't take antacids with your prenatal vitamins, as they decrease vitamin absorption.

Avoiding Infections

Especially during the first trimester, while the baby's major organs and body systems are forming, it's important to steer clear of viruses and bacteria that could imperil that growth. Short of packing yourself in sterile gauze and hermetically sealing yourself away, what can you do? Avoid these dangers:

• **Fever.** This is not an infection itself, but the common result of one. It's the body's way of fighting illness. The problem is that abnormally high body temperatures also pose a risk to the fetus, including organ damage and miscarriage. Practice the obvious: Stay clear of people you know to be sick and wash your hands often, especially during flu season. Always alert your caregiver when you develop a fever above 102 degrees or are feverish for more than 24 hours; a high fever is not something to be "toughed out." Dress lightly and try a lukewarm bath or cool compresses. If you're told to take acetaminophen, do—this medication, by bringing the fever down, will help your baby, not harm it.

• **Rubella (German measles).** If contracted in early pregnancy by someone who hasn't already had it, rubella can damage the developing baby's brain, heart, eyes, ears, and skin. Symptoms in the mother include a rash and swollen lymph glands plus fever, nausea, and vomiting—but some cases are relatively symptom free. Fortunately, up to 90 percent of all mothers-to-be are immune to rubella by having had the disease or having been vaccinated against it, usually in childhood. If you're not sure whether you are immune, tell your doctor. A blood test called the *rubella antibody titer*, conducted at the first pregnancy exam as a matter of course, will verify your status. If you are found to not be immune, you'll want to avoid possible exposure during the first trimester (after that, the risk of congenital malformations is minimal). If a mother-to-be who is not immune to rubella is exposed during the first month of pregnancy, there is a 50 percent chance of birth defects in the baby and a 90 percent chance of spontaneous abortion. Some women exposed this early elect not to continue the pregnancy, or choose to undergo genetic counseling. By the third month, the odds drop to 1 in 10 that a baby born to an exposed, non-immune mother will be affected. Blood tests can confirm whether you have actually contracted the disease. You can't be inoculated during pregnancy because the vaccine contains a live virus, which might harm the fetus. But to prevent problems in future pregnancies, a mother who is not immune should be vaccinated soon after delivery.

• **Chicken pox.** Both its forms, varicella (chicken pox) and herpes zoster (shingles), can cause birth defects in the child of a mother not previously exposed. In addition, a case of chicken pox tends to be more severe in adults, and there is a risk of complications such as pneumonia. The riskiest time to get chicken pox is before the 15th week or within a week of delivery (when the infection can be passed to the fetus, who could be born with it). If you're not already immune, you can be immunized during pregnancy; but it's best to stay clear of people with this highly contagious disease.

• **Herpes simplex.** This virus causes fluid-filled blisters around the genitals (though they can also appear elsewhere on the body), which can result in painful urination. It's caused by intercourse with someone who has active herpes, and the symptoms appear about 3 days to 2 weeks later. If the mother has active lesions when she delivers, the virus can be passed to the baby, jeopardizing its life. But a Cesarean delivery, rather than a vaginal one, would circumvent the problem. Therefore, if you or your partner think you may have ever had herpes, don't worry, but let your doctor know so you can be monitored just in case. Recurrent herpes is not generally dangerous to the baby except at delivery.

• **Cytomegalovirus (CMV).** This hard-to-detect virus can be transmitted by saliva, blood, or sexual contact. It can be symptomless, or you may experience fever, swollen lymph glands, and a sore throat. CMV is common, though rarely contracted during pregnancy. Women who do catch the virus, however, are likely to pass it to the fetus, who then risks developing jaundice or problems with hearing and learning. The best prevention is to avoid contact with known infected people and—as with avoiding all viruses—to wash your hands frequently.

• **Toxoplasmosis.** This infection, caused by a parasite that lives in cats and is also found in raw meats, can pose a threat when a woman is exposed for the first time during pregnancy. (See "IS IT TRUE . . . That pregnant women should avoid cats?" page 26.)

Checklist: What to Watch Out For

Why take risks if you don't have to? Avoid the following throughout your pregnancy. Some are known toxins; others are controversial but have been associated with a possible increased risk of birth defects. Take special care in the first 12 weeks, when the baby's crucial body systems are being formed.

Red Flags: Things to Avoid

☐ *Nicotine.* The ideal time to quit smoking is before you conceive. Failing that, stop now. Don't consider yourself immune if you just puff on the occasional trendy cigar without inhaling, because the dangers are still alarmingly high: snuff the stogies, too. Incentives: Smoking ups your risk of miscarriage, prematurity, or a low-birthweight baby; can cause vision or hearing defects; may slow your baby's mental development; impairs breast milk production; and greatly increases your baby's risk of dying from SIDS (sudden infant death syndrome). To help you think of your familiar cigarettes as the deadly things they are, remind yourself that the U.S. Environmental Protection Agency classifies nicotine as a Group A human carcinogen—putting it right up there with asbestos, radon, and arsenic. (See "MOTHER TO MOTHER: 'How I Quit Smoking,' " page 27.)

☐ *Alcohol.* While the scientific debate rages over how much is too much, there's no disputing that heavy maternal use of alcohol is one of the leading known causes of mental retardation in babies in the United States. Significant drinking can also lead to *fetal alcohol syndrome* (FAS), a pattern of physical and behavioral disorders that can afflict a child for life. But even lesser use (one to two drinks a few times a week) may be linked with some FAS-type problems, such as hyperactivity or learning disabilities, in otherwise healthy kids.

☐ *Nonalcoholic "imitation" spirits.* Near-beers, sparkling wines, and other substitutes for alcoholic beverages sound like the perfect solution for would-be imbibers. While their alcohol content is indeed low (less than .5 percent alcohol for nonalcoholic beers and under 2.5 percent alcohol for near beers, compared with 11 percent alcohol for some wines), medical experts still aren't sure whether *any* level of alcohol is safe. So most prefer to err on the side of caution and nix these drinks, too.

☐ *Marijuana.* Pot remains in the mother's system for a long time, causing prolonged exposure in the fetus. Smoking marijuana releases the gas carbon monoxide, which can deprive the fetus of oxygen.

☐ *Other illegal drugs.* The physical evidence is as clear as the law: danger ahead. Pregnant women who use cocaine have a 25 percent greater chance of a preterm delivery, and should their babies survive, they tend to suffer a constellation of problems, including brain defects. It is *not* true that cocaine can safely induce labor, as some women believe. On the contrary, cocaine crosses into the fetus's circulation within minutes of being ingested by the mother. A single line of coke or one hit from a crack pipe can lead to serious maternal hemorrhage (bleeding) or placenta abruptio, a life-threatening condition in which the placenta tears away from the uterine wall and necessitates an emergency delivery, however prematurely. The fact is that virtually every street drug has been documented to cause birth defects or even fetal death—including heroin and other narcotics, LSD and PCP (angel dust), amphetamines (speed), and glue.

☐ *X-rays.* Exposure can cause birth defects and cancers, especially from weeks 2 through 10. Postpone any screening X-rays (including dental X-rays and mammograms) at least until after the first trimester if possible. Or discuss with your doctors alternative ways to diagnose the problem (such as ultrasound) or protective measures to take during X-rays (such as wearing a lead apron).

☐ *Hot tubs, saunas, whirlpools, Jacuzzis, and hot baths.* High temperatures are associated with decreased fertility in men. After conception, excessive heat can damage the embryo's developing nervous system. One study found that first-trimester use of a hot tub tripled a woman's risk of giving birth to a child with neural tube defects. Avoid soaking in a long, *hot* bath for the same reason. If you're accustomed to hot baths, get a pool thermometer to make sure the temperature stays below 102 degrees and stay in it no longer than 15 minutes. Warm baths are fine—relaxing, too.

☐ *Tanning booths.* Avoid them because too little is known about the possible impact of intense ultraviolet rays on the fetus. At minimum, the high temperature of these booths can cause dehydration and over-heating.

☐ *Certain acne medications.* Definitely out: isotretinoin (Accutane), Retin-A, tetracycline, and ointments that contain steroids. Their effects range from tooth discoloration to serious deformities in the baby.

☐ *Aspirin.* Do not take aspirin unless prescribed to treat a medical problem. Also avoid the nonsteroidal anti-inflammatory drugs (NSAIDs) ibuprofen and naproxin. For head or body aches, aceta-minophen (Tylenol) is preferred.

☐ *Lead.* Some oil paints and housepaints, especially in homes painted before 1978, contain lead. (Since 1996, home buyers and renters are supposed to be told if there is any lead-based paint in the dwelling, but if you've lived in the place longer, regard old paint suspiciously.) If your home has old paint and must be sanded and repainted while you're pregnant, make sure someone else does the work, open the windows, and stay away. Avoid stripping walls or old furniture whose paint may have a higher lead content. If you live in an older home, get the pipes checked as some are lead lined; let cold water run 2 minutes before using. (Ordinary tap water in most areas is safe.)

☐ *Pesticides and fungicides.* Some types are safer than others, but the best course is hands off. Let someone else de-bug the roses or rely on only environmentally friendly pest-control methods (such as a strong blast of hose water in lieu of pesticides). Stay out of bug-sprayed spaces.

☐ *Aerosols.* The chemicals sprayed from cans and bottles this way are more easily inhaled.

☐ *Many chemical products.* Avoid varnish removers, rubber cement, some household cleaning products (oven or toilet cleaners), some wall-paper glues, stains and finishes, and chemicals used for photography.

☐ *Artificial sweeteners and preservatives.* Saccharin should be avoided by all pregnant women. Expert opinion varies regarding aspartame (Nutrasweet, Equal), but small amounts are probably okay—say, a can or two of soda, or two packets of sweetener a day. Exception: aspartame is not safe if you have the disease *phenylketonuria* (PKU, the body's inability to break down an amino acid called phenylalanine). Also beware foods high in nitrates and nitrites, including smoked or salty foods such as lunch meat, hotdogs, and smoked meats, fish, or cheese.

☐ *Vitamin supplements (nonprescription).* If a little vitamin C is good, then a lot must be better, right? Wrong. Doses of vitamins or minerals beyond the Recommended Daily Allowance can poison a fetus, causing birth defects. Some calcium supplements sold in health-food stores are made from ground limestone, which can contain arsenic, poisonous to a fetus. Nor is the quality of vitamins as good in supplemental form as from actual foods. Review your supplement intake with your doctor, and take nothing more than the prenatal formulation prescribed. Avoid protein powders, too.

☐ *Cat litter.* (See "IS IT TRUE . . . That pregnant women should avoid cats?" page 26.)

☐ *Touching or eating raw meat or seafood, or eating raw eggs.* You can pick up dangerous salmonella, toxoplasmosis, or other bacteria and parasites. Off-limits foods include sushi, sashimi, raw clams and oysters, and rare beef such as rare hamburger or steak tartare. Foods that may contain uncooked eggs include Caesar salad dressing, unpasteurized eggnog, French toast that's undercooked, and some health shakes. (No sampling raw cookie dough, either.) Thoroughly cooked shellfish is fine.

☐ *Lobster tomalley.* This green delicacy (actually the lobster's liver) contains high levels of dioxins, which have been linked to cleft palate and other birth defects, even in tiny amounts.

☐ *Douching,* especially with a bulb syringe. Introducing pressured air into the vagina can cause a potentially fatal air embolism.

Yellow Flags: Proceed with Caution

Always check with your doctor before taking or using the following:

☐ *Prescription medications.* Run anything you take past your obstetric caregiver, even if you've been on it for years. Assume nothing. No exceptions.

☐ *Over-the-counter medications.* Cough syrups, antihistamines, and decongestants may pose a health risk to the fetus, especially early in the first trimester. Consult your doctor for exceptions. Antacids and cortisone creams are safe.

☐ *Caffeine.* (See "Healthy Practices to Start Now," page 50.)

☐ *Perms and hair dyes.* There's no scientific evidence that permanent waves or hair dyes cause birth defects, but some of the chemicals that are used are known carcinogens. It is possible for the chemicals in these products to penetrate the mother's scalp and enter her bloodstream, which is why many physicians prefer to err on the side of caution, especially for the first 12 weeks. After that, it's your call. Or use natural coloring products (like henna) or treatments that cover only the hair shaft and not the scalp (like highlights). Be aware that the fumes in hair salons from perms and chemical treatments may be noxious as well.

☐ *Wood-burning stoves, fireplaces, gas heaters, and space heaters.* Heating appliances can leak carbon monoxide if not working properly. A frequently used chimney should be cleaned once a year. It's not a bad idea to buy a carbon monoxide detector to monitor levels in the home.

☐ *Well water.* Private wells are unregulated for safety. The danger is that nitrate from fertilizer or human sewage (when a septic tank is too near a well) can contaminate the groundwater. Excessive nitrate has been linked to miscarriage. If you use well water, have the source checked.

☐ *Some fish.* Eat shark, swordfish, and fresh tuna no more than once a month. These species tend to have the most chemical contaminants.

Checklist: When to Call the Doctor

Pregnancy is no time to suffer stoically when something doesn't seem right. Call your healthcare provider *any* time you have a question about a pain or a nagging doubt. (That's what you pay him or her for.) And definitely check in if you experience any of the following:

☐ *Persistent pain or cramping.* Could indicate something unusual happening with the baby, or something unrelated, such as appendicitis.

☐ *Bleeding*, especially if accompanied by cramping. Could signal miscarriage.

☐ *Severe, constant headaches,* or headaches not relieved by acetaminophen. Sign of hypertension.

☐ *Persistent vomiting or diarrhea.* Can lead to dehydration.

☐ *Swelling of ankles or feet.* Signs of pregnancy-induced hypertension, especially if accompanied by blurry vision or seeing spots.

☐ *High fever* (over 102 degrees), or fever lasting more than 24 hours.

WHAT IF...

I get a cold or the flu? Because colds and flu are caused by viruses, they can't be cured by a dose of antibiotics (the way a bacterial illness, such as some types of bronchitis, can). You've got to wait them out. Avoid cough medicines, which can contain as much alcohol as a 4-ounce glass of wine, as well as antihistamines and decongestants—unless you get a doctor's okay. Try nonmedical tactics: To breathe easier, use a humidifier to add moisture to the air and raise your head slightly with pillows when you sleep. Drink hot broth to open nasal passages. Generally acetaminophen (such as Tylenol) is considered safe in pregnancy for reducing fever (if cool baths or compresses fail) or for body aches. Above all, rest—you don't want to make yourself weaker and more vulnerable to other, more dangerous infections. Menthol rubs, such as Vicks Vapo-Rub, are safe.

Can you outwit the flu? Doctors sometimes advise against flu vaccinations in the first trimester, since they can cause fever, which could be dangerous to the fetus. Exception: women with some chronic medical conditions, including lung disorders and metabolic diseases, who should be vaccinated before flu season starts. The Centers for Disease Control also recommends a flu shot if you'll be in your third trimester during flu season (November to mid-March). There don't appear to be any dangers in the shot itself.

IS IT TRUE...

That it's possible to influence the selection of your baby's sex? You can find entire books written on the topic at your library, or hear women swear that a baking soda douche before intercourse increases the odds of a boy, or that lying on your left side afterward will guarantee a girl. And the odds are that such home remedies will be right—50 percent of the time. However, it's possible in a laboratory to separate the sperm that carry the X (female) chromosome from those bearing the Y (male) chromosome before using them to fertilize an egg through in vitro fertilization. These scientific methods of increasing the odds of successful sex selection are used chiefly for research or to avoid certain female-linked recessive disorders, and are not widely available.

That more morning sickness means it's a boy? The theory goes that a boy causes more testosterone (a male hormone) to be floating around inside you, hence more nausea. For the same reason, some say a mother-to-be with acne must be carrying a boy. Alas, while sickness and acne are indeed triggered by hormones, those hormones are in the mother's system, not the fetus's, where the amount of testosterone would be too minuscule to register any effect on the mother anyway.

The sicker the mom, the hairier the baby? Maybe the folks who tell this one are getting babies mixed up with cats and their hairballs. Totally untrue.

That standing near a microwave is dangerous? Probably not. Microwave ovens are tightly regulated by the Food and Drug Administration and are designed not to operate if there is excessive leakage, so it's highly unlikely that any harm can come to your fetus if you use one to cook. An easy test for slight leakage: Put a dollar bill or a paper towel in the door of the oven and close it. If it fits snugly, with some resistance when you pull on it, your door is okay. If it slides out easily, the door should be serviced. Still nervous? Just step to the side.

That pregnant women should avoid cats? Yes—at least, some cats, and all cat feces. The feces may be contaminated with *Toxoplasma gondii*, a microorganism that can cause an infection in humans known as *toxoplasmosis*. Many people get infected and then develop an immunity. But if you're infected for the first time during pregnancy, the fetus can be affected in ways ranging from premature birth or low birthweight to serious central nervous system defects, even still-birth. A blood test can determine *if* you've been infected, but not *when*. Your cat can be tested for the parasite, too. If the test is negative, feed him store-bought cat food and keep him inside. (Cats contract the parasite from rodents, birds, and raw meat.) To be really safe, ask someone else to change the litter box. But if the test is positive, you're wise to avoid touching the cat, keep it off your bed or chair, and *definitely* stay clear of the litter box. Since strange cats or strays are especially likely carriers, avoid touching them, and always wash your hands after gardening (where they may have contaminated the soil). It's also prudent not to eat raw home-grown vegetables until they've been thoroughly washed.

Note: You can also get toxoplasmosis from eating or touching raw or under-cooked meat or shellfish.

MOTHER TO MOTHER:
"How I Quit Smoking"

Zaida Gonzalez, 30
Flushing, New York

Zaida first lit up 13 years ago for that age-old reason: peer pressure. By the time she conceived, her first smoke had become a pack-and-a-half-per-day habit. At her doctor's urging, she tried to quit cold turkey. Haunted by "giving birth to a baby with three heads," she taped pictures of healthy babies to her refrigerator as incentive. But her addiction proved too strong.

At her 12-week checkup, Zaida first heard the baby's heartbeat. Because her partner couldn't make it to the appointment, she chanced to record it for him—which proved to be her turning point. "Every time I had the urge to light up, I reached for the recorder instead," she says. Having tangible evidence of life inside her was especially useful in the first trimester, before she could feel the baby move. When she caved in to her craving to smoke, she'd take just a few puffs, then snuff it out. In a few weeks, she was able to lower her daily cigarette count from twenty down to just one.

Not that it's fun, coping with nicotine withdrawal on top of hormones already gone haywire. "I was nervous, anxious, and grouchy all the time," she says. At work, she posted a sign on her desk asking colleagues not to talk about her vanishing habit, which only stokes her desire. "But nothing can outweigh the good I'm doing for my baby," she says.

Some 1.3 million smokers a year successfully quit smoking, nearly three-fourths on the first or second try. One good tactic is to keep a smoking diary, noting what you were doing or eating when you smoked, and how badly you felt you needed it. Then try to eliminate those cues. Exercise helps divert many pregnant smokers, too.

Zaida's tips for kicking the habit:

• *Accentuate your progress.* "Don't worry about the cigarettes you smoke, so much as congratulate yourself for the ones you don't have."

• *If you can't quit smoking cold turkey, quit buying.* It helped Zaida to have to ask someone for a cigarette first.

• *Bribe yourself.* "Say things like, 'I didn't smoke for five days, I can do it for five more, then treat myself to one.' " You may find you don't even want that.

• *Get professional advice.* Zaida relied on March of Dimes booklets. You can also find information and support at hospitals, the local American Cancer Society office (call 800-ACS-2345), or the American Lung Association (800-586-4872).

What's Going on in Your Head

Conflicting Thoughts

Being pregnant, you may feel as thrilled as if you've won the lottery, and rightfully so. But even the sunniest mamas have their gray moments. With every facet of your life about to change, it's only logical that your mind should feel as transformed as your body. Often pregnant women are expected to wear a happy face, despite morning sickness, worries about the baby's health, and fears of their own possible inadequacies. There's an unwritten expectation that if you say anything negative about how you're feeling, you must be a bad mother. Or that negative vibes can somehow penetrate the uterus and depress your unborn baby. Don't believe it.

The truth is, you'll probably be stirring a crazy soup of emotions for the next 9 months. Part of the reason is biological: fluctuating estrogen and progesterone fuel some of pregnancy's infamous mood swings. Moreover, your psyche (and your partner's) need time to adjust to the profound changes taking place. Your relationship to your partner, your parents, your own body, and possibly to your job, friends, and older children or stepchildren are all teetering on the brink of change. Don't let anyone intimate that pregnancy is no big deal or nothing to get worked up about.

The first weeks can be especially intense. The reality of the pregnancy is still sinking in, for one thing. There's a strange "unrealness" about the delay between when the home test dipstick first turns pink or blue and when you get tangible confirmation of the baby's presence in the form of an ultrasound image, a heartbeat, or a swift kick to the ribs. Especially if you haven't broadcast the news yet, the time of not-yet-showing, not-yet-telling can be an exquisite private trip—or a maddening wait.

If the pregnancy was unplanned, you may need extra time to absorb the shock. Often women whose pregnancies were a surprise find they embrace the idea quickly, while mothers-to-be who planned the event suddenly find themselves out-of-sorts. Everyone—and every day—is different.

Possible first-trimester reactions (many of which your partner may share) include:

• *Awkward ambivalence.* You go back and forth between excitement and panic. Or you're not really sure how you feel. You might even be sad, as if mourning your old life before you can make way for the new one, and then feel guilty on top of that because it seems like a peculiar emotion at such a stereotypically happy time.

Peculiar, yes. Unusual? Not at all. Uncertain feelings are partly caused by the purely academic sense of the pregnancy just now, especially if you don't have severe morning sickness or some other constant reminder of the baby's presence. But ambivalence is also a healthy sign that you're taking the pregnancy seriously, contemplating the enormity of it all. Face it—there's plenty to be excited about, and plenty of legitimate reasons to be nervous, too. Ambivalence doesn't mean you're unfit for parenthood or won't be very good at it.

• *Moody blues.* Especially in the first weeks, you might find yourself bursting into tears at a television commercial or snapping at your partner for passing the salt too slowly. Introspection, detachment, and self-absorption are common. Hormones feed some of these mood peaks and plummets, as can fatigue, restless sleep, nausea, and severe morning sickness (hard to be cheery when you spend half the day hanging over the toilet bowl). Your psyche is also deeply preoccupied, making you less tolerant than usual.

• *Self-doubts.* Even the most elated prospective parents may wonder, "Are we really ready?" "How will we afford it?" "How is the baby going to change our household routines and our weekends in the country?" One or both of you may feel unprepared for parenthood, especially if you've had limited experience around young children. Luckily, you have 8 months or so to ease into the role, and even then you may be second-guessing your skills or your budget on the drive to the hospital on D-day. Fortunately, parenthood unfolds one minute at a time, and anyone can handle that.

• **Out of control.** First you notice your body speaking to you: "Put out that cigarette." "Get me some water!" "Quick, to the toilet!" "I need to sleep—*now.*" It's a compelling, almost unavoidable voice. But it's annoying, too, especially if you're a control freak who's used to calling all the shots in your life. Nevertheless, *listen.* Your body knows what it's doing. And you'll feel a lot better by giving in to these signals and making them your priority than if you try to fight them. Let other pressing matters slack off a little. Enlist the help of your partner, your friends, and your colleagues as best you can.

• **Mother smother.** Many women see their own mothers in a new light once they're pregnant. Often it's a "welcome to the club" sort of shift, in which you understand a new dimension about your mom, and the shared experience brings you closer. On the other hand, an eager grandma-to-be (on either side of the family) may not be able to resist doling out her own advice. Even one who never meddled before may consider your pregnancy to be an open door for laying on the reminiscences, old wives' tales, nags, and plans—in other words, driving you crazy. Some moms can't give up old habits of competition or overprotectiveness with their daughters, which now get channeled into pregnancy talk. ("I only gained 15 pounds with you." "Shouldn't you quit your job now?")

Even though pregnancy should be a selfish time for you, try to see the situation from her point of view. Grandparenthood is a thrilling passage, and given the delayed childbearing of many baby boomers, it's a life event many of these older women have been waiting a long time for. Others may be grappling with the idea of themselves as grandmas. Indulge the stories and advice as best you can, and reserve your combat responses for what really matters, such as her insistence on some dietary practice you know is unsafe or her nursery purchases that don't suit your tastes.

• **Miscarriage misgivings.** Paranoia about the baby's health is another common refrain that lasts throughout the pregnancy. At first, you may berate yourself about getting drunk at a party before you knew you were pregnant; for unwittingly taking allergy medicine; for smoking pot back in college. At every new twitch or symptom, you fear the worst. Even tests intended to allay your anxieties can have the opposite effect, as you imagine what *might* be discovered. And if you've had a prior miscarriage, the on-eggshells worry is magnified. (See "MOTHER TO MOTHER: 'I Worried About a Prior Miscarriage,' " page 33.)

Remind yourself that some 97 to 98 percent of babies are born without serious defects. The advice you're given about nutrition and hazards is intended to create the optimal conditions for a healthy pregnancy, but beating yourself up for having a beer is probably more destructive than the brew itself. You're smart to be vigilant about what you eat, do, or feel. Pay attention, ask questions, and get the facts. But if your worries consume every waking moment, you'll be missing many of the sweet joys of pregnancy. Don't let vigilance turn into obsessiveness.

More Ways to Feel Good

Aside from reassuring yourself that you're not crazy or alone, there are a few practical steps you can take right now:

- To help make the baby seem more real, flip through the miraculous photographs of first-trimester fetal development like those found in Lennart Nilsson's classic book, *A Child Is Born*.
- Read ahead in pregnancy guides like this one to arm yourself with full knowledge about the enormity of these 9 months.
- Start a pregnancy journal in which you record your thoughts and actions. It can be as simple as a factual record of your prenatal visits or as easy as a tape-recorded monologue.
- Buddy up with another woman who's at your same stage of pregnancy. It might be a coworker or neighbor you never had much in common with before—but rest assured, you do now.
- Join an on-line support group for women who are delivering the same month as you.
- Make a point to do something nice for yourself every day—give yourself a foot massage, buy fresh flowers, reread a favorite book, order take-out, *nap*.
- Go with the flow. Learn to let new experiences and setbacks roll off your back with less resistance than you might have allowed in the past. Change is a constant in pregnancy; nothing stays exactly the same, so get used to it.
- Avoid the Pregnant Pollyanna trap—thinking you must act grateful and grin all the time. So much of pregnancy is magical, even spiritual. But it can also be uncomfortable and worrisome. Allow yourself to be real about it.

GOOD ADVICE: SPREADING THE NEWS

To tell or not to tell. And when. And who. And how. Sharing your pregnancy with the outside world is an intensely personal decision. Some things to consider are:

• *Do you want time as a couple to absorb or savor the news?* Some expectant parents find the secret draws them especially close. Some worry that sharing the news too early will jinx their odds of a successful pregnancy. Other couples say they'd tell friends and family about a miscarriage anyway.

• *How will you feel if you miscarry?* For some, the idea of a miscarriage is so private, they'd rather be safely past the first trimester before risking telling their friends, in case they must go back to reverse the information. Would that be too hard? Will you feel uncomfortable fielding condolences?

• *What kind of reactions are you expecting?* Brace yourselves for a possible letdown if the news doesn't bowl over relatives, or if someone gives a more understated "Congratulations" than you'd hoped for. You might feel strangely crowded by the crowing and cheering of others sharing your joy. If you're nervous about telling a close friend who's struggling with infertility, choose a time when you're alone and you know she hasn't just received more bad news. Be sensitive and low-key. Don't avoid her—what would that say about your friendship?

• *Are there professional advantages to keeping mum?* You may worry about being shortchanged good assignments at work or being treated differently if you tell too early. Or, on the other hand, a long lead time may provide the smoothest transition for you and your employer to plan for your leave time.

• *Will you want to talk to other women and compare notes?* If you're torn, consider telling just one confidante, ideally a mother, so you'll have an outlet beyond the baby's father for early venting and planning.

WHAT IF ...

I have older children—when do I tell them? Let your child's age be your guide. Under age 2 or 3, the news of a baby registers no more significantly than a visit from the Easter Bunny, nor does the child have a real concept of time. Holding off until your last trimester is fine; if the child asks about your belly, tell the truth but don't expect the news to stick in his head meaningfully. If you need to move the older child out of a crib, do so as many months before the baby's arrival as feasible so he or she won't feel displaced. By age 3 or 4, a child will start asking questions when you show, especially if she has seen baby cousins or neighbors, making this an opportune time to tell. Begin to explain, in an everyday way, what living with a baby is like. Older school-age children are uncannily perceptive; tell them before you spread the news beyond the family circle. Reading age-appropriate books about babies—and they are plentiful in libraries and bookstores—helps children of all ages prepare.

MOTHER TO MOTHER:
"I Worried About a Prior Miscarriage"

Sharon Heaps, 24
Berwyn, Pennsylvania

The thrill of a positive pregnancy test was dampened for Sharon by lingering thoughts of a miscarriage she had suffered a year earlier at 7 weeks. *Would it happen again?* she worried. "I was on the phone with my doctor almost every day to ask what to expect and to get moral support," she recalls. "I was constantly looking to see if there was blood when I went to the bathroom."

Then at 7 weeks, she began spotting. Certain that history was repeating itself, she informed her doctor. He gave her an hCG blood test, which showed that her hormone levels were still rising appropriately. His honesty helped, too. He told her that most early miscarriages happen for a reason beyond the mother's control, and that while she certainly could miscarry again, the signs appeared unlikely this time. In 2 days the bleeding stopped.

At 2 months, she told friends and family she was pregnant. "If you're going to have another miscarriage, you're just going to have it," she reasoned. By the fourth or fifth month, as she could feel the baby move, she found herself fretting less about losing it and focusing more on delivery. Daughter Marissa was born perfectly healthy.

Sharon's tips for coping with a prior miscarriage:

• *Do all the "right" things you can so you won't blame yourself.* "Miscarriages are so unexplained, you just have to keep the faith. Don't smoke, don't drink, eat healthy. That's all you can do."

• **Communicate your concern to your doctor.** "Tell him how you feel and what's going on to get an added sense of comfort." In addition to verbal reassurance, you may receive extra tests such as ultrasounds or hCG measures, especially if you bleed.

• **Remind yourself about the facts of miscarriage.** "Read a lot and talk to others who have gone through it." Learn the warning signs and remind yourself how great the odds are that the first time was a fluke.

• **Focus on the present—and the future.** "Worrying takes away from your happy time."

MOTHER TO MOTHER:
"Going It Alone"

Kim LoSchiavo, 26
Hicksville, New York

Divorced and facing a pregnancy that was unplanned, many of the 9 months' usual ups and downs were magnified for Kim. (She and the father are no longer together.) For example, the stress of her situation made it hard for her to quit smoking right away. She also developed premature labor in her seventh month and had to leave her job early to go on bedrest. She worries about childcare and finances. "I feel like I've given up my life," she says. "But keeping the baby is a decision I made and have to live with."

Even single moms-to-be who planned their pregnancies need financial, physical, and emotional support. Kim found that pregnancy was an isolating experience, so staying engaged with others helped her outlook a lot. Her doctor and friends advised her to look into prenatal exercise classes, childbirth education, and the Internet to find other women in similar situations with whom to share ideas, complaints, and thrills.

Kim's tips for single expectant moms:

• **Build a support network.** "Don't be shy about asking friends and family to go with you to doctor's appointments, run errands, or help you plan. It's never too early to decide who you'd like to be your childbirth coach."

• **Find single-mother role models.** "You can listen to stories about how they pulled through and find out how they're handling their situation."

• *Conserve your cash right from the start.* "I could have been tighter on the wallet at the beginning to save for later expenses, like daycare and formula."

• *Don't neglect your health.* "Worry about yourself and the baby first and foremost."

• *Focus on the future.* "Try to forget about your immediate situation if it's less than ideal, and get excited about the baby. You don't want to bring the baby into an unhappy home."

For More Help: Single-Mother Resources

• The National Organization for Single Mothers, P.O. Box 68, Midland, NC 28107; 704-888-6667.

Checkups and Tests

Choosing a Caregiver

Before you begin an obstetric relationship with a health professional, you need to decide who it will be—an ob-gyn, a primary-care doctor, or a certified nurse-midwife.

• *Obstetrician-gynecologist (ob-gyn).* They deliver the majority of American babies. Most women already have a gynecologist and choose to stick with that person during the momentous months ahead. If he or she doesn't handle obstetric cases—or if you've been itching to make a switch—ask your gynecologist for an OB referral. Better yet, ask friends who have recently had babies. If you're new in town, one smart bet is to ask around at a good childcare center or local mother's group. Labor and delivery nurses may also make reliable firsthand recommendations; call the maternity department at your local hospital. You may also wish to choose your doctor based on the hospital or birthing center with which he or she is affiliated.

Consider the size of the practice. In a one-doc office, you can build a good rapport but may have long waits for exams. Some MDs in larger practices rotate checkups, giving you little continuity, while others stick to a specific patient load. Some obs work with nurse-practitioners and certified nurse-midwives, who may handle the routine screenings.

Definitely select an ob-gyn if your pregnancy is high-risk or you're over age 35, in case unexpected medical emergencies arise (though you can still have a nurse-midwife, too).

• *Family practitioner (FP) or general practitioner (GP).* If you see a generalist for your routine care, you may wish to continue using that primary caregiver during pregnancy. Almost all are qualified for the job, since it's their role to oversee your general health and to refer you to specialists (including an obstetrician) on an as-needed basis. Both FPs and GPs are trained in obstetrics and gynecology.

Some primary-care physicians automatically refer their pregnant patients to an ob-gyn because they lack the higher insurance coverage required of that branch of medicine. Or, if your pregnancy deviates in any way from the norm (such as you're carrying multiple fetuses, you're diabetic, or you've had previous gynecological problems), your doctor may feel that an ob-gyn is better positioned to handle your case.

• *Certified nurse-midwife (CNM).* Registered nurses with an additional 1 to 2 years of clinical training in childbirth, CNMs (also known simply as *midwives*) are one of the fastest-growing components of the healthcare system. They attended more than 200,000 hospital births in 1994—up from 19,600 in 1975. Often based in obstetric practices, where they may work as part of a team of physicians, they specialize in the prenatal care and deliveries of low-risk patients. (Also trained in preventive care, CNMs can provide gynecological exams, Pap smears, and counseling on everything from contraception to lactation to menopause.)

Studies show that CNM-supervised births feature less anesthesia, fewer episiotomies, quicker recoveries, and dramatically reduced odds of a C-section, compared with doctor-assisted deliveries. Part of this impressive contrast can be explained by skewed statistics, since CNM patients have fewer complications and risk factors to begin with. Beyond that, however, they're trained to view pregnancy as a natural, healthy process. They tend to act as partners with the patient, taking emotional concerns and lifestyle issues into great account. And the average midwife tends to provide greater one-on-one care and moral support during labor than the average doctor, who may rely on labor-and-delivery nurses to monitor and coach you through much of the delivery. (Exceptions abound, of course.) Also, whereas L&D nurses may change shifts several times during your labor, the midwife will stay with you. She also has a more personal relationship with you than the labor nurses, by virtue of having provided all your prenatal care. And most midwives are women, which many mothers-to-be prefer.

If you're a high-risk pregnancy, however, your medical needs will be beyond the scope of most certified nurse-midwives. And though CNMs practicing in hospitals have physicians in easy reach should something go wrong during delivery (say, an emergency C-section was warranted), those who practice at some birthing centers or at home do not have the necessary backup immediately at hand.

While selecting a healthcare provider, also think about what kind of delivery you imagine. Ask where your candidate has delivery privileges. Babies are born today (1) in traditional labor wards at hospitals, where you might labor in one room, be transferred to somewhere else for delivery, and move to yet another room for recovery; (2) in hospital maternity centers with all-in-one-place LDR (labor-delivery-recovery) rooms, also called family birthing rooms, which resemble hotel rooms; (3) in independent maternity centers (that often favor natural childbirth and may have restrictions, say, against epidurals or C-sections); or (4) at home. Evaluate how well you like the hospital where your doctor would deliver you. What's the birth experience typically like there? Poll friends for their input, too. And think about convenience: how far are the doctor or midwife, and the birth facility, from your home?

The First Exam

Knowing you're pregnant as early as possible gives you more time to absorb the news. More urgently, it allows you to make health and lifestyle changes in time for them to ensure your baby's odds of healthy development. That's why the first person you should call as soon as you suspect a pregnancy (other than your mate) is your doctor. In addition to assessing your health and providing timely advice, an early appointment also enables the doctor to accurately assign your due date, which may be important later if you have preterm labor or are overdue.

Most physicians recommend scheduling the first prenatal visit between the sixth and tenth weeks of pregnancy. Earlier than that, many pregnancies are naturally and inevitably lost. (See "Early Miscarriage," page 81.) Later than 10 weeks is much too late to provide you with useful counseling for the period while the embryo is forming.

What will happen at your initial appointment, which is usually the longest and most comprehensive checkup?

• *A detailed medical history.* Covers your parents and grandparents as well as background on your menstrual history, previous pregnancies, lifestyle (do you smoke? drink? where do you work?), and diseases, birth defects, or genetic problems in either family.

• *An external physical exam.* Evaluates your overall health, including breasts, lungs, and heart. Your blood pressure and weight will also be recorded as a baseline comparison for later changes.

• *An internal physical exam.* Assesses your reproductive system, looking for any problem with your cervix, vagina, uterus, fallopian tubes, or ovaries. It also determines the size and position of your uterus, relative to how many weeks pregnant you are.

• *An estimation of your due date.* Usually based on the first day of your last menstrual period, so arrive with that date in mind.

• *Various lab tests.* (See next section.)

After the initial exam, you'll return once a month until the last trimester. From about 28 weeks, you'll be seen once every 2 weeks, then from 36 weeks, once a week. If yours is a complicated or high-risk pregnancy, you'll probably come in more often to be monitored or to have extra tests.

First-Trimester Tests

Prenatal tests help keep tabs on your general health (and, in turn, your baby's) and screen for problems that may be treatable if caught early. It's smart to be an active participant in the process. Develop the habit of asking a test's purpose at the time it's taken. Your doctor may be keeping mum so as not to make you worry unduly, but you have a right to know. Even more important, follow up on the findings at your next visit if the information isn't volunteered.

In the first trimester, you may encounter the following routine and optional exams:

• *Pregnancy test.* (routine) A blood or urine test to confirm your pregnancy is often done first. This may not be necessary, though, if a home test was positive and an internal exam verifies the result.

• *Blood pressure.* (routine) Taking this reading at the beginning of your pregnancy will establish your normal figures. Further readings can be compared with them. Small changes in blood pressure during pregnancy are normal; your doctor will look for sudden increases, which could indicate pregnancy-induced hypertension or *preeclampsia.* (See "Preeclampsia," page 190.)

• **Urinalysis.** (routine) Your sample will be taken and tested each checkup for protein, blood, or bacteria that may signal a bladder or kidney problem, including urinary tract infections. Sugar in the urine can also be a sign of diabetes, and a protein called albumin may indicate the presence of preeclampsia or kidney disease. A urine test is also used to measure levels of the hormone hCG.

• **Pap smear.** (routine) Cells will be scraped from your cervix to check for precancerous or cancerous changes. Vaginal swabs are also used to detect chlamydia, gonorrhea, and bacterial vaginosis, an infection that could lead to preterm birth if untreated.

• **Blood and Rh type.** (routine) This first-visit blood test determines your type (A, B, AB, or O) and your Rh status (positive or negative). It will also screen for the presence of Rh antibodies. The *Rh factor* is a protein on the surface of the red blood cells. Whether or not you have it matters only when you are pregnant. If the mother doesn't have the Rh factor (meaning she is Rh-negative) and her fetus does (having inherited the Rh factor from an Rh-positive father), the mother can become Rh-sensitized, or *isoimmunized*, when their blood mixes. This almost always happens at delivery but sometimes occurs earlier. During a subsequent pregnancy with an Rh-positive fetus, the mother's body will produce antibodies to combat what it perceives to be a foreign substance. These antibodies can cross the placenta and destroy the future fetus's Rh-positive blood cells, putting it at grave risk. This is called *Rh disease*. Typically the first child born has no problems, whatever its blood type. But if the first baby is Rh-positive, the antibodies left behind in the mother will endanger future Rh-positive babies.

If you are Rh-negative—and approximately 15 percent of women are—you'll be given an injection of *Rh immunoglobulin* (or RhIg; trade name: RhoGAM), a naturally occurring blood product, between 28 and 29 weeks and, if your baby is Rh-positive, again within 72 hours of delivery. This shot almost always prevents the mother from producing antibodies against Rh-positive cells. It may also be given after the tests CVS or amniocentesis, any abortion or miscarriage, an ectopic pregnancy, or following some vaginal bleeding. The shot must be repeated at delivery and again during each successive pregnancy.

Also available is a newer Rh immune globulin called WinRho SD. This product works exactly the same way but, unlike RhoGAM, has been treated to render viruses such as HIV and hepatitis C inactive. No Rh shot has even been implicated in the spread of a disease, but because it is a blood product some people may still worry.

Rh disease used to cause problems ranging from severe newborn jaundice and the need for blood transfusions to late miscarriages and stillbirths. Thanks to the development of RhoGAM, however, complications from having Rh-negative blood pose little threat. If a pregnant woman is found to be Rh-sensitized (that is, she has already produced antibodies that will fight Rh-positive cells), her doctor will monitor her throughout her pregnancy. The prenatal tests amniocentesis or CVS can reveal the fetus's blood type. If it's Rh-negative, nothing further needs to be done. If it's Rh-positive, or if no prenatal testing is done to disclose the fetus's blood type, the level of antibodies in the mother's blood will be monitored throughout the pregnancy and the baby can also be evaluated in utero for signs of Rh disease. Treatment may include an intrauterine blood transfusion to the umbilical cord to minimize danger to the baby.

• *Anemia.* (routine) A blood test for anemia (iron deficiency) measures the amount of hemoglobin, an oxygen-carrying protein, in your red blood cells. If you have too little, you are anemic. Most anemias can be easily treated. Iron deficiency is the usual cause; you'll probably be prescribed an iron-rich diet and iron supplement pills. Because your blood volume doubles during pregnancy, it's easy to tax your iron stores. Iron-deficiency anemia is fairly common, especially by mid-pregnancy. This is a major reason most pregnant women are prescribed special prenatal vitamins and retested in midpregnancy for anemia.

• *Rubella immunity.* (routine) Having rubella (German measles) during the first trimester of pregnancy can cause birth defects, so a blood test is performed to determine whether a woman is immune—that is, whether she's had the illness previously or has been vaccinated. If you aren't immune, it's vital to avoid exposure.

• *Sexually transmitted diseases, or STDs.* (optional) Chlamydia, syphilis, gonorrhea, herpes, and other such STDs can be passed from the mother to the fetus, with potentially serious consequences. If detected early, some effects of these illnesses can be treated and minimized, preventing the baby from being at risk of infection. Always be candid about your past history with a new physician.

• *AIDS.* (optional) This is a relatively new addition to the blood-test roster, and doctors recommend it for all expectant patients. That's because a pregnant woman with the AIDS virus can lower the chance of her fetus becoming infected by two-thirds if she is treated early with the drug AZT.

• *Genetic disorder screens.* (optional) Depending on your racial, ethnic, or family background, your doctor may suggest that you and your partner consider blood tests for genetic problems that are found more often in certain population groups. Tay-Sachs disease, for example, which causes nervous-system degeneration and eventually death, occurs more often in descendants of Middle European Ashkenazi Jews. African Americans run a higher risk of sickle-cell anemia, a deformity of the red blood cells that can have mild to life-threatening consequences.

• **Ultrasound.** (optional) To most expectant moms, this word has come to mean: "Our first baby snapshot!" and "Is it a boy or a girl?" There are actually several types of ultrasound exams, whose purpose is medical, rather than gender revealing.

Ultrasound is energy in the form of sound waves. A *Doppler* ultrasound reflects motion—such as the fetal heartbeat—in the form of audio signals. A handheld device called a *transducer* is placed over your abdomen. The reassuring, rapid "whoosh, whoosh" of your baby's heartbeat, which will be audible to anyone in the room, is one of the highlights of the first trimester. A Doppler first picks up the heartbeat around 11 weeks and can be done at any time in pregnancy. It's also used to monitor the fetal heart rate during labor and to measure blood flow within vessels of the uterus, fetus, and umbilical cord.

In an ultrasound you see on a screen (also called a *sonogram*), grainy, jerky pictures are formed by sound waves reflecting off organs and being read by scanners. Another type of transducer is moved across your abdomen, scanning the area to produce an image of your baby and the placenta. It's painless, and a bit like a computer mouse gliding across a mousepad. The image produced can help to ascertain the baby's age and rate of growth, to locate the placenta, to check fetal movement and heart rate, to assess the amount of amniotic fluid in the uterus, to count the number of fetuses, and to diagnose some birth defects.

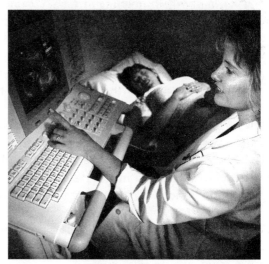

Ultrasounds can be performed abdominally or vaginally. A *vaginal ultrasound*, which uses a wandlike transducer that's inserted into the vagina, is most

Your baby's first photo opportunity may come by way of ultrasound—grainy pictures of the fetus formed by sound waves reflecting off his or her organs.

common in the first trimester because it produces a better image. It's used to help date a pregnancy, to diagnose an ectopic pregnancy, to find the cause of bleeding or pain, or to spot certain types of birth defects. Any discomfort you feel is mild; a vaginal ultrasound feels like having a Pap smear, though it lasts longer.

You may be given an ultrasound in your first trimester if the doctor has reason to suspect a multiple pregnancy or if there are possible complications, such as bleeding or a history of miscarriage. An early sonogram may also be warranted if the heartbeat cannot be picked up by a Doppler.

Ultrasounds have become a standard part of prenatal care because of the wealth of information they provide at little risk to the mother or baby. Despite early concerns about how much ultrasound is advisable, the medical community has found them safe in some three decades of regular use. Still, some insurance companies, doctors, and scientific studies question their usefulness. One major study of more than 15,000 women in low-risk pregnancies concluded there was little benefit to routine sonograms because, while they detected more anomalies, these problems couldn't be addressed before birth anyway. Also, some insurers may pay for only a limited number of ultrasounds (excluding Doppler use) or cover them only for high-risk patients.

• **Chorionic villus sampling or CVS.** (optional) CVS is usually performed at 10 to 12 weeks. Along with amniocentesis (a similar test done at 15 to 18 weeks), CVS is one of the most informative invasive screening tests for birth defects. (An invasive test involves going into the mother's body, unlike a noninvasive blood or urine test, in which fluid comes out of the body.) *Chorionic villi* are tiny, fingerlike extensions of the chorion, a fetal membrane that is part of the placenta formed from the fertilized egg, giving them the same genetic makeup as the fetus. In the procedure, developed in the last decade, a small sample of these cells is removed and grown for examination in a lab.

There are two ways to collect the cells. In a *transvaginal* CVS, a speculum (the same device used in a Pap smear) may be inserted in the vagina, followed by a thin plastic tube, which is guided in place with the assistance of an ultrasound. Alternatively, a needle may be inserted through the abdomen to the placenta for a *transabdominal* CVS. The discomfort you're liable to feel will come primarily from the full bladder you may be asked to bring to ensure a good ultrasound picture, although some women complain of cramping similar to their periods. The risk of miscarriage as a result of the procedure is 1 percent, or roughly double that of amniocentesis. There is also a very slight risk of limb deformities. (See "CVS or Amnio?" page 46.)

• *Embryoscopy.* (optional) This new procedure allows doctors to examine a fetus as early as 6 weeks, though more typically around 10 weeks. Guided by an ultrasound, the doctor inserts a thin needle into your abdomen. Next, an *endoscope* (a tiny medical telescope) is threaded through the needle and into the uterine cavity, and a video camera is attached to the end outside the body— revealing a head-to-toe picture of the embryo or fetus on a video screen. Not yet widely performed, embryoscopy is used only when there is reason to suspect certain problems (say, early ultrasounds hint at malformations or the mother took a medication linked to birth defects). The procedure's risk of miscarriage is 1 percent when done between 10 and 12 weeks—about double that of amniocentesis.

• *Fetoscopy.* (optional) In rare cases (such as when a serious blood or skin disorder is suspected), a miniscule telescope is passed through the abdomen or cervix to examine the fetus or embryo. Done at 18 to 22 weeks, there is a 3 to 5 percent chance that the procedure will cause a miscarriage.

Cautions on Prenatal Testing

Despite the modern craving that many parents have to find out their baby's sex in advance, most admit, "I just want my child to be born healthy." The prospect of learning more about your baby's health before birth can be tantalizing, reassuring—and unnerving, too. Not all results are conclusive. False-positives (in which a test result suggests a problem when there isn't one) and false-negatives (in which a test result suggests everything's fine when in fact a problem exists) are frequent for tests such as ultrasound or alpha-fetoprotein (AFP). Some procedures, such as amnio or CVS, introduce potential dangers, albeit rare ones.

Before giving you any prenatal test, your doctor should lay out the pros and cons and be able to explain what he or she hopes to learn from it. Many tests (such as urinalysis) are no risk, high gain, and therefore highly recommended and considered routine. Others (such as AFP or amnio) are recommended for specific medical indications and are performed with the patient's explicit consent. Together, you and your caregiver can weigh the risks and benefits of each test for your individual pregnancy.

But be forewarned that, while it's a huge relief to know that a certain test turned up nothing wrong, there is a flip side. Waiting for results (and imagining the horrors that might be unearthed) can be nerve-racking. So can deciding what to do next if a test indicates the possibility of a problem, but the doctor isn't certain. (See "Test Anxiety," page 111.) You'll also want to consider, ahead of time, what actions you'll take following bad news. If you know you wouldn't terminate the pregnancy for any reason, there are certain tests, such as amnio, that you may *not* want. On the other hand, knowing in advance about a problem gives you time to absorb the news and learn all you can about it before making a decision. If you continue with the pregnancy, knowing about a problem in advance also enables you to arrange for delivery at a hospital with pediatric specialists best poised to handle it. Depending on the abnormality, you may even elect to undergo treatment in utero.

Genetic Counseling

Before having any prenatal tests (especially invasive ones), you may be advised to see a genetic counselor (someone who has advanced training in genetics). You may also be referred to such a specialist if you are over 35 or 40, have a family history of birth defects or genetic disease, or have had a child with those conditions, or have had multiple miscarriages or a stillbirth. Inherited disorders include Tay-Sachs disease (which afflicts French Canadians and Middle European Ashkenazi Jews); sickle-cell anemia (African Americans; some Mediterranean Caucasians); thalassemia and Cooley's anemia (Mediterranean Caucasians and some Asians). Genetic-defect disorders include Down's syndrome, muscular dystrophy, hemophilia, spina bifida, epilepsy, and cystic fibrosis.

To assess your specific risks, you'll be asked for detailed family histories and may be given special tests. You'll also be advised on your options (though genetic counselors do not make any decisions for you). Such counseling is entirely optional. For many couples, however, the information offered in genetic counseling offers reassurance and potential courses of action in the face of uncertainty.

Checklist: Questions to Ask at Your First Visit

Your caregiver should make time to talk about his or her policies and philosophies at your first prenatal encounter—preferably before you change into an examining gown. Bedside manner counts, too. Is he or she forthcoming with explanations and up-to-date in his or her thinking? Does he or she seem interested in you personally, or does the individual rarely look up from his or her charts? You want a healthcare partner, not a dictator. Learn the answers to questions such as:

☐ *How do I reach you if I have an emergency or an urgent question?* Find out whether the practice posts an on-call doctor 24 hours a day (more likely in larger group practices than in two-doc operations). If there's an answering service after hours, how long does it usually take before a health professional responds? If you call the office, can you talk directly to the doctor? Some physicians return all calls at a certain point in the day, while others reserve a special line for messages or staff it with a nurse who can answer basic questions or act as a go-between with the doctor for other information. There's no single best setup, so long as you can get a prompt response.

☐ *What are the odds that you—rather than an associate—will deliver my baby?* Many group practices rotate on-call duty, so the likelihood of your regular doctor's being present for your labor may only be 1 in 5 or 1 in 10. Nor is a solo doc likely to be available 24 hours a day, 365 days a year. If having a familiar doctor deliver matters to you, you may be happier with a smaller practice (where you get to know a handful of MDs) or with a nurse-midwife. On the other hand, few physicians hold your hand throughout labor. But you'll want to know how the medical partners' views compare with your doctor's, and whether your wishes will be communicated to the physician on-call.

☐ *Where do you deliver?* Which labor procedures (IVs, enemas, pubic shaves, continuous fetal monitoring) are routine there? Tour the hospital now, so you're familiar with its requirements. Most women make the mistake of waiting until the third trimester, when making a change can be a hassle.

☐ *Under what circumstances do you induce labor? How often and why do you give epidurals? Episiotomies?* You obviously can't predict what your individual case will require, but you'll get a sense of the caregiver's outlooks from his responses.

☐ *How do your patients usually approach pain management, and how does the decision for pain relief in labor get made?* The best answer, of course, is that the patient's wishes are respected going into labor and she's consulted throughout.

☐ *What's your C-section rate?* Recognize that doctors specializing in high-risk patients will, necessarily, have higher percentages. In what circumstances does the doctor perform them? Can your husband or coach be with you at all times, even in surgery?

☐ *Additional questions for a nurse-midwife:* How do you reach her when you're in labor? Who is the backup physician? Under what circumstances would the midwife call in a physician? How quickly can he or she get to the place you're delivering? If you need a C-section, will the midwife stay with you?

GOOD ADVICE: GETTING THE MOST OUT OF CHECKUPS

"I looked forward to my appointment for a month, and then I was in and out in five minutes." Don't leave your checkups with that common lament. Here's how to feel better about your visits:

- Between appointments, jot down questions that occur to you on a sheet of paper kept in some handy place, like your purse or the refrigerator door. Bring it with you.
- Speak up. Your caregiver's not a mind-reader and may not know what's bugging you just by looking at your physical stats.
- Consider *nothing* too small ("There's this twitch in my side") or too embarrassing ("I think I've got hemorrhoids") to mention.
- Bring evidence. Show your doctor the labels of vitamins, herb teas, or medications whose safety you're doubting.
- Don't tolerate a doctor who won't give you complete answers, show reasonable compassion, or bestow his or her full attention. After all, that's what you're paying for.
- Question anything you're told—it's your right.
- At the same time, be open-minded. State preferences, rather than make demands. And listen. Your provider has gone through a lot more pregnancies than you have.

CVS or Amnio?

Deciding which, if any, prenatal screenings for birth defects you'll choose can be wrenching. Your provider will probably lay out the pros and cons of each course and interpret them according to your age, lifestyle, stage of pregnancy, and other factors. But ultimately, the choice is yours. Or you may elect to skip a test, regardless of your age or whether your insurance will cover it. Some considerations regarding the two most common invasive screens are given in the table on page 47.

	GENERALLY RECOMMENDED IF	HOW IT WORKS	WHEN GIVEN	RESULTS ARRIVE	MISCARRIAGE RISK	WHAT IT SHOWS
CVS	You're over 35, want results as early in your term as possible, have a family history of birth defects or other reason to suspect them.	A thin needle is inserted in your abdomen or through your vagina to collect chorionic villi cells from the placenta, which are then tested.	Usually 10 to 12 weeks, sometimes sooner.	Usually within 7 days, but may take up to 3 weeks.	About 1 percent, probably because it's done so early and removes material located nearer the fetus; possibly less if done by an experienced technician. CVS has also been linked to .03% risk of causing limb defects when performed before 10 weeks.	Certain major birth defects; some genetic diseases; sex of baby. Cannot detect open neural tube defects. Not as widely available as amniocentesis because it requires special training.
Amniocentesis	You're over 35, have an abnormal reading on your alpha-fetoprotein (AFP) blood test (given at 15 to 18 weeks), have a family history of birth defects or other reason to suspect them.	A thin needle is inserted into your abdomen and uterus to remove a sample of amniotic fluid, from which cells will be grown and tested.	Usually performed at 15 to 18 weeks, but can be done as early as 11 weeks by someone with special training.	In 7 days to 2 weeks. Some information available within 24 hours at certain major medical centers.	About 0.2 to 0.5% at 15 weeks, and 2.2% at 11 to 14 weeks.	Certain major birth defects, including 95 percent of neural tube defects; some genetic diseases; the baby's sex. Is 99% accurate in detecting Down's syndrome and other chromosomal abnormalities.

I don't like my healthcare provider? Find a new one, fast. Pregnancy is an emotional time anyway, and your comfort level is a lot more important than harboring anger or disappointment. Remember you'll be seeing this person once or twice a month (or more). Don't feel guilty. You don't even have to give a reason, unless you think articulating the reason for your discontent might benefit other patients. After you've chosen a new doctor, write to the old one requesting the quick transfer of your medical records.

I don't want certain tests? It's your right to refuse prenatal tests, although doing so can affect the level of care you receive. Many tests (including urine screenings, blood pressure checks, and many blood tests) are virtually risk free and have become simply standard practice; some may be required by state laws. Common, but less routine tests (such as amniocentesis or the alpha-fetoprotein screen) may be recommended, though the decision to take them should be made jointly. If you're over 35, for example, amnio may be advised, but if you would not act on possible negative findings (for example, have an abortion) or wouldn't want to know about them ahead of time, there's no reason to take the test. Always speak up with questions or reservations about any exam.

For More Help: Prenatal Care Resources

- The American College of Obstetricians and Gynecologists, Resource Center, AP109, P.O. Box 96920, Washington, DC 20090-6920. Send a business-size SASE to request the brochure "Your Ob-Gyn: Your Partner in Healthcare."
- The American College of Nurse-Midwives, 818 Connecticut Avenue NW, Suite 900, Washington, DC 20006; 202-728-9860. For information on nurse-midwife referrals.
- The National Association of Childbearing Centers, 3123 Gottschall Road, Perkiomenville, PA 18074. For information about freestanding maternity centers.

What Should I Eat?

Why This Trimester Is Unique

For now, forget about "eating for two" or forcing down green veggies. During the first 3 months, the fetal *formation stage*, the vital organs and body systems are unfolding in a carefully calibrated, preordained order. The fetus needs little from you to accomplish this task other than a generally healthy and well-hydrated environment, a few key nutrients, and protection from poisons. Despite all the action taking place within you, your caloric needs barely rise—only by 100 to 200 calories a day, the amount in a glass of milk! By contrast, the last 6 months of gestation, the fetus's *growth stage*, will demand an extraordinary amount of calories and nutrition of you. (More about that in the next chapter.)

Therefore it makes sense to think about food differently during the first trimester. That may be easy, especially if you're having any degree of nausea. Spinach salads or trout amandine may be impossible to stomach no matter how well-intentioned you are. That's okay. Pregnant women are so deluged with information (and misinformation) about proper diet that it's easy to become paranoid about counting fat grams and guilt-ridden over an innocent muffin. The reality is that a healthy, balanced diet is fairly easy for the average American to obtain, with a little special attention but not necessarily much effort.

That's not to say you have 12 free weeks to gorge on garbage. Nutrition *is* important throughout pregnancy, perhaps more so than at any other time of your life. Right now, what the "trust your instincts" message means is that you don't have to be a slave to the food pyramid or force yourself to eat things you can't stand. Some women also find that they develop preferences for certain types or textures of foods, especially salty or crunchy ones, and for fruits. The sane way to view your diet in the first trimester is to aim for the optimum, but don't berate yourself if you fall short.

Recent research in evolutionary biology suggests that in early pregnancy, we're actually programmed to avoid certain types of foods because they present potential dangers to the developing fetus. Not all doctors subscribe to this theory, so you're still apt to get drilled on the basic food groups at your first prenatal visit. But the idea does bear a certain logic.

It goes like this: The food aversions, changes in smell, nausea, and vomiting that make up pregnancy sickness (or "morning sickness") during the first trimester serve to protect the developing embryo from naturally occurring plant and bacterial toxins, which can cause birth defects and miscarriage. The expectant mother temporarily loses her appetite for these potentially dangerous foods, even those she once counted as her favorites, and avoids them. It's a primitive safeguard dating to the days when our ancestors hunted wild animals and gathered wild plants.

According to the theory, many (but not all) of these toxins pose no threat to the fetus once its major organs and body systems are in place. That timing coincides with the passing of the mother's natural aversion for their odors and tastes—by the end of the first trimester. A woman who experiences very little pregnancy sickness may lack a natural defense against these substances, but should try to avoid them even if she can tolerate them well. These include pungent, bitter foods (such as broccoli or garlic); fried, burnt, or barbecued meats; most condiments (such as horseradish and mustard); potatoes (the skins, especially, have been linked to neural tube defects); and beverages made from bitter plants (coffee, tea, cola).

Healthy Practices to Start Now

• *Aim for nutritional variety.* Give your usual eating habits a close inspection. At the very least check your typical diet against the USDA's recommended Food Pyramid, the ubiquitous black triangle found on food packaging, which is a general guide on how much to eat from the basic food groups. Even if you can't stomach all the food groups in perfect harmony, certain vitamins *are* worth aiming for now. Folate, for example, can prevent spinal-cord defects, making it vital before conception and through the first 10 weeks. Iron is needed to fuel the extra blood cells manufactured during pregnancy.

• *Wean off caffeine.* To brew or not to brew? The scientific jury is still out on the advisability of caffeine during pregnancy. Some studies have linked its consumption to miscarriage, low birthweight, and birth defects such as cleft palate. Other researchers believe the methodology in such research was flawed (risk factors such as smoking and alcohol were not always taken into account) and that if caffeine is risky, it's only a problem at very high doses. On the other hand, caffeine has no obvious benefit to the fetus, either. It's a stimulant, which increases your heartbeat and metabolism, adding stress to the fetus. It's also a diuretic, which causes you to lose valuable fluids and calcium needed to maintain a healthy pregnancy. Caffeine also inhibits the absorption of iron.

The general medical consensus is that moderate amounts are probably okay—between 150 and 300 milligrams per day, or one to three cups of coffee, depending on the blend. Still, if you're a java junkie, you know it's easy to quaff six or more cups in a day. Factor in after-dinner espressos and lattes, a Coke, and some chocolate, and a day's caffeine consumption can climb quickly. (See "How Caffeine Adds Up," page 51.) Some over-the-counter medications that contain aspirin (such as Anacin, Excedrin, Dristan) also contain caffeine. If you want to get off caffeine but can't quit cold turkey, try brewing coffee and tea more weakly than usual. Letting a teabag steep in a cup for 30 seconds, rather than 2 or 3 minutes, more than halves the caffeine content. Also, your taste buds may do the cutting back for you, since a bent for coffee often evaporates in the first trimester. When caffeine's natural bitterness is masked by sweeteners in cola and candy, however, your body may not reject it as readily.

How Caffeine Adds Up
What's the caffeine content of your favorite beverages?

BEVERAGE	AMOUNT	CAFFEINE
Coffee	5 ounces	80 to 120 mg
Latte, mocha, or cappuccino	5 ounces	60 to 180 mg (depending on coffee blend)
Nonherbal tea	5 ounces	20 to 100 mg (depending on tea and how long it steeps)
Iced tea	8 ounces	30 to 60 mg
Cola	12-ounce can	22 to 45 mg
Dark chocolate	2 ounces	40 mg
Milk chocolate	2 ounces	12 mg
Coffee ice cream	1/2 cup	20 mg

• *Junk the junk food.* A Big Mac or a bag of Fritos is harmless enough. Sometimes, in fact, it might feel like just the thing to save your sanity. Generally, though, junk foods and fast foods are high in fat and low in nutrients, compared to other foods. Depending on how often you indulge, you might pull up short on the necessary nutrients that are more easily found in whole foods like fruits and breads. Highly processed junk foods are also slower to digest than whole foods, and thus can cause bloating and gassiness.

Luckily the newer low-fat, fat-free, and baked-not-fried snacks help make cutting back on the fat content (if not the gassiness) of snack foods less traumatic. Even drive-through menus offer more diverse choices than ever before, including salads and grilled sandwiches. If you eat fast food every day for lunch, try to cut back to just once or twice a week. Order menu choices that haven't gone into the fryer. Best bets: the salad bar, grilled chicken, roast beef sandwich, chili, pizza with vegetable toppings. Ask the server to hold the mayo. And bring along a banana, carrot sticks, or other raw fruits and vegetables as a side dish to your sandwich order. They may taste better than greasy fries or onion rings to your pregnant palate anyway.

How Much Weight Gain?

The usual recommendation today is 25 to 35 pounds. If you're very athletic or have spent half your life counting fat grams and doing step aerobics in a cellulite battle, that may sound like a huge amount. But in truth most of those pounds make up the baby, the placenta, amniotic fluid, your enlarged uterus and

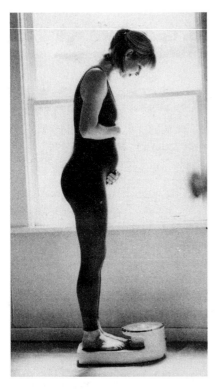

breasts, and your increased blood volume. (See page 110.) And what's really "yours" isn't idle fat; it helps ensure a well-nourished baby. In the first trimester, for example, the typical gain is just a few pounds, much of that the result of your increased blood volume.

Your pre-pregnancy size influences weight gain, too. The American College of Obstetricians and Gynecologists recommends that women who weigh less than the ideal for their height and build put on 28 to 40 pounds, but overweight women should gain just 15 to 25 pounds. Obese women, defined as 20 percent above the ideal, are urged to gain just 15 pounds, but also require closer monitoring by their caregiver since they're at higher risk for many complications. Women expecting twins should add 35 to 45 pounds.

The typical pace for gaining is 3 to 5 pounds in the first trimester, then about ½ pound to 1 pound per week through the eighth month, with a slighter gain in the ninth month. This is just a rough rule of thumb, though. You may find that you gain just 3 pounds one month, then 6 or 8 the next. In very hot weather, you may retain more water weight. In general, your doctor will be monitoring you for gradual gain, without sharp increases or drops. It's best for most women not to gain too much in the first trimester, however. Most of those pounds go to you, not the fetus, and will be harder to shed after delivery. What's more, women "wear" their pregnancies differently, depending on their bone structures, heights, and builds. The two most common archetypes are the "pumpkin" (who carries all in front) and the "box" (who gets a little bigger all over). Two pregnant women at the same stage may look quite different, even if they weighed the same when they conceived and proceeded to gain at the same pace.

If you gain more than the recommended amount, then what? In fact, there are some risks. Gaining too many pounds in pregnancy can up your risk of gestational diabetes, hypertension, varicose veins, backache, preterm labor, and Cesarean delivery. Only about 10 to 12 pounds will be shed at delivery in the form of the baby, placenta, and amniotic fluid. You'll lose several more pounds in the weeks after childbirth in the form of bodily fluids, and sometimes a little more if you breastfeed. What's left you'll need to work off after postpartum recovery, or live with.

Gaining too little, on the other hand, can interfere with normal fetal growth and development, a condition known as *intrauterine growth retardation* or *intrauterine growth restriction*, or IUGR. (IUGR occurs when a baby is smaller than expected for its gestational age, and can happen for many reasons.) A fetus denied necessary nutrients will try to get them from the mother's muscle and body fat, which may sound handy but in fact can lead to a condition known as *ketonuria*, a metabolic reaction in which dangerous compounds are released into the bloodstream that can further retard fetal growth. Without sufficient carbohydrate intake, the calories taken in from protein get burned for energy, rather than being applied to fetal brain and muscle development. Finally, underweight babies (less than 5½ pounds) statistically have more health problems than those at normal weights.

All that said, however, don't let a preoccupation with the scale (or a preachy doctor) ruin this thrilling time of life. Pregnancy is a time to gain weight, not worry about losing it. The fact is, you're going to get bigger during the next 9 months—no matter what. Many expectant women eat more vigorously than ever and gain just 20 pounds. Many more mamas-to-be gain 50 or more pounds, experience no complications, deliver healthy babies vaginally, and then lose the extra padding over the next year through breastfeeding and chasing after a growing baby. *Everyone's different.*

If you're gaining weight too quickly, your doctor may want to review your nutritional know-how as well as your estimated date of delivery. It's possible your dates may be wrong, or even (rarely) that you're carrying undiagnosed multiple fetuses. In addition to talking to your doctor, you should check your diet with the special expertise of a nutritionist or a health educator, who may be able to point out diet pitfalls you hadn't noticed and work out a healthy eating plan for the rest of your pregnancy.

More ways to not make yourself crazy over this culturally charged issue:

* *Don't* compare yourself to other pregnant women.
* *Don't* obsess over numbers (or bother mapping your weight gain against a curve on a chart that indicates the optimum).
* *Don't* even look during weigh-ins at checkups, if you find it upsetting.
* *Do* take off your shoes and bulky sweater before you step on the scale, if doing so makes you feel better.

- *Do* try to make the most healthful food choices you can, exercise regularly, and eat an occasional ice cream cone if you feel like it.
- Above all, *don't* attempt to diet while you're expecting.

If You're Overweight at the Start

Many women are substantially overweight when they conceive—what, if anything, should they do differently with regard to their diet? First, a woman in this situation should consider the reason she's overweight. Very likely, she has less than ideal eating habits and may not exercise regularly. Fortunately, pregnancy provides greater motivation to make healthful changes than at any other time in her life. And the revved-up metabolism of pregnancy can help her.

If you've started your pregnancy heavy, begin keeping a journal of everything you eat for an entire week—the type of food and how much you consumed. Be brutally honest and include snacks as well as meals grabbed on the run. Then take this record to a knowledgeable childbirth educator, nurse-midwife, or nutritionist. (Call a hospital or maternity center for references to people qualified to give dietary advice to pregnant women. Your doctor may not be the ideal source of this information unless he or she has had additional specialization in applied nutrition, since research has shown that most doctors don't have enough specific training in nutrition.) A nutrition expert can help you pinpoint trouble spots, such as too-large portion sizes, calorically dense foods, or an overreliance on junk foods. He or she can also suggest easy changes you can make.

Your baby's body is being formed from the foods you eat every day. As much as possible, you need to make the food you eat count for your baby. While the occasional cookie is no problem, eating a whole bag of them (or other foods that rob your appetite and provide little or no nutrients) is a big problem because such habits shortchange your baby.

If you revise your old habits during pregnancy, you'll not only be doing your baby a favor but you may find that you shed fat yourself. Women who were overweight before they got pregnant but took steps to improve their eating habits during their terms have found that they wore smaller-size clothes after they gave birth than before they conceived. Regular exercise, such as walking every day, helps a lot, too, and has such side benefits as reducing or eliminating gestational diabetes, which obese women are particularly vulnerable to.

The only caveat: *Never* diet or try to lose weight during pregnancy. Rather, your goal should simply be to reform your eating habits by making more careful choices about the foods you eat. That, in fact, is wise advice for all pregnant women, regardless of their weight at conception.

TRY THESE RECIPES!

The following recipes take into account the fussy palate characteristic of the first trimester, while serving up nutrients.

Yogurt Fruit Smoothie

Preparation time: 5 minutes

This quick drink, made in a blender or food processor, combines low-fat yogurt with fresh fruit and juice—without the addition of sugar. It makes an ideal quick breakfast or a nutritious, soothing snack. It can also be a great antidote to an unsettled stomach. Substitute whatever type of fruit is in season. Other great combinations: peach-cantaloupe, raspberry-blueberry-orange, or plum-peach.

1/2 ripe banana
1/4 cup sliced strawberries, fresh or frozen
2 tablespoons orange juice, fresh or bottled
1/2 cup plain or vanilla low-fat yogurt

Place the banana, strawberries, and orange juice in the container of a food processor or blender, and puree. Add the yogurt, and puree until smooth. Serve in a tall glass. Yield: about 1 1/4 cups, or 2 servings.

Fruity Spritzer

Preparation time: 5 minutes

This fresh, fruity drink is more interesting than drinking glass after glass of water. Experiment with your favorite juice and fruit.

1/2 cup seltzer or sparkling water
1/3 cup cranberry juice (with no sugar added)
2 tablespoons orange juice, preferably fresh-squeezed or not-from-concentrate
Ice cubes
2 tablespoons fresh raspberries
1 thin slice fresh orange

In a large glass, mix the seltzer, cranberry juice, and orange juice. Add the ice cubes and mix well. Add the raspberries and place the orange slice along the edge of the glass. Yield: 1 serving.

Sweet-Potato Chips

Preparation time: 10 minutes
Cooking time: about 13 minutes

If you crave something crunchy and comforting, these sweet and meaty chips are positively addictive. They're also loaded with fiber, beta-carotene, and vitamin C.

> 1 large sweet potato, peeled and very thinly sliced
> 2 tablespoons vegetable oil
> Salt and freshly ground black pepper

Preheat the oven to 350 degrees. Brush a very light coating of oil on a baking sheet. Lay the potato slices on the sheet, being careful not to overlap them. Using a pastry brush or the back of a spoon, brush the slices lightly with oil. Sprinkle with salt and pepper, and roast for 8 minutes.

Flip the slices with a spatula and brush the other side lightly with oil. Sprinkle with some more salt and pepper. Roast the chips another 5 minutes, or until they are cooked throughout and slightly crispy. Drain well on paper towels. Yield: 4 servings.

Cheese Frittata

Preparation time: about 20 minutes
Cooking time: 10 to 15 minutes

A cross between an omelet and a soufflé, this frittata can be made with any cheese or vegetable combination you like. In this version, folate-rich spinach and calcium-rich cheese are used.

> 2 cups fresh spinach
> 1 1/2 teaspoons olive oil
> 1 medium onion, thinly sliced (optional)
> 8 to 10 thin strips raw or roasted red bell pepper (optional)
> 1 tablespoon chopped fresh basil, or 1 teaspoon dried
> 1 1/2 teaspoons chopped fresh thyme, or 1/2 teaspoon dried
> 5 eggs
> Salt and freshly ground black pepper
> 1 cup crumbled soft goat cheese or grated hard cheese

Wash the spinach leaves well and place in a medium saucepan with the water still clinging to them. Bring to a boil, cover, and steam about 4 to 5 minutes, or until soft and tender. Drain and press the spinach between 2 small plates to remove excess moisture. Chop fine and set aside.

Preheat the oven to 400 degrees. In an ovenproof medium skillet or shallow casserole, heat the oil over moderate heat. Add the onion slices and sauté, stirring frequently, for about 8 minutes or until golden brown. Add the pepper—if raw, sauté about 3 minutes; if roasted, sauté for 1 minute. Add the cooked spinach and half the basil and thyme, then remove the vegetables to a plate and set aside.

Meanwhile, whisk the eggs with the salt, pepper, and remaining basil and thyme.

Place the skillet or casserole over moderately high heat. Add the eggs and top with the sautéed vegetables. Sprinkle with the cheese and let cook 1 minute. Remove from the heat and place on the middle shelf of the oven. Bake for 10 to 15 minutes, or until puffed and golden brown. Serve immediately. Yield: 4 servings.

Is It True...

That "eating for two" means I should double my portions? Sorry. That old adage refers to the nutrients you're passing along to your baby, not the serving sizes. The average pregnant woman requires just 150 extra calories a day in the first trimester, and an extra 250 to 300 calories per day thereafter. On the other hand, your calcium and zinc needs increase by 50 percent, and the amount of iron and folate you should consume doubles.

That decaf coffee and tea are bad, too? For a while, the agents used to decaffeinate coffee were themselves suspected of causing cancer. Today the trend in decaffeination is to use natural filtering agents, such as water, carbon dioxide, oils, or a fruit extract called ethyl acetate. The best advice is to ease your consumption of coffee altogether, especially in the first trimester. After that, occasional decaf beverages are probably fine (decaf coffee has 97 percent of its caffeine removed). Exception: some herbal teas, including sassafras, comfrey, pennyroyal, yarrow, goldenseal, and tansy, which have no caffeine but are not recommended for expectant mothers. Two safe herbal teas are peppermint and chamomile. Most brand-name herbal teas sold commercially are also okay, but always check the labels.

That chocolate milk provides less calcium? The calcium content is the same in chocolate milk and white milk (284 milligrams per 8 ounces) and is absorbed just as well, though the fat content is a little higher when milk is not skim. As for caffeine—a cup of chocolate milk has just 5 milligrams.

Checklist: Best/Worst Foods for the First Trimester

What to eat when you're chronically queasy—not to mention uneasy about unsafe choices—during the fetal-formative stage?

Best

☐ bland cheese (such as mozzarella)
☐ 100 percent whole wheat breads or toast
☐ cold cereal
☐ cottage cheese
☐ crackers
☐ fish if well cooked and minimally seasoned
☐ fruit
☐ juice
☐ lemonade
☐ lean meat (well-cooked)
☐ milk
☐ pasta

Worst

☐ broccoli
☐ bell peppers
☐ brussels sprouts
☐ chocolate
☐ coffee
☐ mushrooms
☐ onions
☐ potatoes (especially the skins)
☐ raw meat, fish, shellfish, or eggs
☐ seasonings (including garlic, mint)
☐ tea

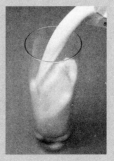

Filling in the "Problem Four"

Of all the nutrients your body needs right now, most pregnant women's diets are notoriously low in four. Make a point to stoke up on these vitamins and minerals:

RDA*	*WHY YOU NEED IT*	*WHERE TO GET IT*
Iron		
30 milligrams.	Helps manufacture hemoglobin, a component of red blood cells that carries oxygen in the bloodstream (and, in turn, to the fetus).	Dried fruits such as raisins, figs, apricots, and prunes; organ meats such as liver and kidneys; whole-grain breads; dark leafy vegetables; dried beans and peas; blackstrap molasses. Cooking in an iron skillet and eating vitamin C–rich foods (such as orange juice) with those that contain iron enhances iron absorption.
Folate (Folic Acid)		
400 micrograms (though some researchers recommend 800 micrograms).	Produces the extra blood you and your baby need; in early pregnancy helps prevent neural-tube defects and cleft palate. Can also reduce odds of a preterm delivery.	Leafy green vegetables, liver, asparagus, lean beef, lentils, oranges, peanuts, chocolate, fortified breakfast cereal. As of January 1998, the FDA requires manufacturers to fortify enriched grain products (bread, pasta, rice) with this B vitamin.
Calcium		
1,200 milligrams.	Builds fetal teeth and bones without depleting your resources; may help reduce high blood pressure.	Skim milk, yogurt, cottage cheese, hard cheese, dark leafy vegetables (kale, collard greens), dried figs, dried beans, canned salmon and sardines.
Zinc		
20 milligrams.	Aids conception and ensures fetal growth.	Fish, oysters, shellfish, eggs, meat, milk, wheat germ.

*RDA=Recommended Daily Allowance (for pregnant women)

Good Advice: How to Drink More Water

Aim for six to eight 8-ounce glasses of H_2O a day (that's 48 to 64 ounces) to keep your body well hydrated. This reduces constipation and dry skin, too. You'll probably find yourself parched more often then usual in early pregnancy. Don't worry that drinking extra water will send you to the bathroom more—you'll spend plenty of time there regardless. The advantage of lots of water later in pregnancy is that it wards off dehydration, which can trigger preterm labor.
Try these tricks:

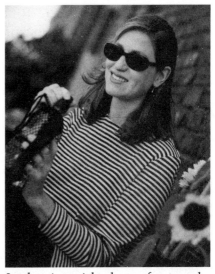

• Chill a gallon (64 ounces) of water at the beginning of the day and draw your consumption from it all day long to be sure you get the total amount.
• Carry a quart-size plastic sports bottle with you throughout the day.
• Have a glass with every meal.
• Substitute water for your customary cup of coffee or tea, and drink it out of your favorite mug.
• Try sparkling or flavored waters if you can tolerate the carbonation, but only as a supplement, not as your main water source.

It takes six to eight glasses of water a day to keep an expectant mother well hydrated.

• Dilute fruit juice with half water to make one or two of your daily glasses more palatable.
• Leave a full glass in the bathroom at night to sip when you get up to urinate.

What If...

My prenatal vitamin makes me sick? If your doctor agrees, you can postpone starting your prenatal vitamin until the second trimester, when your queasiness subsides. Or try to take it on a full stomach. Sometimes iron is overprescribed—say, if a supplement is recommended before your blood workup reveals whether you're anemic or not—which can cause nausea and constipation. If your vitamin is making you sick, ask whether it's possible you may be taking too much iron.

I can't keep *anything* down? During the first trimester, calorie intake is less important than just keeping yourself generally healthy and hydrated. When you can eat, make your choices as healthful as possible and drink lots of fluids, particularly salty ones like soup or potassium-refueling beverages like Gatorade. But if you're vomiting persistently, contact your doctor, especially if you can't even tolerate liquids, have cottonmouth and dry skin, and notice your urine getting darker. Though rare, dehydration is a serious risk to you and your baby. (See "Common Aches and Pains: Pregnancy sickness," page 13.)

MOTHER TO MOTHER:
"Eating Vegetarian"

Elizabeth Sinnott, 23
New York, New York

A year and a half before her second pregnancy, Elizabeth became a vegetarian. She eats fish, seafood, eggs, and dairy products, but no red meat or chicken. Going into her pregnancy her aim was to deliver at a birthing center, but because Elizabeth was slightly anemic (she had a low iron count), her risk of hemorrhaging during labor was increased. Therefore, the birthing center told her to increase her iron levels.

To help gauge Elizabeth's specific needs, her midwife asked her to keep a complete food diary for 3 days. The results showed that she got plenty of protein, especially from the nuts and seeds she likes to snack on and because she eats seafood, but she needed to eat more fruit and drink more milk. In particular, Elizabeth needed ample iron. She tried to eat six daily servings of iron-rich foods from a list provided by her midwife, and took a prescribed prenatal vitamin and iron supplement.

Typically, pregnant vegetarians run low on protein, calcium, iron, and B_{12} (which is found mainly in animal foods). True vegans (who eschew all animal products, including dairy) need to be especially vigilant about adequate intake of these nutrients. To keep her diet interesting *and* nutritious, Elizabeth gleans recipes from vegetarian cookbooks and magazines, friends, even food boxes. "By experimenting you can come up with something great," she says. Read labels to learn more about nutrient contents, too, she suggests. Vitamin B_{12}, for example, is found in fortified breakfast cereal.

Elizabeth's tips for vegetarian moms-to-be:

• *Try every idea you get.* "Being a vegetarian sometimes narrows your diet, but there are so many wonderful recipes."

• *Be adventurous.* "I've looked into other protein sources, such as tofu, which is a form of soy. I also try to cook the same dish different ways by changing the spices."

- **Vary your diet to make it more interesting and get more nutrients.** "If I eat one apple, one banana, and one orange, I feel better than if I just eat three apples. I also try for two different colored vegetables on my plate."

- **Play Popeye.** "In terms of iron, spinach is the most versatile. You can have it in a sandwich, a salad, lasagne—cooked or raw."

- **Do what's best for you and your baby.** Evaluate your diet with a nutrition professional to be sure that you're meeting the special dietary demands of pregnancy. "I'm very happy staying a vegetarian throughout my pregnancy, but I would switch to meats if it were a question of nutrients for my baby."

MOTHER TO MOTHER:
"I Was Overweight at the Start"

Jenny Smith, 33
Laurel, Maryland

Jenny carried 198 pounds on her 5-foot, 6-inch frame when she became pregnant the first time. Though she delivered a healthy daughter without complications after gaining 30 pounds, she developed chronic high blood pressure. Now, three years later, she started a second pregnancy, weighing 215. Because her hypertension and excess weight make her a high-risk patient, she sees a specialist ob-gyn every other week. He has advised her to keep her weight gain under 20 pounds this time.

How to accomplish this without becoming counterproductively obsessed—and stressed—about pounds? "I eat only when I'm hungry," Jenny says. She cut out caffeine and tries to follow her doctor's guidelines for nutrition, especially eating enough servings of fruits and vegetables. She walks wherever she can for daily exercise. And weighing herself only at doctor's visits helps minimize the tyranny of the scale.

Doctors monitor overweight patients closely because of their increased health risks. They may also call for more ultrasounds to check fetal growth more closely than is possible by palpating the abdomen (feeling it externally). Jenny was also taught to take her own blood-pressure readings to help monitor this dangerous condition. When her readings spiked in late pregnancy, she was advised to stay off her feet and rest on her side. In all, she gained a respectable 30 pounds.

Jenny's tips for overweight moms-to-be:

• *Stay connected with your doctor.* He or she is there to help you deliver a healthy baby, not judge you as a person. "Ask a lot of questions. Be realistic and don't be afraid of what you might hear."

• *Shake old ideas about dieting.* "You're not supposed to lose weight now. Focus on eating healthily and on what's good for your child."

• *Make it a point to exercise.* "I didn't start any major weight-loss program, but I took a swim class for the first time since I was 12, and I walk everywhere on my errands with my older daughter."

• *Keep your self-esteem high.* "Pass along details of your pregnancy to other people in your life, and talk to other moms in similar situations. Be comfortable with who you are—big women get pregnant, too."

Fit for Pregnancy

Why Be in Shape?

Back in the nineteenth century, pregnancy was considered a delicate condition that required confinement to the chaise longue in one's private sitting room. Twenty-first–century wisdom is quite the opposite: get-up-and-go is not only harmless to you and your baby, it can do you both *good*.

A mother who exercises is bound to weather the physical stresses and strains of pregnancy better. Physical activity helps you fight fatigue more effectively and motivates you to eat more nutritiously. The endorphins (a feel-good substance produced by the pituitary gland) released during exercise help you maintain a more chipper outlook even as your hormones whip you through the roller coaster of mood changes. By strengthening back and abdominal muscles, you can help ease back pain, a common complaint as ligaments stretch and your weight load increases.

Some ob-gyns have also found that expectant mothers who exercise regularly have an easier or shorter labor. In one study, moms who worked out three times a week had 21 percent fewer Cesareans and quicker recoveries. (Don't let the dream of a perfect delivery be your only motivation to be fit, however: the notion that prenatal exercise makes for better labors remains controversial, since many divergent factors influence the length and course of labor.) Whatever the nature of your delivery, it certainly stands to reason that mothers accustomed to physical exertion are better prepared for the rigors of labor going into it. In terms of physical stress and oxygen consumption, the average labor is equivalent to jogging 12 miles!

Rating the Workouts

Which exercises best suit mothers-to-be? The factors to consider include your pre-pregnancy conditioning, the risk of accidents, and the progress of your individual pregnancy.

	WHY	NOTE
Worst (*Highest danger of injury to mother or baby*)		
Skiing	Danger of violent falls and collisions.	Risk increases after 20 weeks as balance fails. Cross-country skiing okay on mild terrain (no hills) for experienced skiers and at elevations below 10,000 feet.
Horseback riding	Danger of severe falls.	
Water skiing	Speed makes falls especially dangerous.	
Scuba diving	Decompression may harm fetus.	Especially *not* advisable in first trimester, possible link to birth defects.
Contact sports (football, basketball)	Risk of jostling, hits by balls, falls too great.	
So-So (*Best for those who participated in the sport pre-pregnancy*)		
Jogging	Aerobic, but risks overheating and jarring.	Best for seasoned runners, and then not in last trimester.
Light weight training	Strengthens muscles and can prevent lower-back pain in moderation, but experience necessary.	Certain lifts can be dangerous; ask for modification advice from a doctor or trainer.

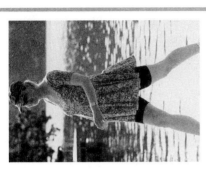

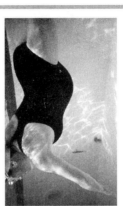

| Tennis | Aerobic, but risk of falls. | Beware of overexertion; agility gets awkward by last trimester. |
| Cycling | Risk of falls. | Okay to ride until balance worsens mid-pregnancy; shift to stationary bike. |

Best (Generally safe for anyone expecting)

Swimming	Low risk of injury, little impact on the joints, keeps the body cool.	Drink lots of fluids; you can sweat or get overheated in water without knowing it.
Walking	Easy to do, good overall conditioning.	Use good posture and wear low shoes, ideally those made for walking.
Low-impact aerobics	Cardiovascular workout, stretches muscles.	If you haven't done it before, stick to routines designed for pregnancy.
Stationary cycling	Easy to sustain, non-weight bearing.	Back strain possible in late pregnancy.
Yoga	Improves flexibility, muscle control, breathing, and body awareness—all useful in labor.	Most classes not aerobic.

Walking is one of the best ways to stay in shape.

Swimming is particularly enjoyable late in pregnancy because it will make you feel lighter, and the water will keep you cool.

One thing you *shouldn't* use an exercise program for right now, of course, is weight control. Losing weight by any means is not recommended during pregnancy.

Expect Differences

Even if you're accustomed to regular exercise, don't expect to sweat in exactly the same way you did pre-baby. Your heart rate is higher during pregnancy, for example, meaning you won't have to work out as vigorously to get the same kind of aerobic result. In fact, because of this change you'll want to take care not to overexert inadvertently. It's much easier to get overheated now. The strain on your respiratory system may make you feel winded faster than usual, too. As the months go by, the hormone relaxin causes your joints and ligaments to soften and become more easily stretched, leaving you more prone to falls, sprains, and other muscular injuries. The risk of accidents swells right along with your belly because your center of gravity gets thrown off, affecting balance.

What do these changes mean for your current routine? It's hard to issue a one-workout-fits-all dictum for expectant women. Too much depends on your pre-pregnancy condition, the nature of your activities, and how your pregnancy proceeds in terms of complications or health risks. Always—make that a capital A—review your exercise plans with your caregiver. In general, however, the following guidelines apply.

How Much Is Enough?

Moderation is the operative word. Overdoing any exercise can divert blood and oxygen away from the growing baby. Most experts recommend keeping your heart rate below 140 beats per minute. (To find your heart rate, locate your pulse at your neck or wrist, count the beats for 6 seconds, then multiply by 10.) Listen to your body; if you're too breathless to talk while you work out, you're pushing too hard. Never exercise to the point of exhaustion. If you feel tired or achy the next day, ease up. It's also important not to become overheated, which, like having a high fever, can affect the development of the fetus.

Stop immediately if you experience the following: rapid heartbeat, dizziness, faintness, pelvic pain, a cramp, bleeding, or shortness of breath. Alert your caregiver immediately.

Even well-conditioned athletes usually need to make modifications. In fact, vigorous workouts are controversial even for the ultra-fit because of the risk of too-high body temperature and concern about the oxygen supply to the baby. Distance runners, for example, are often advised to cut back on runs or to quit jogging altogether. Contact sports should be given up immediately, while activities such as cross-country skiing may be all right until about 20 weeks, when precision balance becomes an issue and falling down becomes increasingly dangerous. An experienced athlete should get her caregiver's blessing on heavy workouts before continuing them.

Good Habits to Start Now

• *Always warm up and cool down.* Take 5 to 10 minutes to gradually ease your heart rate up (and back down). Stretches also help prevent joint injuries and leg cramps by improving the flow of blood and oxygen to your muscles. Bonus: stretching relieves tension. (See "The Tip-Top Ten," page 129.)

• *Dress lightly.* Your body temperature is already warmer than usual, thanks to the hormone hCG and the internal combustion taking place in your midsection. To stay comfortable and avoid overheating while exercising, wear loose, cool clothes, ideally made from a moisture-wicking fabric, such as cotton. (Don't forget a supportive maternity or sports bra.) If you can swim without wearing a cap, do so; swim caps hold in heat.

• *Stay cool.* If the weather outside is very hot or humid, limit your activities to cooler mornings or evenings, or move inside. Make sure the room you're in is well ventilated (you'd be surprised—not all gyms are).

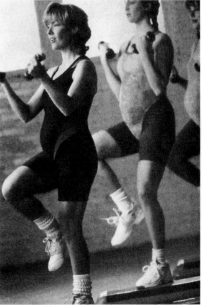

• *Take breaks.* You're not training for a marathon; you're trying to thrive as healthfully as possible to safely deliver a healthy baby. Anyway, even marathoners know the value of pacing and resting.

• *Replenish liquids and calories.* Eat and drink both before and after workouts. Go for snacks like crackers or fruit that give energy and are easily digested. Lots of water—before, during, and after—helps ward off dehydration and maintain amniotic fluid levels.

Exercising regularly during pregnancy is not only emotionally and physically satisfying, it improves the health of you and your developing baby.

• *Be careful.* Don't take risks or try anything your body doesn't feel ready for.

• *Be consistent.* You'll get more benefit from exercising three to five times a week—or better yet, taking moderate exercise (like walking) every day—than you will from one big workout once or twice a week.

Prenatal Exercise Class

How about a workout that takes your pregnant body to heart in terms of stretching, strengthening, and safety—and helps you meet other expectant moms with whom you can compare notes? Prenatal exercise programs abound at fitness centers, YMCA/YWCAs, pools, dance studios, and hospitals. There are even national franchises of pregnancy workout facilities, called Pregnagym. (They're great for new moms, too.)

Check out the instructor's credentials. You'll want to be sure he or she is sensitive to and knowledgeable about pregnancy. Even in a class designed for pregnant women, though, know your limits and stick to them.

Checklist: Who Should Exercise Caution?

Always run your workout routine by your healthcare provider. Depending on your pre-pregnancy fitness and on complications that may develop, modifications may be recommended.
Get your provider's okay first if . . .

☐ You've had repeated miscarriages
☐ You have high blood pressure or diabetes
☐ You are extremely overweight or underweight
☐ You have never exercised before

Back off exercise altogether if . . .

☐ You develop pregnancy-induced hypertension (preeclampsia)
☐ You're at risk for preterm labor or you've experienced preterm labor during this pregnancy or a previous one
☐ You have a history of incompetent cervix
☐ You're carrying more than one baby
☐ You develop vaginal bleeding

I'm just not athletic? Don't think you need a drawerful of lycra or a natural tennis swing to be fit. Every adult woman should get a minimal workout (30 minutes, three times per week) regardless of whether she's pregnant or not. The 9 months of pregnancy are not the time to kick off an ambitious new program, but there are easy things most everyone can do now. Consider a walking regimen, for example. Start slowly—try parking your car farther from the office and walking the difference or meeting a friend for a daily after-lunch stroll (the buddy system is a powerful reinforcer). Or use your pregnancy as a motivator to try an easy class, such as swimming for beginners or a prenatal exercise program.

That the baby can drown if I swim in water over my navel? Impossible. In fact, the fetus is already safely swimming—in the amniotic fluid of your womb. This myth gets an F, but swimming is A+ exercise for expectant moms.

The Pregnant Look

Early Changes

The test is positive, and there you are, eager to be transformed into a beatific, blooming icon of expectant motherhood. Instead you see—zits on your chin. Or the greenish cast of nausea. The first trimester can be frustrating in that *you* know you're pregnant, but to strangers on the street you look like any ordinary, tired woman who might be having a bad day.

Before trimester's end—and more likely, just a few weeks into it—you'll detect some definite changes:

• *Your breasts.* Right away they'll feel different—the word *ouch* comes to mind—and soon after they'll look different, too. In preparation for breastfeeding, your milk glands and ducts enlarge and fatty tissue begins to form. In fact, your breasts will gain as much as 2 pounds and your bra size may increase by three cup sizes or more before you deliver and expand still more after your milk comes in. The areolae (the pinkish-red areas that encircle the nipples) become larger and deeper-hued, and develop raised bumps called *Montgomery's tubercles.* These small glands on the surface of the areolae begin producing an oily substance that helps protect the nipples from cracking and drying. They become raised and more bumpy during pregnancy. You might notice a new lumpiness, too—these are milk ducts and glands. Your rib cage may also expand as it lifts to accommodate your growing uterus. In fact, by the end of the third month (for many women, much sooner) you'll probably need to retire your old bra and get a larger one. (See "GOOD ADVICE: Buying Comfortable Lingerie," page 73)

• *Your skin.* While some women get the maternal glow right away, others are stuck with the return of adolescent-style acne. Your face, neck, shoulders, back, even random patches of skin all around your body can break out. Blame hormonal changes—the influx of estrogen and progesterone tend to change the activity of sebaceous glands, causing them to clog more easily. (Some lucky women find that their customary pimples disappear altogether.) You may need to switch to less greasy formulations of moisturizer and makeup base. Look for water-based types. Try a gentle cleanser to remove oil without overdrying the skin and be sure to drink plenty of water. Just don't pick, poke, or fight back with *any* acne medication you haven't cleared with a doctor first. Even adolescent drugstore standbys like benzoyl peroxide are suspect. Specifically avoid Accutane and Retin-A.

That legendary glow, by the way, reflects more than a blissed-out countenance. It's caused by the increased blood flow in the mother's system. Most women—even acne-riddled ones—experience this maternal flush by the second trimester.

If you appear "wiped out" courtesy of nonstop nausea, a few things can help you look (and feel) fresher. Rinse your face with cool water as often as possible. You may need to reapply makeup more frequently, but rest assured that a little mascara and blusher (and for that matter, powder and base) are perfectly safe. A short hairstyle, or hair pulled off your face, helps you look neater even if you feel like you're coming apart at the seams.

• *Your hair.* The topline: mostly pleasant surprises. By the end of the trimester, you'll probably notice that your hair is growing faster, feels thicker, and just looks healthier than before. Skip the heavy deep conditioners, which only weigh down this new lushness.

Of course, in pregnancy, exceptions abound. A minority of women will find that hormonal shifts have the opposite effect on their locks: fine hair becomes thinner, oily hair oilier, or the texture is drier than ever. Sometimes blondes even turn dark or naturally curly 'dos go straight. Since today's hair-care products are as varied and occasion-specific as pantyhose, coping with the changes may be as simple as switching to a shampoo, conditioner, mousse, gel, or spray that better meets your changing needs.

Hold off on permanents, dye jobs, relaxers—even prescription dandruff shampoos—until after the first 12 weeks. Biological changes enable the scalp to more easily absorb the chemicals these products contain, and it's just a short trip from there to your bloodstream, through the placenta, to the developing fetus. There's no scientific proof linking these chemicals to birth defects, but extra caution in the first trimester can't hurt. After that, hair coloring and perms are considered okay by many doctors.

• **Your waist.** "What waist?" you say. Before the trimester is out, most first-time moms notice that pants and skirts feel tight even though they still lack any sign of a pregnant belly. A vanished waistline is often the first shape change you'll experience because your organs are beginning to shift around to accommodate the growing uterus, but the uterus hasn't yet risen above the pelvic bone.

When should you start wearing maternity clothes? Most women don't begin to acquire the right proportions until the fourth month, but there is no hard-and-fast rule. Generally, your hems will start to rise a little in front, pants get tight, and tops stretch across the chest. Even before those sartorial signals appear, by the second or third month you may find that a more forgiving pair of maternity leggings simply feels better, even though you continue to wear your other clothes just fine, or at least the looser-fitting ones. (Because maternity leggings look like the ordinary kind, but are cut narrower than maternity pants, they're often the first special clothes women slip into undetected. You may need to roll the waistband over at first, or wear it pulled up to your bra, but under the looser, tails-out shirts you'll probably also begin reaching for, no one can really tell.)

Since you'll probably need to shop for a new bra during the first trimester anyway, make that your excuse to go ahead and browse in the local maternity shop. They won't laugh you out of the store if you reveal a due date that seems impossibly far away.

If this is not your first pregnancy, or if you're expecting twins, you may find yourself ready for some maternity clothes as early as the second month. (See "Maternity Clothes: A Buyer's and Borrower's Guide," page 133.)

NO-WAISTLINE DRESSING TRICKS

You're still concealing the news, but how can you hide the physical evidence? Here are a few ways to get around the disappearing-waist dilemma:

• Vests. They let you sneak by with an open button or two at your waist. (In cool weather, a long cardigan sweater works, too.)
• "Long over lean." A big shirt or long straight jacket atop narrow pants, a straight slim skirt with matching tights, or leggings.

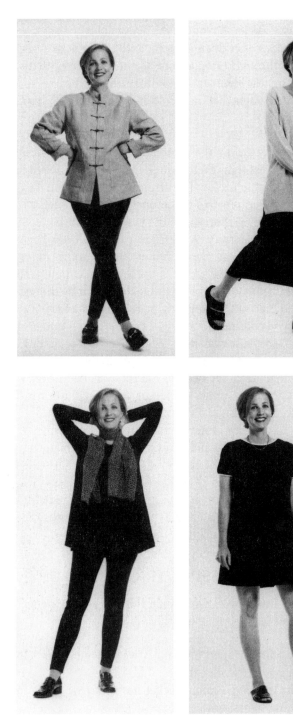

Even as you start to show, long tops over lean pants (or a skirt) help you wear your condition with flair.

An elastic waistband allows for added girth—without letting anyone in on your secret.

A long, flowing scarf artfully draws attention away from an expanding middle.

An A-line dress, which narrows at the shoulders and flares below the bustline, camouflages a vanishing waist.

- Elastic waistbands. Provide extra room without raising suspicion.
- Long scarves. Oblong-shaped scarves especially draw attention to your neck while obscuring the midsection. Shawl-style scarves also can be draped to conceal, provided they're not so large as to overwhelm you.
- Waist-free shifts. If they skim the body without darts or clinginess, they're great to wear after your waist is gone but before your pouch appears. Depending on the current fashions, look for A-line or empire-waist cuts.

GOOD ADVICE: BUYING COMFORTABLE LINGERIE

Good-bye Wonderbra, hello maternity model. Granted, most pregnancy lingerie emphasizes comfort over style and sex appeal, but you'll be grateful for the easy fit soon enough.

Some shopping tips:

- As early as possible, switch to underclothes made of 100 percent cotton, which feels soft and won't seal in moisture. (If you're an E cup or larger, a cotton-nylon blend will provide better bra support.)
- If you don't want to splurge on special maternity underpants (which feature an expanding panel across the abdomen), choose a regular bikini style that rests *under* your belly. You may need to go up a size.
- Look for a terrycloth crotch or double-layered cotton to help absorb vaginal discharge.
- Unless you're starting out in the A-cup range, don't try to make do with regular fashion bras in bigger sizes. Maternity bras are engineered with broader straps and better support that ease back strain, too.
- A good alternative for accommodating growth in the first trimester (and for sleeping more comfortably) is a seamless athletic bra.
- Buy your first maternity bra in the same numerical size you usually wear (or one size up if that seems more comfortable), and one to two

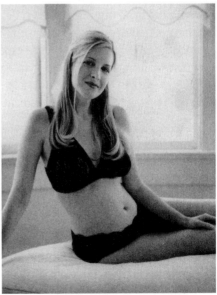

Many expectant moms appreciate the expanding tummy panels on maternity underwear, not to mention the wider straps and all-around support of maternity bras.

cup sizes larger. You'll grow into it as the months wear on and spare yourself the necessity of buying new ones every few weeks.

- If the bra is comfortable when fastened on the tightest rows of hooks, it'll fit longer as your rib cage expands.
- Be careful when fitting underwire styles—if the wiring presses on any breast tissue, you could be setting yourself up for clogged milk ducts. Given the support engineered into today's maternity bras, even large-busted women may feel comfortable skipping underwires altogether.
- By the second or third trimester, consider buying nursing bras, which have the support you need but feature convenient openings you can use later. Bonus: many nursing bras let you adjust the cup size.
- When it comes to maternity hose, ignore the usual maternity clothes advice about buying your pre-pregnancy size, and go one size up unless you're very small. Maternity hose are cut roomier in the tummy and longer in the crotch, though the legs are unchanged. Still, you don't want to feel like sausage in a casing.

IS IT TRUE...

My feet are going to grow? You won't be buying new shoes at the same rate you'll be replacing bras, but most women do find that before the 9 months are out, their feet have expanded. That's because hormones released in pregnancy loosen your ligaments, causing feet to spread, especially under the weight of some 30 extra pounds you'll be adding. More than half the women in one recent study reported *permanent* growth of up to one whole shoe size. Wearing sturdy, flat shoes that fit well will help prevent the development of more serious foot problems.

That when a mother-to-be looks worse than usual, she's having a girl? Wise grannies like to say that acne or pallor indicate a girl baby "stealing your beauty." Sexism aside (there are, after all, plenty of mighty pretty newborn boys), who knows any woman—pregnant or otherwise—who looks terrific *every day?*

What About Sex?

Libido Lost and Found

Expectant couples usually brace for plenty of changes on the road to parenthood. Still, changes in their *sex* life often catch parents-to-be off guard, especially when impatience (usually his) or guilt (usually hers) sets in. It hardly seems fair, not to mention more than a little ironic, that something so pleasurable as sex—the very thing that gets the miracle of life rolling—should so often get squelched by that same little life as it grows.

In fact, fluctuations in desire vary widely from trimester to trimester—and from woman to woman or pregnancy to pregnancy. "Normal" is hard to define. There are certain predictable patterns to a pregnant woman's libido, however, and common issues at stake.

At first, morning sickness may render you unable to get out of bed—or you may suddenly find yourself hopping randily into it. Either way, your hormones get the credit. From the moment of conception, estrogen and progesterone levels begin to surge to several times normal levels. These happen to be two of the hormones that fuel passion. Estrogen, for example, increases blood flow to the breasts, vagina, labia, and clitoris, making them softer, swollen, and hypersensitive. In a way, pregnancy mimics carnal readiness. There's also a certain randiness that freedom from birth control may inspire. Alas, all that potential sexual energy is often zapped by the body's other adjustments to this hormonal rocket launch: vomiting, moodiness, overwhelming fatigue.

Mental adjustments to pregnancy affect *amour*, too. You might proceed more tentatively if it has taken a long time to conceive, you're starting a family late in life, or you have had a previous miscarriage. Some nervous couples feel better forswearing sex altogether. Men may feel hesitant out of awe or fear. First-time mothers-to-be are most apt to lose interest in sex during the first trimester. Medically, however, there's usually no reason to forgo intercourse. Your baby is snug and away in the amniotic sac—and oblivious, too. (For exceptions, see "CHECKLIST: When to Abstain," page 76.)

Staying Close

One thing that helps keep intimacy on track—even if making love suddenly holds about as much appeal to you as ice fishing—is candid communication with your partner. It's important for him to know you're not rejecting *him*, but that there are physical reasons you've lost interest. Likewise, he may have fears and frustrations that need your ear. In the first trimester, the novelty of the pregnancy may make it easier for both of you to cordon off sex without much thought. But as the months wear on, intimacy is too vital a resource to your relationship to be ignored. Don't forget that sex and closeness are about more than vaginal intercourse. Touching, handholding, massage, and even nonerotic activities such as planning the baby's nursery together can be powerful ways to express caring and love. If your breasts are not only supersized but also supersensitive, educate your partner about how to massage them gently, starting from the outer fleshy part before working his way in to the most tender areola (oil helps). Other erogenous zones right now are your back, your inner thighs or buttocks, and your navel on down.

Checklist: When to Abstain

Sex is considered quite safe during an uneventful pregnancy, but doctors may recommend abstinence if:

☐ You have a history of either preterm labor or premature ruptured membranes.

☐ You've had a previous miscarriage (you may be asked to wait out the first trimester while the pregnancy establishes itself, though it's unlikely sex will have any effect on the developing embryo).

☐ You or your partner has a sexually transmitted disease (such as herpes) that has not fully cleared up after treatment.

☐ You have *placenta previa*, in which the placenta covers the cervix instead of being higher in the uterus. There is a danger of damaging the placenta, and therefore the fetus's nutrient delivery system.

☐ You are spotting or experiencing vaginal bleeding. Always check with your caregiver.

☐ Your water has broken.

Is It True...

That thrusting during sex can hurt the baby? No, the fetus is well protected in the amniotic sac where, thanks to the angle of your vagina, not even deep penetration can reach it.

That mothers of twins shouldn't have sex? No studies support this old wives' tale. Because multiple fetuses place you in a high-risk pregnancy, however, it's a good idea to get your caregiver's opinion.

Special Situations

Who's High-Risk?

A high-risk pregnancy is any that deviates from the norm. Some women begin a pregnancy in that category; others become high-risk as certain circumstances develop. If you're high-risk, you'll be more closely monitored during your term, perhaps with extra tests and special counseling about nutrition, medication, or lifestyle.

Each doctor may interpret the label differently. It used to be that all first-time mothers over 30 (ego-rippingly known as "elderly primagravidas" in the medical literature) or all women with Rh-negative blood were considered high-risk. Today, neither of those cases fall in that category. Chronic illnesses or gynecological histories that are more typically high-risk include:

• *High blood pressure.* Elevated blood pressure readings before pregnancy (hypertension) can cause kidney damage to the mother or prematurity and low birthweight in the baby. Not all medications used to treat hypertension are safe during pregnancy, including diuretics. You may be able to quit drugs altogether if you have a minor case. If carefully monitored throughout pregnancy by both you and your doctor, mild hypertension may pose little risk to your baby. Severe hypertension (greater than 160/105) requires even greater care, possibly including bedrest and special diet.

The condition can also develop during the second and third trimesters, when it's called *preeclampsia*. (See "Preeclampsia," page 190.)

• *Diabetes.* Insulin-dependent (Type I) and chronic (Type II) diabetics are no longer advised to avoid pregnancy, thanks to advances in control of the condition. Starting to reduce blood-sugar levels up to 6 months before conception reduces nearly all the risks (which can range from urinary tract infections to miscarriage, stillbirth, and birth defects). During pregnancy, a strict regimen of eating right and exercising, coupled with constant monitoring of glucose levels, is required to control the disease.

Another kind of diabetes—known as *gestational diabetes*—can develop in the second and third trimesters. (See "Gestational Diabetes," page 142.)

• *Rheumatoid arthritis.* RA can't harm your baby, and joint pain typically disappears during pregnancy. Often, however, it returns full-scale within a month or more after delivery. The usual medications—aspirin and steroids—aren't advised for most expectant mothers, but have been used in special medical circumstances with close supervision. Check with your obstetrician and/or a specialist so that your dosages can be adjusted to the lowest possible safe dose, and look for other relief measures, including rest. During pregnancy, line up advice and assistance for coping with postpartum flareups. You'll probably need help with household and baby care.

• ***Epilepsy.*** A lot of good news on this front. Some studies show that half of all epileptics do not have seizures during pregnancy; a quarter have them less frequently; and a quarter have them more frequently, especially toward the end of the last trimester when progesterone levels are highest. Luckily, doctors now have a better understanding of how to control brain seizures in pregnancy. Although birth defects have been linked to some antiepileptic drugs, the risk is relatively low, only 2 to 6 percent higher than normal. Your doctor may recommend safe levels to which dosages can be cut back or dropped. If you've had seizures within the past 2 years, don't stop taking your medication without consulting your doctor. Folic acid is frequently prescribed before conception to reduce the risk of drug-induced birth defects. And during pregnancy, sleep and stress avoidance have been shown to help some women avoid epileptic episodes.

• ***Being 40 or older at delivery.*** Some doctors use 35 as the marker. While age doesn't automatically boot you into a high-risk category, certain risks do statistically increase with age. These include the odds of developing high blood pressure, fibroids, and diabetes, and an elevated incidence of birth defects. Your care will generally be no different unless a condition seems to warrant it.

• ***A history of repeat miscarriages.*** You may be monitored more closely, especially in the early months.

Multiple Pregnancy

You'll also be considered a high-risk patient if you are carrying more than one fetus. This may be discovered in the first trimester if your uterus is growing faster than normal, if more than one heartbeat is detected, or if you're particularly nauseous. It will be suspected and looked for if you were taking fertility drugs. Many cases of twins, which account for 1 in about every 40 to 45 births, are picked up by routine ultrasounds in mid-pregnancy. Births of triplets or more, known as higher-order multiples, account for 1 in 860 births (four times the rate in 1971). Like twins, they're growing in prevalence because of the increased use of fertility treatments and because more women over 30 (who are more likely to conceive multiples) are becoming mothers.

Most twins and triplets are born healthy today. There are some increased health risks, however. For the mother they include greater odds of developing hypertension, anemia, placenta abruptio (in which the placenta tears away from

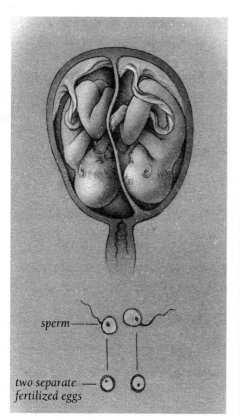

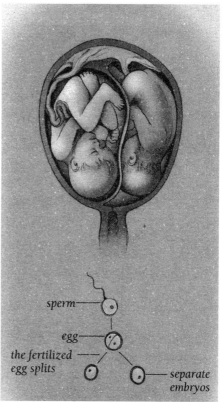

sperm

two separate — fertilized eggs

sperm

egg

the fertilized egg splits

separate embryos

Fraternal Twins: *When two eggs are released from the ovaries and both are fertilized by different sperm, the resulting embryos have individual genetic characteristics—they look different and can be different sexes.*

Identical Twins: *When a fertilized egg splits into two, the embryos are genetically indistinguishable.*

the uterine wall prematurely), and preterm labor (before 37 weeks). Half of all twins are born prematurely, as are nearly all other multiples. Babies born prematurely tend to have low birthweights and may have related disabilities, though not necessarily serious ones. The mother also experiences more physical discomfort during her term. For these reasons she has more frequent checkups and more prenatal tests than someone expecting a singleton. She may also be advised to eat more, gain more weight, take additional vitamin supplements (especially iron), and exercise less (or at least with greater precaution).

Fraternal twins (the kind who don't look the same and can be of the opposite sex) are conceived when two eggs are released by the ovary instead of just one, each fertilized by a different sperm. Each has its own placenta and amniotic sac. *Identical twins,* which occur once in every 250 births, develop when a single egg, fertilized by a single sperm, splits in early pregnancy and develops into two fetuses. No one knows why this happens. They usually share a placenta and most often have individual amniotic sacs. More significantly, they shared the same genetic material at the start, causing them to look remarkably similar.

Triplets, like twins, are formed by the fertilization of multiple eggs, by a single egg splitting several times, or by a combination of the two.

First-Trimester Bleeding

The sight of blood on your underpants or toilet tissue provokes just one response: panic. Calm yourself long enough to ascertain as much as you can about it: Is the color bright red, pinkish, or brownish? Are there any noticeable clots? How much is there—just a staining of your usual vaginal discharge, a small amount, or a continuous flow? Can you tell whether it's coming from your vagina, rectum, or bladder? Are you experiencing any other symptoms, such as cramping, fever, or painful urination? The answers to these questions can help your caregiver assess the cause. Call immediately to report any bleeding, as it can be a sign of a serious problem.

While bleeding in pregnancy is not normal, it's not unusual, either. As many as 20 percent of pregnant women do. It's most common in the first trimester. In about half of these early-bleeding episodes, it stops and the pregnancy progresses to term without further problem. The other half end in miscarriage.

What might cause bleeding? Some cases go unexplained, almost always when the blood is not accompanied by any cramping. When it occurs in early pregnancy, the uterus may be shedding some tissue the way it does every month at your period, but to a lesser extent, and for unknown reasons. Here are other possible causes:

• *Implantation bleeding.* Sometimes this occurs when the fertilized egg attaches to the uterine wall, at roughly the same time you would normally be expecting a period. This produces just very slight spotting (usually pale) with no cramping.

• *Cervical abrasions.* After a bleeding episode, you'll usually be asked if you've recently had intercourse. That's because the penis can rub against the tender cervix in such a way that produces a slight irritation or inflammation. A little blood is produced and that's the end of it. It *doesn't* mean that sex is unsafe or that you should abstain, because the bleeding is caused simply by the skin abrasion. Less commonly, a cervical infection can cause bleeding.

• *Placental tears.* Occasionally it's possible for a small bit of the placenta to tear away from the uterine wall, causing bright red bleeding. The cause is usually unknown. Such tears are not thought to be caused by the mother's actions. Nor is this kind of bleeding the same as *placenta previa*, in which the placenta lies low on the cervix and can cause painless bleeding as the cervix dilates, or *placenta abruptio*, in which more than a quarter of the placenta tears away from the uterine wall. (See pages 191–192 for details on these conditions, which are very serious and usually occur later in pregnancy or at delivery.)

• *Threatened miscarriage.* When there is prolonged early bleeding in the first trimester, whether or not accompanied by cramps, the situation is termed a "threatened miscarriage." Because miscarriage is so common this early in pregnancy, bedrest is sometimes the only course of action advised (and that's more to make you feel better than to actually stop anything from happening). Cruel as it sounds, whatever will happen, will probably happen. Your doctor may do an ultrasound to determine if there is still a heartbeat or give you a blood test to see if your hCG levels have dropped off rather than continued to rise as they normally do when you are pregnant. In about half the cases, by the time bleeding begins, the embryo or fetus has already stopped forming and the situation is then termed an *inevitable miscarriage*.

   Note: You may feel some painful stretching along your sides as the uterus expands. This is common and *not* the same as cramping, which is usually more rhythmic and internal, like menstrual cramps.

• *Ectopic pregnancy.* (See page 83.)

Early Miscarriage

You'll cringe if you see the medical phrase on your chart, but a "spontaneous abortion" is a miscarriage, or a pregnancy that terminates itself naturally before the first 20 weeks. As many as one-quarter to one-third of all pregnancies are thought to end this way, especially before 12 weeks. Don't let that high figure alarm you, however; the percentage has gone up in recent years as accurate home pregnancy tests have verified pregnancies earlier than ever, when in the past many such pregnancies were lost before ever being detected. While miscarriage is a normal fact of reproductive life, most women don't experience it more than once or twice, if at all.

The signs of miscarriage include prolonged bleeding accompanied by cramps; eventually larger clots of blood or grayish or red tissue are passed. (There is no recognizable fetus or embryo.) The body reverts to its pre-pregnancy state: nausea, breast tenderness, and fatigue disappear. Always alert your doctor if you feel cramping. He or she can assess the situation through ultrasound and blood tests, and by checking your cervix for signs of dilatation. If it is a pregnancy loss, you may be instructed to do nothing more until everything has been expelled and the cramping and bleeding stop. This may take a week to 10 days if you were in the seventh or eighth week, and perhaps longer if it happens later in the first trimester. Afterward, you'll be checked again to make sure no tissue remains. The doctor may perform a D&C (*dilatation and curettage*), a minor surgical procedure in which the cervix is widened and the uterine tissue is gently scraped or suctioned to reduce your risk of infection or hemorrhage from retained products of the pregnancy.

What causes miscarriage? There are many possible reasons, though it's usually hard to pinpoint the cause of early loss. In all probability, it wasn't anything you did. That's the main thing to remember. Most early miscarriages are random acts of biology: chromosomal abnormalities right from the start probably caused the embryo to develop poorly. Hormonal deficiencies and exposure to infection or toxins account for a smaller percentage. Don't berate yourself for being slow to kick your Starbucks habit or for having jogged too far one afternoon. While it's true that a healthy lifestyle helps ensure a healthy pregnancy, miscarriage in the first trimester is simply too common an event to point fingers over.

That's not to say you won't grieve. It's breathtaking how swiftly you can become attached to your unborn child. After thinking "Why me?" and "What did I do?" you'll probably find yourself mourning over the lost picture of pregnancy you had painted in your head and, even more painfully, over the child who might have been. You may feel withdrawn and moody. Telling people may loom as an awkward, unwelcome task, and you may find their expressions of sympathy hard to take. It does help to talk to people about what you've experienced, especially other mothers who have also miscarried. (You may be surprised how many stories you'll hear from mothers, cousins, coworkers, and friends that you had never known about.) Give yourself time to heal and to mourn, including taking time off from work even if you feel physically fine. It's not uncommon to experience persistent symptoms of major depression (such as insomnia, lethargy, and difficulty concentrating) after a miscarriage; such signs should be mentioned to one's doctor at the post-miscarriage checkup. Counseling can help. Perhaps the very best advice is to keep reminding yourself that a miscarriage, however unfortunate, is a relatively common experience. In all likelihood it doesn't mean you'll never be a mother.

On the contrary. After a first miscarriage, your odds of another one are just the same as they were before, and even after two miscarriages, your risk of a third increases only slightly. Because miscarriage is so commonplace, most doctors don't consider you high-risk or initiate investigative tests until you have had two or more. This may seem frustrating, but it's also sensible. It sometimes takes a series of miscarriages to produce a pattern that provides important clues. Moreover, chances are good that your first miscarriage was a biological fluke, and extensive testing now can delay your next pregnancy or cause you unnecessary worry and cost. In most cases you're advised to wait until your next menstrual period comes and goes before trying to conceive. While some women are urged against planning another pregnancy right away, there's rarely a physical or psychological benefit to waiting 6 months or a year after a first-trimester miscarriage. The best course is to begin again.

Ectopic Pregnancy

In rare instances, the fertilized egg nestles somewhere outside the uterus and begins to grow, usually in a fallopian tube. (Implantation in the abdominal cavity or an ovary is also possible, but very rare.) The pregnancy test turns positive, and at first all the usual symptoms unfold. Within a few weeks, however, the embryo grows bigger than the fallopian tube can accommodate. The woman may feel sudden, sharp abdominal pains or cramps, vaginal bleeding,

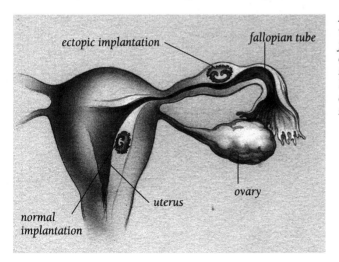

ectopic implantation

fallopian tube

normal implantation

uterus

ovary

An ectopic pregnancy—which occurs when the fertilized egg implants and starts to grow outside the uterus—can be life threatening, and the embryo must be removed surgically.

and faintness. Most ectopic pregnancies (also called tubal pregnancies) are diagnosed before 8 weeks, sometimes even before the woman knows she's pregnant, or right after she's found out. About 1 to 1½ percent of all pregnancies are ectopic.

Early diagnosis is important so that the embryo can be surgically removed before the tube ruptures. If a rupture occurs, a woman risks hemorrhaging, and sometimes the entire tube must be removed, impairing fertility. Laparoscopic surgery is done through the navel and leaves very tiny scars. For later-diagnosed cases, a laparotomy is performed with an incision through the abdomen. Doctors rely on pelvic exams, blood tests, and ultrasound to rule out tubal pregnancies.

You're at risk for ectopic pregnancy if:

- You've had pelvic inflammatory disease (PID) or endometriosis, which can damage the fallopian tube and make it easier for the fertilized egg to become trapped there.
- You conceived with an IUD in place.
- You've had a ruptured appendix.
- You've had previous tubal surgery (such as reversal of having your tubes tied).
- You've had a previous ectopic pregnancy. (Even then, your odds of a normal pregnancy are only slightly lower than someone who's never been pregnant; after two ectopic pregnancies your odds of a successful pregnancy are just slightly less than 50 percent.)

Checklist: Could I Be Expecting Multiples?

Clues that you're carrying more than one fetus include:

- ☐ A family history of fraternal twins (mother's side)
- ☐ You've taken fertility drugs
- ☐ You've conceived via in vitro fertilization
- ☐ Your uterus grows more quickly than expected
- ☐ You're of African-American heritage (African Americans have a higher rate of twin births)
- ☐ You're over 35 or 40, which may cause you to release more than one egg at ovulation

WHAT IF ...

I take allergy medication? Most medications are safe, including allergy shots, but check with your doctor. Allergies usually worsen during pregnancy because of hormonal changes, but sometimes they clear up. Ask also about cortisone nasal sprays, which are not absorbed into your blood.

I have asthma? About half the time, pregnancy has no effect on asthma; one-quarter of the time it gets better, and one-quarter, worse. Most newer inhalers are safe to use in pregnancy; check with your physician.

I get migraines? You may be surprised to discover your headaches disappear during pregnancy, partly owing to hormonal changes. If they do continue, or if you experience migraines for the first time during pregnancy, nondrug approaches are preferable: consider lying in a dark room with a cool compress over your eyes, walks in fresh air, avoiding known food triggers, and relaxation techniques, including meditation and Lamaze–type breathing exercises. Acetaminophen is safe for occasional use, but most standard migraine drugs are not. Check with your doctor.

I'm taking Prozac? The most widely prescribed antidepressant doesn't appear to cause serious birth defects, but some studies have linked it to premature deliveries and later subtle behavioral and IQ problems in children whose mothers took the drug. Other major studies have not found such risks, however, and suggest problems associated with Prozac may have been due to the mothers' underlying conditions instead. Also, many doctors believe that the danger of going untreated for significant depression is far greater than any risks presented by the medication. The best advice is to get your doctor's opinion. Do not quit taking the medication without consulting your obstetrician and the prescribing doctor first.

For More Help: Resources for Special Situations

- American Diabetes Association, 1660 Duke Street, Alexandria, VA 22314; 703-549-1500. Advice for pregnant diabetics, including an information hotline.
- Sidelines National Support Network, P.O. Box 1808, Languna Beach, CA 92652; 714-497-2765. A support network for women in high-risk pregnancies, including advice for women on bedrest.

continued

- Arthritis Foundation, 1330 West Peachtree Street, Atlanta, GA 30309; 404-872-7100. Advice for coping with arthritis during and after pregnancy.
- Pregnancy and Infant Loss Center, 1421 E. Wayzata Boulevard, Suite 30, Wayzata, MN 55391; 612-473-9372. Offers miscarriage, stillbirth, ectopic pregnancy, and infant death support and resources.
- National Organization of Mothers of Twins Clubs, Box 23188, Albuquerque, NM 87192-1188; 800-243-2276 or 505-275-0955 or http://www.nomotc.org/. Information and referrals to local chapters.
- The Triplet Connection, Box 99571, Stockton, CA 95209; 209-474-0885 or http://www.inreach.com/triplets. National clearinghouse for education, referrals, and support.
- Twin Services, P.O. Box 10066, Berkeley, CA 94709; 510-524-0863. Hotline, referrals, publications and counseling.
- Mothers of Supertwins, P.O. Box 951, Brentwood, NY 11717-0628; 516-434-6678 or http://www.mostonline.org. A national support network for mothers of triplets or more.

MOTHER TO MOTHER:
"It's Twins!"

Lisa Billhime, 27
Orlando, Florida

"There's two!" Darin Billhime shouted as he and Lisa peered at the video monitor during her routine 12-week ultrasound. "Darin, just let the doctor do her job," Lisa replied, thinking he was joking. But her husband was right, and in that moment, the course of her prenatal care—and, indeed, her whole life—changed.

"I was completely shocked," says Lisa, who has no family history of twins. "I miscarried the previous July, so it seemed like a true blessing. That evening my husband just kept rubbing my belly and I kept saying, 'Can you believe it?' "

The next day, reality set in. Her doctor explained that she'd require more frequent visits, including weekly fetal monitoring in the last trimester to make sure the boys were both growing well. She also would have an ultrasound every 3 weeks. Swimming was the only exercise she could indulge in, and her recommended weight gain was 50 to 60 pounds. (She gained 60.) The couple worried about finances, too. "We will go from a two-person, two-income family to a four-person, one-income family." Twins Austin and Ethan were delivered 3 weeks early, weighing in at a healthy 5 pounds, 3 ounces, and 6 pounds, 6 ounces, respectively.

Lisa's tips for expecting multiples:

• **Listen to your body.** "If I was tired, I sat. I ate more and slept more for both of them. Twins are twice as taxing on your body."

• **Indulge yourself now.** Take leisurely baths, plan a mid-pregnancy getaway. "Maintain your sanity."

• **Ask a lot of questions.** "Test results may be skewed when you are pregnant with twins." For Lisa, both a glucose screen and an AFP test indicated suspicious results that worried her until this was explained.

• **Know you're not the first person to go through it.** "Do some research, read books, start talking to other people, or join support groups. You realize that having twins is a do-able thing."

Work Worries

Telling Your Colleagues

The wisest rule: when you're ready to tell your good news, tell your boss first. It's just good politics that the leader not hear your big news from the office grapevine or, worse, from a competitor or a client outside the company. And you certainly don't want your bulging belly to tell the tale before your lips do. That's not to say, however, that your supervisor needs to know as soon as your spouse and your mom do.

To decide when to make the announcement, consider your individual pregnancy and your current work situation. The conventional wisdom is to keep your lips zipped through the first trimester, until the greatest risk of miscarriage is past. (The rationale being that in case you lose the baby, you'll spare yourself and your colleagues a lot of needless planning and anxiety—not to mention hubbub over your loss.) Or you may choose to postpone the announcement until you show, just to spare the distraction of coworkers asking all day whether you've picked out a name or how you're feeling.

If you're in a job where the work is cyclical, such as teaching or retail, you may want to time the announcement to give your employer ample notice to fill your spot while you're away. Or there may be a big project slated right around your due date that warrants your colleagues' knowing as far ahead as possible that you may not be around for it. Or you may anticipate special health needs (frequent doctors' appointments, the specter of prolonged bedrest) if, say, you're carrying twins or have had preterm labor in the past, that necessitate spilling the beans. Let common sense and good faith be your guide.

Don't assume your employer will be as thrilled as you are. On a personal level, he or she may be genuinely happy for you. On a professional level, though, the boss's gut response may be pure panic. In fact, you may want to have two conversations with your supervisor about your pregnancy. In the first one, you simply announce the news, then suggest a follow-up meeting in a week or two to begin hammering out your plan for leave or replacement, once you've both had a chance to absorb the implications and options.

Planning Your Leave

Do some homework even before you approach your boss. Consult your employee handbook and insurance papers about your rights and your company's policies. (If you need to call the personnel department, rest assured that they're obligated to keep the news confidential.) What length of leave is covered with pay? How long can you take without pay? How many vacation days can you include? Is your company covered by the Family Medical Leave Act? Check your insurance coverage as well.

Be prepared to give your employer some sense of your plans. Will you work up until your water breaks or would you prefer to establish a quit date? Some women start leave on their due date, or a week before, to make the transition more clear-cut for all and to use the time to rest and mentally shift gears to motherhood; others find that work distracts them from the interminable waiting of the final weeks. Health permitting, it's up to you.

More urgently, do you intend to return to your usual duties and hours after your leave? Would you prefer a modified schedule (say, part-time)? Or do you know already that you don't plan to return? Being honest about your intentions helps everyone: you and your boss can plan realistically, you don't have to feel deceptive, and future moms-to-be in your department will benefit from your candor, since it sets a bad tone all around if you insist you'll come back full-time, then up and quit after delivery. What if you really don't know yet what you want to do? Admit it. Then begin researching the options. It's a tough call—and impossible to predict how you'll feel about work with a baby in tow. Even if you know financially that you need to work, you may choose not to return to your same job. (See "Seeking Work-Family Balance," page 197.) But it's far better to be up front with your employer about your uncertainty, if that's the case, than to be evasive.

Present the news in as confident and upbeat a style as you can muster. Pick a quiet time when a good mood prevails. (Friday afternoons work well, and they let your boss have the weekend to digest the news.) Give your supervisor reason to be on your side when it comes to supporting your health needs throughout the pregnancy and devising a leave strategy that's satisfactory to you both. Frame your discussion in terms of your value to the company. Toot your horn about your past responsibility and performance. Lay out for your boss a possible action plan for who will cover your duties in your absence and how that shift will be managed. Will your job be divided among several coworkers, and if so, can you suggest the best candidates? Will you hire or train a temp? Can certain projects be pushed ahead and others postponed? What you propose may not turn out to be the final plan, but being preemptive reassures your supervisor's lurking worries and shows that you're on top of things. Taking the initiative also reveals your thoughtfulness and goodwill— transforming an event your boss may nervously view as a potential liability into further proof of you as an asset. (See "GOOD ADVICE: Negotiating a Better Leave," page 91.)

Avoiding Hazards on the Job

Dangers—both proven and suspected—lurk in many workplaces. Not all are obvious. As soon as you know you're pregnant, make a quick inventory of your surroundings for possible threats to your baby's health. Remember that the first trimester, when the baby's vital organs are forming, is a crucial time to avoid potential hazards. Think about the materials you work with as well as the smells you may inhale. Review the substances in "CHECKLIST: What to Watch Out For," page 20. If you have *any* questions, ask your doctor. He or she can also provide advice based on the National Institute for Occupational Safety and Health guidelines. In some cases, you may be legally entitled to a safer position at comparable pay.

Here are some other potential dangers:

• Auto-exhaust fumes (tollbooth attendant, auto-shop mechanic). Take frequent fresh-air breaks or try for reassignment to more open work areas.
• Chemicals (hair stylists, manufacturing). Learn about the substances you

handle and whether they're safe during pregnancy. Wear protective clothing, avoid fumes, take frequent breaks.

- Lead (printing, pottery glazing). Determine exactly how you encounter lead and take steps to avoid direct contact.
- Infectious diseases, colds, and flu (teaching, daycare, nursing home and healthcare workers). Wash hands often. Get a flu shot.
- Prolonged standing or lifting (manufacturing, some retail). Get a physician's input on how much of these activities are advisable at various stages of pregnancy. Put up your feet whenever possible.
- X-rays (healthcare workers). Leave the room or wear a lead apron. Keep your dosages monitored.

Staying Productive

You may feel like you're leading a double life if you're not telling coworkers your news yet, while running to the ladies' room every hour and struggling to stay alert during meetings. The first trimester can be surprisingly taxing. Some survival tactics:

- *Plan your day according to your body rhythms.* Schedule meetings, important phone calls, or your most grueling tasks around your best times of day (usually mornings).

- *Stock your desk with snacks.* The hungry-all-the-time phase doesn't usually kick in before 12 weeks, but you'll want to arm yourself with foods that stave off nausea, such as saltines, pretzels, bananas, raisins, or grapes.

- *Try to get early-morning or late-afternoon doctors' appointments.* You'll miss a minimal amount of work. Lunchtime is convenient, too, but the rushing there and back can leave you more tired, feeling as though you didn't get a break at all that day. Try booking several appointments ahead with your doctor in order to grab the most convenient time slots.

- *Use your lunch break to rest.* Break old habits like dashing out to run a dozen errands, working at your desk while you nosh, or meeting colleagues or clients for business lunches. Instead, use this time to sit quietly and recharge. (One enterprising woman went so far as to put a curtain up for a cubicle door, unroll a futon, and take a short nap.)

GOOD ADVICE: NEGOTIATING A BETTER LEAVE

First the bad news: The United States lags behind almost every other Western nation when it comes to maternity leave. Assuming you can't move to Finland (where you'd get a 3-year leave at 80 percent pay), what's the good news? Only that you have a groundswell of growing sympathy for your plight, and with a little research and a lot of tenacity, you might be able to negotiate better than the minimum your company offers. Some tactics:

• *Know what the law allows.* The Family Medical Leave Act requires employers with more than 50 workers to provide women and men with 12 weeks unpaid leave for the birth or adoption of a child. You're required to give 30 days' notice to take advantage of this leave (unless you deliver prematurely or are adopting); remind your partner to put in for some leave time, too! Your employer must maintain your health insurance coverage during your leave, and you cannot be penalized in terms of seniority or any other benefits.

Another law, the Pregnancy Discrimination Act, requires employers with more than 15 workers to treat pregnant workers the same as disabled ones. That means that if the company provides paid leave or job security for an employee to have surgery, it must do the same for pregnant women. It also prevents firms with 15-plus employees from firing workers just because they're pregnant.

• *Learn not just what your company offers but also what other workers have wrangled.* Every case is different, but it helps to know how much latitude you may have and under what circumstances exceptions have been made. Investigate not just new mothers but also workers with other disabilities, such as someone who needed time off for gallbladder surgery or to care for an aging parent.

• *Take as much time as you can.* The standard 6 weeks might sound like a long vacation now, when you're feeling tired and overworked, but it will pass by in a flash. At 6 weeks postpartum, you may be healed from the physical stress of delivery, yet getting up all night to feed your baby.

• *Bid for a gradual return.* If you can't get a leave that's as long as you'd like, perhaps you could ease back to work, say 3 days a week for a month, or half-days at first.

• ***Don't make promises.*** Be honest and well intentioned—but be flexible. You can't foresee any medical complications that may arise for you or your baby, for example. You can't be sure now how you'll really feel about working motherhood.

• ***Don't offer to work while you're on leave.*** Not even to take phone calls or review light paperwork. You'll be busy enough.

• ***Put it in writing.*** Draft a memo highlighting your agreement and get your boss to sign off. Make it sound like a thank-you note: "I appreciate your meeting to discuss the birth of my baby in April. As we agreed, I plan to do such and such."

Checklist: Insurance Questions

Reviewing your benefits package is a little like trying to cozy up with *War and Peace* in Latin. A good way to start is to reread your policy, highlighting with a marker everything that relates to prenatal care, delivery, and newborn care. If there's anything you don't understand, ask for clarification from your personnel department or your insurance rep. Issues to be clear about are:

☐ *Is the pregnancy covered?* Sounds obvious, but some insurance policies cover only prenatal care for patients who develop a "life-threatening" condition or who require surgery. If you changed carriers while pregnant, you may discover that the plan won't cover a preexisting condition until a period of time (often 9 to 12 months) after you've signed on.

☐ *Is my chosen doctor or midwife covered?* Especially if you're changing providers, don't forget to check.

☐ *What kind of preauthorizations are necessary?* Some plans automatically pay for any tests. Managed-care plans may specify that you need advance approval for certain kinds of tests (such as amniocentesis or CVS) or for certain numbers of tests (such as any ultrasounds after the first).

☐ *What if my pregnancy is high-risk?* Your policy may reimburse you only for a "normal" uneventful pregnancy. If you have conditions that require added care, such as preterm labor or "advanced maternal age," your insurer may balk at paying for extra tests or exams.

☐ *Will my baby be covered?* Many insurers provide automatic coverage for a newborn for a preset amount of time, such as 30 days. After that, it's up to you to arrange additional insurance. Figure out now what you'll do for your child's insurance and set the wheels in motion. Remember that some children's health plans do not cover well-baby visits and immunizations, so search for a plan that does, or budget accordingly.

IS IT TRUE...

That VDTs can cause miscarriage? Not likely. Though some studies have found a link between VDT (video display terminal) use and miscarriage, it's well documented that terminals built since the mid-1980s emit only minuscule amounts of radiation—less than could harm a fetus even at 8 hours a day of exposure. The more likely culprit, researchers now believe, is *how* the terminals are used. Heavy users may sit cramped into their seats for long periods of time. If you use a computer, take frequent breaks, sit in an adjustable chair an arm's length away, and intersperse your on-screen work with other tasks. Exception: If your computer is more than 15 years old, it may emit higher magnetic fields (a kind of radiation) than a newer VDT; ask for a newer model if possible.

That stress can cause miscarriage? Not the ordinary modern working woman's stress—commutes, deadlines, boorish bosses, crazy clients. Though you're wise to make taking it easy your mantra in the face of such annoyances, it's amazing what the pregnant body can endure. On the other hand, severe chronic stress, such as that brought about by a death or divorce, has been associated with preterm delivery and lower birthweights. A possible reason is that stress increases the levels of hormones linked with starting labor while reducing blood flow to the placenta and decreasing the fetus's supply of oxygen and nutrients.

> **For More Help: Pregnant Workers' Resources**
>
> • The Women's Bureau, U.S. Department of Labor, 200 Constitution Avenue NW, Room S-3311, Washington, DC 20210; 800-827-5335. Booklets on pregnancy discrimination.

Other Big Deals

Dealing with the "Pregnancy Police"

"Is that coffee you're drinking?" "Have you taken a nap today?"

Once the word is out that you're with child, don't be surprised to find that everyone is an expert on your health needs. (And once strangers can plainly see your condition, too, look out.) Aim for the state of Gracious Obliviousness. How to pull this off?

- Avoid answering directly, since giving a response will only invite further lecture.
- Turn the question around and ask the inquisitor the same question.
- Say "I'm doing fine, thanks," and change the subject.
- Smile blandly and walk away.

Traveling

In the first trimester there are really no restrictions for health reasons. You may not want to be too far from home in the event of miscarriage, since the odds are highest now. (For specific advice, see "Going Out and About," page 154.)

Choosing Baby Names

It's one of the first major decisions you'll make on your child's behalf, and one he or she will bear the effects of for a lifetime. What pressure! Some questions to ask yourselves are:

• *How original do you want to be?* While monikers with flair (Uma, Keanu) can give a child individuality or emphasize his or her heritage, research suggests that kids with common names (Michael, Jessica) tend to be more popular and enjoy greater peer acceptance.

• **Is it a he or a she?** Giving traditional boys' names (Drew, Dylan) to girls is so trendy that some have lost their masculine sound altogether (Ashley, Leslie). Some critics of the practice say that giving a girl a boy's name sends the subtle message that boys are better, while other research hints that male names give girls greater leadership potential.

• **How will you spell it?** Resist the temptation for unusual spellings (Jaymz, Karollynne). Rather than lending distinctiveness, you may unwittingly be burdening your child with confusion and annoyance.

• **Will the name have an appropriate ring throughout the child's life?** Try to picture how the name will look or sound in a school roll call, atop a résumé, or on a campaign billboard. "Bunny" might make a cute toddler and a sweet granny, but it could slow your child on the path to CEO.

• **Do you want to spill the beans early?** One way to avoid criticism or second-guessing of your final picks is to vaguely tell questioners that you're "still thinking" until after the baby's arrival. Once the name is attached to a real baby, friends and family are more apt to react positively and not try to talk you out of it or foist their own ideas.

For inspiration, turn to:

• The family tree (look back two or more generations; old-fashioned names are sounding fresh again).
• Historic or present-day public figures (preferably someone with character worth aspiring to).
• Your favorite characters from literature or movies.
• The Bible.
• The telephone directory.
• Baby-name guides (try basing a choice on the name's original meaning in Latin or Greek).
• A map. Or consider place names that hold special significance for you.
• The birth announcement listings in your local newspaper. (Scan the announcements for couples celebrating golden anniversaries, too—men and women wed 50 years ago tend to have names that are oldies but goodies.)
• Pregnancy and parenting Web sites, which offer hundreds of names and their meanings.
• Special baby-naming computer software programs such as Namease, which lists 12,500 names by categories such as ethnicity and religion.

IS IT TRUE...

That I should make a will before I go into labor? Every adult should have a will. There's nothing morbid about it. It's not expensive, and you can even buy software such as Willmaker that lets you do it yourself. A will tells your heirs how you want your estate handled. Without one, the government might end up making that decision and perhaps even taking a larger share for itself.

Once you have children, a will is particularly important because it ensures that they will inherit your estate. Moreover, it can specify who will raise your children, how the estate will be held in trust until they reach adulthood (if that's what you desire), and in what manner you'd like your child raised. Your odds of dying in childbirth, of course, are extremely remote these days. Legal experts advise planning ahead *now* on this crucial issue so you don't forget or postpone it—and so your child won't have to live one day without this vital legal protection.

MOTHER TO MOTHER:
"Mum's the Word"

Caroline Wyman, 27
St. Louis, Missouri

Not everyone gets on the telephone the minute her pregnancy test turns up positive. Foremost, Caroline worried about miscarriage. "Having to go back and tell everyone who knew I was pregnant 'Well, no, I had a miscarriage,' would be harder than keeping a secret," she says. She also felt she needed private time to get childcare and other plans in order, to change her diet, and to just share this special secret with her partner, Andrew. What's more, a colleague at work was further along and very excited. "I didn't want to take away from her," she says.

Caroline was aided in her secrecy by her build (she didn't show until about 5 months) and a lack of morning sickness. Even so, she took no chances. She'd drink her requisite 16 ounces of lunchtime milk in the bathroom or out of sight by the office refrigerator. She explained her new appetite by saying that she was trying a new diet plan that required her to eat more during the day. She also dressed to conceal.

"It was easy. Time passed quickly," she says. She only slipped once: "I was having a baby shower for the pregnant woman in my office and, while showing people around the house, I said, 'And this is where the nursery will be. You know—in a couple of years.' I think the excitement of the evening went to my head." Except for telling her mother, in whom Caroline confided at one month, she kept mum until her sixth month. ("I kind of thought you were letting yourself go," commented one woman.) Son William was born 3 months later.

Caroline's tips for keeping pregnancy a secret:

• *You can't be wishy-washy.* "Get it in your head that you aren't going to tell anyone and then it will be easy to stick to."

• *Give yourself a D (for declaration) Day.* "Set a certain time, like a specific month or week, to tell everyone. It's fun to have something like that to look forward to."

• *To quell suspicions, alter your wardrobe before you need to.* "I started putting loose clothes into my wardrobe even before I was pregnant because I knew it would make it easier to mask my condition later."

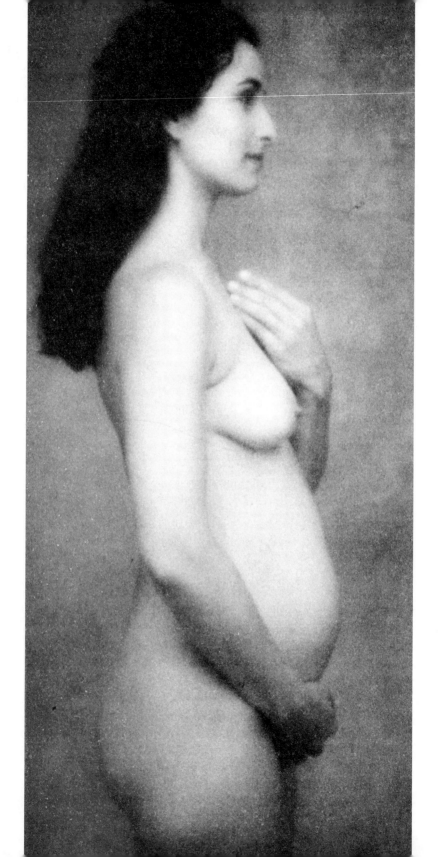

YOUR SECOND TRIMESTER

THIRTEEN TO TWENTY-EIGHT WEEKS

Welcome to the stage of pregnancy that mothers tend to remember most fondly. The body's early unpleasant reactions—nausea, fatigue, frequent urination—start to subside. Energy and buoyancy pick up. On top of feeling good, you'll probably look great. You're unmistakably ripe for maternity clothes now (and let's face it, it's fun to let your belly proclaim your news to passersby). Hormonal shifts make skin and hair more lustrous. Last trimester's painful breasts feel more comfortable and take on a sexy voluptuousness.

Best of all, some of pregnancy's most thrilling milestones are at hand. You'll feel the baby kick. You'll probably see him or her via ultrasound. You may even be able to find out the sex, if you want to. With this new concrete proof of life inside you, and with the greatest odds of miscarriage behind you, you can dwell more wholeheartedly on plans for the baby. What kind of childbirth preparation class should you take? What to buy? How will you decorate the nursery?

That's not to say that the middle stretch is free of discomforts, dangers, or worries. No part of pregnancy is immune from those things. But, overall, you'll find yourself reveling in the delightful combination of feeling more like your old self, but enjoying the novelty of your new self, the one with life growing inside.

All in all, the second trimester (weeks 13 to 28) is a time of blooming expectations.

Week-by-Week Highlights

Here's a peek at how you and your baby will grow, and what you can anticipate during the second trimester:

Week 13: Just 2½ to 3 inches long, the fetus looks like a fully formed, tiny human now, albeit with a head that's still alien-big in relation to the body. The

99

fetus will squirm if your abdomen is prodded, though you cannot feel the movement. The top of the uterus (called the *fundus*) can be felt low in the abdomen.

Week 14: The baby is 3 to 4 inches long (about as big as a large goldfish). Already in place are its facial features and unique fingerprints.

Week 15: The parchment-thin fetal skin is covered with *lanugo*, ultrafine down that usually disappears before birth. Eyebrows and hair on top of the head begin to grow, though this hair may fall out after birth and its color or texture may change. Triple-screen maternal serum screening tests (to measure levels of alpha-fetoprotein, hCG, and estriol) are scheduled between 15 and 20 weeks. Amniocentesis is usually performed around 15 to 18 weeks.

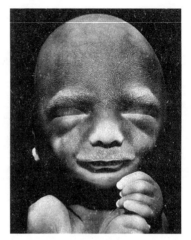

By week 15, a fetus's body is usually covered by fine downy hair that is usually shed before birth.

Week 16: Whither thy waist? Most women need maternity clothes by now. Although you've probably gained a few pounds, the baby accounts for less than 3 ounces.

Week 17: All systems are go: the baby's lungs begin to exhale amniotic fluid, the circulatory system is operating, and the urinary tract works.

Week 18: Most mothers-to-be begin to feel their baby move (a phenomenon called *quickening*), usually between 16 and 22 weeks. The fetus is 5 inches long and weighs 5 ounces, about the size of a small hamster. Its skeleton is mostly rubbery cartilage, which converts into hard bone later.

Week 19: A mid-pregnancy ultrasound is often done around 18 to 22 weeks to assess fetal growth and development, screen for some defects, check the placenta and umbilical cord, and verify the due date. You may see the baby kick, flex, roll, or even suck its thumb. The genitals are distinctive (if the baby is in the right position to show them). If it's a girl, your potential grandchildren—in the form of eggs—are already present.

Week 20: Halfway to Delivery Day! The top of your uterus now reaches your belly button and will grow about 1 centimeter each week. The baby weighs 9 ounces and is 6½ inches long. To get a sense of how much growth lies ahead, compare that to the average newborn's birthweight of 7 pounds, 7 ounces and the average length at birth of 20 inches.

Week 21: The fetus is steadily gaining fat (to stay warm) and has grown a whitish coat of waxy vernix (to protect skin during its long submersion in amni-

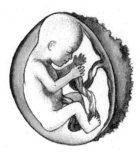 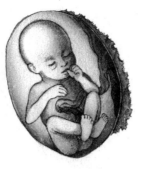 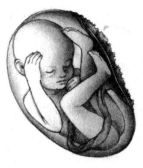

Month 4: The heartbeat is getting stronger. The fetus wakes, sleeps, kicks and moves. When he swallows the water around him, he can eliminate it by urinating.

Size: 6 to 7 inches long
Weight: 5 ounces

Month 5: The fetus is growing rapidly, sleeping and waking and turning from side to side according to a regular pattern, and the genitals are now defined enough that through ultrasound, you can often identify what sex your baby will be.

Size: 8 to 12 inches long
Weight: 1/2 to 1 pound

Month 6: Internal organs continue to develop. The skin is less transparent, and the body is now covered with soft fine hair called lanugo.

Size: 11 to 14 inches long
Weight: 1 to 1 1/2 pounds

otic fluid and to ease delivery). Look into childbirth education classes, if you haven't already. You'll want to complete a course before your ninth month begins.

Week 22: Muffled sounds of your growling stomach, your beating heart, and your voice (albeit a distorted version) can all be heard in the womb. Loud bangs may cause a startle reflex in the fetus—the heart rate rises and the limbs flail.

Week 23: The fetus now weighs about 1 pound and is proportioned like a newborn, though still scrawny. Its newborn "baby fat" hasn't yet developed. You'll begin to gain weight more steadily.

Week 24: At a little over 1 pound, the fetus is now similar in size to a box turtle. Hearing is well established. Glucose screens for detecting gestational diabetes are given between 24 and 28 weeks.

Week 25: If you feel repeated blips in your midsection that bring to mind the steady persistence of a drippy faucet, that's the baby having hiccups. (It's very common and doesn't mean anything.)

Week 26: The baby's weight is now about 1½ pounds. Nine inches long, he or she is comparable in size to a small rabbit. It's extremely rare for a baby born this prematurely to survive, but each day after this point, the chances for a healthy baby grow exponentially.

Week 27: As your uterus expands to accommodate all the growth, stretch marks may appear. Most women have gained 16 to 22 pounds.

Week 28: Imagine a small kitten—that's the size of the fetus now (11 to 14 inches long, with a weight of just over 2 pounds). The eyelids have opened, after being fused shut since their formation in the first trimester. Light-sensitive, the fetus will try to shield its eyes with its hands if a fetoscope with a light is shone inside the uterus. If born early, the baby probably will survive now in a neonatal intensive-care unit, with a 50 percent chance of no serious complications. At 28 weeks, women with Rh-negative blood get an Rh immunoglobulin shot, which will be repeated within 72 hours of delivery if the newborn is Rh-positive.

What's Going on in Your Body

Common Aches and Pains

Physically, the news is mostly rosy in the second trimester. You may first notice that certain smells no longer irritate you, and that your stomach accepts a broader range of foods. (Some aversions, such as to coffee, can last the full 9 months, though.) As your energy revs up, the need to nap may wane and you may find yourself once again able to stay up late enough for prime-time TV. You'll also begin to sleep better at night with fewer interruptions to use the bathroom as the growing uterus begins to lift off the bladder, returning it to its previous size (at least until the weight of the baby begins to squash it again around the seventh and eighth months).

The catch is that these changes do not happen the instant you cross the second-trimester threshold. Shaking off the early symptoms of pregnancy happens gradually, mostly the result of the body's adjusting to the hormonal flood that conception had unleashed. Not every woman gets relief from every symptom, however. For a minority, nausea and even morning sickness linger on. Fatigue may dog you, especially if you have older children. (It's hard to nap with kids afoot.)

Your weight gain until now has probably been slight—under 5 pounds in the first trimester and usually 10 to 15 pounds by the midway point, 20 weeks. After 20 weeks you'll begin to add ½ to 1 pound weekly. Your body is priming to nourish the pregnancy. The baby has most of its growth ahead. As a result, your appetite returns with gusto.

What else might you experience?

• **Heartburn (dyspepsia, or acid indigestion).** If you thought your swelling womb was wreaking havoc on your innards before, just wait. From the 14th to the 28th weeks, the uterus expands exponentially. One effect is to press the stomach, causing its acidy contents to back up to the esophagus and leaving an unpleasant burning sensation in the throat and across the chest (hence the name). Heartburn tends to worsen as the baby grows bigger. Progesterone adds to the problem by relaxing the valve that normally closes off food from the stomach to the esophagus. Digestion is twice as sluggish as normal.

Prevention is the best cure. Eat slowly and chew thoroughly so that food will pass through your system more efficiently. Small, frequent meals continue to be kinder to your system than three large ones. Some foods cause more heartburn, so try to identify and avoid them. Common triggers are carbonated beverages (sodas and waters), beans, bologna and hotdogs, citrus, spicy foods, and greasy foods. A little yogurt as a before-meal appetizer eliminates heartburn for many women. Smokers often have more heartburn than nonsmokers—another incentive to quit, if you haven't already.

Once heartburn ignites, resist the temptation to lie down. Standing up (or propping yourself up if you're in bed) allows gravity to help the irritants move through your system. Avoid drinking large amounts of fluids with meals. Over-the-counter antacids containing magnesium, aluminum, and calcium (Maalox, Mylanta) can safely be taken in pregnancy, or you can try a simple nonmedical solution, a cup of mild hot tea (like chamomile). Check with your doctor if you have chronic heartburn.

• *Constipation/hemorrhoids.* The same conspirators behind heartburn and indigestion can stop up your digestive system entirely. The three main ways to prevent the discomfort of constipation are to: (1) eat ample fiber in the forms of whole grains, fruits, and vegetables; (2) drink eight to ten 8-ounce glasses of water a day; and (3) exercise regularly—at minimum, doctor permitting, take a brisk half-hour walk each day.

Hard-to-pass bowel movements can lead to painful hemorrhoids (also called *piles*), which are swollen veins in the rectal area. Alarming to discover and painful to endure, these clusters of grape-size tissue can occur inside the anus (internal hemorrhoids) or herniate just outside it (external hemorrhoids). They may itch, bleed, or make it hard to sit or walk. Hemorrhoids are especially common in pregnancy because of the increased blood circulating in the pelvic area.

To soothe, apply ice packs or witch hazel. Or try a sitz bath, which is soaking your bottom in a special, shallow pan of hot water that fits over your toilet (ask at a healthcare supply store). Special pillows called hemorrhoid rings or doughnuts provide temporary relief but may actually worsen pressure on the area. Your doctor may prescribe a stool softener or suppository medication. Don't take laxatives or mineral oil.

• **Varicose veins.** Though every pregnant woman worries about stretch marks, those red or silvery lines are usually less traumatic than seeing a bulging blue snake suddenly appearing along your calves. Varicose veins occur when the walls of the blood vessels stretch so much that their valves don't close properly, causing blood to pool. They appear as a purplish blotch or a raised welt along a vein line. Thank pregnancy's increased blood volume, plus the weight of the uterus, which affects lower-body circulation. The legs are the most common site, though you can get them anywhere, even your neck or vulva. (Hemorrhoids, in fact, are technically varicose veins of the rectal area.)

About 40 percent of pregnant women develop varicose veins. If your mom had them, you're more likely to get them, too. You're also at higher risk if you're overweight or if you sit or stand still for long periods during the day. Varicose veins may itch or hurt, or merely scar your vanity. Chronic circulatory problems or blood clots resulting from varicose veins are unlikely.

Exercise and stretching can minimize varicose veins. Avoid crossing your legs or wearing knee-high or thigh-high stockings, which cut circulation. Elevate your feet when you're sitting, avoid standing or sitting for long periods, and take breaks several times an hour just to move your legs around. Rest in bed on your side to keep your legs level with your head. Some doctors advocate the gentle pressure of support hose or elastic stockings. Put them on while you're still lying down, before blood gets a chance to pool. Check maternity stores or ask your doctor about prescription-strength hose, obtainable from pharmacies or medical supply stores. Note, though, that hose can be uncomfortable (especially in summer) and a hassle to use, and are not a surefire cure. Most varicose veins subside after pregnancy, though they increase in severity with each successive pregnancy. In worst-case scenarios, they can be removed surgically or shrunk medically postpartum.

• **Softening ligaments.** Your belly isn't the only thing growing—your hips are widening, too, as part of the body's grand scheme to make delivery as easy as possible for your baby. The hormones relaxin and progesterone begin to soften your joints so that the pelvic bones will separate more easily. Alas, the whole body is affected, making you feel a bit more rubbery than usual as the months wear on. Your balance may be affected, and your grip loosens. There's not much you can do to prevent this inevitable change, though regular exercise will improve overall muscle tone. Take care to pick up breakable objects more slowly and deliberately than usual.

• **Backaches.** Not even your spine is spared the effects of your bulging uterus and relaxed musculature. Its natural curve increases, which, combined with the added weight it's supporting at your breasts and your shifting center of gravity, can lead to an achy back. The best defense is good posture. That includes when you're sitting, standing, walking, or exercising. (See "Fit for Pregnancy," page 185.) It also helps to sleep on a firm mattress (if yours is more than 10 years old, it may be ready for retirement). Wear low shoes, either supportive sneakers or sturdy lace-up shoes with a wide, slight heel. If you sit at a desk for long periods, tuck a firm pillow between the small of your back and the chair back, and elevate your feet on another chair, a box, or even a stack of books.

Pelvic tilts throughout the day also minimize discomfort. Stand with your back against a wall. (Place your hand in the small of your back; you will feel a hollow. Then let your hand drop.) Tip slightly forward so that your stomach comes in and up. Tighten your abdominal muscles. Then bring your shoulders back against the wall. To do it in a chair, sit up straight, round your shoulders, and tip them slightly forward. Your stomach will come in and up. Simultaneously tighten your abdominal muscles, then straighten up. Try 40 in the morning, 40 at noon, 40 at dinnertime, and 80 before bed.

• **Leg cramps.** Suspected causes for these sudden, annoying, and painful muscle seizures are a shortage of calcium or magnesium, or a circulatory glitch. To increase your intake of calcium, look for ways to add dairy foods and dark-green vegetables to your diet, and talk to your doctor about calcium supplements. (A Swedish study found that oral magnesium supplements may reduce the severity of leg cramps, but check with your healthcare provider before taking any supplements.) To avoid leg cramps when you stretch, flex your foot flat in the air while pushing your heel away from your body (rather than pointing

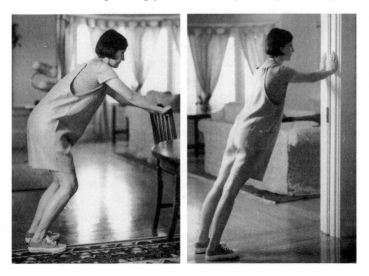

Gentle stretching—against a chair or a wall—helps stop painful cramps in their tracks.

your toes). Sometimes you can use this stretch for a cramp that's just beginning. Try gentle massage to ease a slight cramp, too.

For full-blown cramps, stand and stretch the backs of your legs. Do this by hanging forward slightly from the hips and gently bending and straightening your knees; breathe deeply and evenly. Hold on to a chair back for support. Alternatively, lean toward a wall, with your feet flat on the floor and your arms outstretched so that the palms are flat on the wall, and gently lean in.

• *Dry eyes.* If you notice that your eyes feel gritty, are more light-sensitive than usual, look red, or produce a lot of mucus, you may have a condition called dry eye. The hormone prolactin dries out the corneas, making them more sensitive. The cure is simple: use an over-the-counter "artificial tears" solution that replenishes moisture. Beware that not all eye drops are alike; those designed only to clear up redness won't relieve dry eye and can even make it worse. Dry eye usually disappears after pregnancy but can become a chronic condition.

Changes in your cornea can affect the fit of your contact lenses, too. If you notice dry eye or changes in focus, reduce wear time and rewet your lenses frequently. Don't bother getting a new prescription, since eyes return to their normal refraction once your baby is weaned. If wearing contacts becomes simply intolerable, you may need to switch to glasses for the duration.

The Kick-off Kick

If pregnancy is a landscape of peaks and valleys, then one of the highest highs is surely the day you feel the baby moving inside you. Quickening can occur as early as 15 or 16 weeks for slender women or for second-time mothers who know what to expect, or as late as 21 or 22 weeks (sometimes even later). For a few weeks beforehand, you may guess at every episode of indigestion or each muscle ache: *Was that it?* But one day, you'll just know. Either the same feeling will repeat itself unmistakably and often, or all at once you'll experience a series of unfamiliar flutters very low in your abdomen (below the navel) that can't be anything else. Most women make analogies to butterflies, bubbles, and bumps to describe this wonderful feeling. It's not constant or painful (though the intensity of these movements gets stronger as the baby grows). But once you get used to these fetal movements, it'll be hard to remember when you *didn't* have them. The baby becomes infinitely more "real," an unforgettable buddy whose internal presence you may come to miss after delivery.

Be forewarned: once the fetal acrobatics begin, the show doesn't close until delivery day, nor does it pause when you go to bed. (The baby is beginning to fall into regular sleeping and waking cycles, but they won't match yours.) At first, only you can sense the movements, most often when you're resting. But soon your partner will be able to lay a hand on your belly and feel them, too. By trimester's end, you may even see stray elbows and feet rippling the surface of your ever-firmer abdomen.

Dental Care

One of the most common self-care bloopers is to ignore your oral health during pregnancy. In fact, your mouth deserves special attention right now. Gums may bleed just from ordinary brushing—no cause for alarm; hormonal changes and increased blood volume make them swollen and prone to inflammation, a condition called *pregnancy gingivitis*. Rather than avoiding brushing altogether, switch to a softer brush. Continue to floss despite any blood, and don't postpone your biannual checkup (at least one will fall during your term). A tooth infection now could harm the baby if left untreated.

At your exam, let the dentist and hygienist know that you're pregnant. Don't be unduly alarmed if you need care beyond a regular cleaning that involves anesthetics or antibiotics or if diagnostic X-rays are suggested. While X-rays should generally be avoided if possible, after the first trimester many doctors will okay them if needed and if you wear a protective lead shield. If you develop something like an impacted wisdom tooth that requires oral surgery, it's possible for an experienced anesthesiologist to administer safe dosages of painkiller without endangering your fetus's oxygen supply. Always involve your obstetrician before any such dental work is done, however.

Sleeping Smart

Though you're no longer thinking about sleep at every opportunity, you do need to rethink some sleep habits. For one thing, lying on your stomach is no

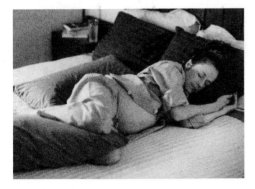

COMFORTABLE, SAFE POSITIONS FOR SLEEP.
Best bet: *Lie on your left side, which most safely shifts the uterus away from the vena cava, with knees bent slightly. Place a soft pillow between your legs and also, if you like, alongside your belly and/or behind your back for support.*
Next best position: *Lying similarly on your right side.*
If you do turn on your back: *Prop your upper body with pillows and place another one under your right buttock so that you're tilted to the left.*

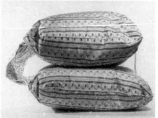

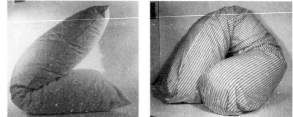

A maternity pillow is actually two pillows attached with fabric and adjustable Velcro tabs to provide simultaneous support for your front and back.

Wrap your body around a column-shaped pillow—which come in several styles and shapes—for both stomach and back support.

longer comfortable. What's more, after the fifth month, you should avoid lying flat on your back (supine). In this position, the heavy uterus compresses the *vena cava* (a major blood vessel that returns blood to the heart) and, in turn, decreases blood flow to the fetus. Don't panic if you wake up to discover that you've moved into this position in your sleep. Everyone shifts around in slumber; just change to a better position and try to train yourself, over time, to automatically choose these positions.

IS IT TRUE...

That raising my arms over my head can cause the cord to strangle the baby? The thick umbilical cord is an amazing creation. Slightly spiraled like a telephone cord, it contains three interlocked blood vessels that bring nutrients to the fetus and carry waste away. It's long enough to allow the fetus plenty of freedom to move. Often at delivery, the cord is looped around the baby's neck, but usually can be easily lifted off. Tight knots or strangulation are very rare. Rest assured, though, that your arm muscles are nowhere near the cord and therefore cannot influence its position.

That I shouldn't lift anything heavier than a newborn? Mothers with older children often worry needlessly about this. And women with some conditions, such as preterm labor, may have their movement restricted. But if you're having a normal pregnancy, you can lift away as usual until the final months. Just be sure to use correct posture: kneel before you lift so the strain is borne by your legs, not your back. One trick is to get a child to stand on a chair before you pick her up. Avoid extreme lifts (such as moving furniture) and consult your doctor first if your job or a weight-training routine involves lots of heavy lifting.

That if I have a lot of heartburn, my baby will be born with lots of hair? Despite the persistence of this belief, the only link between heartburn and hair is that both words start with the letter *h*. Even moms who endure the severest acid indigestion give birth to baldies.

What's Going on in Your Head

Smooth Sailing

The general well-being of mid-pregnancy tends to extend naturally to your emotional state. The ability to eat better, sleep better, and exercise again can't help but boost your mood.

In many cultures, feeling the first kick is considered a major turning point in pregnancy. Once you sense the baby surfing inside you, or see its black-and-white reflection on an ultrasound screen, the bonding process gets fully under way. No longer is your baby an abstract notion; now it's a bona-fide personality. Suddenly, there's greater incentive to drink more milk and to take it easy. You may begin unconsciously to rub your belly, or talk or sing to it. Go ahead and bond—and encourage your partner to do the same. Feeling your baby within you is a rich, once-in-a-lifetime (or at least, just-a-few-times-in-a-lifetime) experience that every expectant couple should revel in. One caveat, though: some women give this ever-more-real baby more personification than it deserves. Rest assured the fetus will *not* be affected by bad moods and anxiety. So go ahead and indulge in your full range of emotions during pregnancy. If you feel like kicking a wall or bursting into tears, don't hold back now. Also common is feeling especially private and self-protective, or like you need extra nurturing and protection yourself.

Take advantage of this overall feel-good phase to get as many preparations out of the way as you can, such as signing up for childbirth classes or planning your nursery and layette. Now's the time to tackle big jobs you've been putting off, too, like clearing out the spare room closet. If you're contemplating a move or a vacation, you'll enjoy the experience most during this trimester. Many doctors (and some airlines) restrict flying after the eighth month.

Body Image

Even the most contented mother-to-be can feel twinges of distress about her changing shape. Those breasts! Those hips! Those dimpled thighs and puffy ankles! You may wonder if you'll ever be able to bounce back to your old self. You may question how alluring your partner finds you now. And in a culture ob-

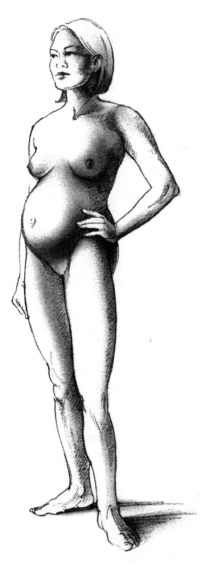

WHERE THE WEIGHT GOES
Pregnancy is no time to be a slave to the scale. Eat healthily, exercise regularly, and allow yourself to indulge in occasional cravings. Beginning in the second trimester, you'll begin to add weight at a steady pace. Here's how a typical 30-pound gain over 9 months breaks down:

baby: 7.5 pounds

amniotic fluid: 2 pounds

placenta: 1.5 pounds

mother's fat and nutrient stores: 7 pounds

fluids and blood: 8 pounds

breast growth: 2 pounds

uterus: 2 pounds

sessed with thinness, some women simply have a hard time accepting a larger self, as if they are somehow "bad" or less worthy because their reflections look less like the mannequins in *Vogue* and more like something distorted by a funhouse mirror.

Hard as it can be to give in to a rounder shape after a lifetime of counting calories, remind yourself every day that you're not looking at random accumulations of fat cells—you're looking at your baby. Respect your body for what it's accomplishing and surrender to its cues (including hunger and fatigue). Find a maternity look that accentuates your figure without overwhelming you in tent-like yards of fabric. Flip through art books of seventeenth-century paintings, with their voluptuous, fleshy women, to remind yourself how arbitrary standards of beauty really are. And don't assume that your partner will think you resemble a whale. Most men find their blossoming wives a turn-on.

Test Anxiety

Women typically undergo prenatal tests for reassurance that everything's okay. There's an added peace of mind that comes with knowing you can cross some major problems off your worry list. But the knowledge provided by such tests can be a double-edged sword. First, there is the fear of the test itself. Then, the stress of waiting for results. A suspicious but inconclusive result—common with screening tests—often leads to unfounded worries or to soul-searching about what to do next. Decisive bad news on a diagnostic test also leads to "Now what?" anxiety and, indeed, alters the entire tenor of the pregnancy. Such concerns are particularly common with tests offered in the second trimester.

You can meet test anxiety halfway by arming yourself with enough knowledge to determine which tests you really want to take, and why. You have the right to have every test explained to you, as well as to refuse any test you're uncomfortable with. (It's called "*informed* consent.") You also have the right to be informed of the results. Some doctors don't alert patients if everything looks fine, or wait until the next visit to tell them. But if you're concerned, know that you can ask when the results are expected and then call the doctor's office directly to obtain them. Another key to allaying panic is feeling comfortable in your relationship with your doctor. The more forthcoming and responsive he or she is, the better. Your peace of mind is as important as the quality of care you're receiving.

MOTHER TO MOTHER:
"Being Pregnant Made Me Finally Like My Body"

Beth Andersen, 33
Evergreen, Colorado

Like many women, Beth never felt satisfied with her appearance. "I thought I was too flat-chested and flabby," she says. At 5 feet 7 inches, she normally weighed about 120 pounds, with narrow hips and a thin frame. She never felt 100 percent comfortable with the skin she was in. She fretted that having a baby would mean she could never wear a bikini again.

During her pregnancy, she gained 40 pounds. But straying even further from the lean-but-curvaceous feminine ideal celebrated in our culture didn't upset Beth. Instead, she was surprised to discover a new respect for her body—which has lasted long after giving birth. "I remember looking at the slim women on television and thinking that their bodies appeared so boring. They weren't building a little life as mine was," she says.

"It was shocking to see my stomach grow big, but also exciting at the same time," she recalls. Her growth made the pregnancy seem more real than the positive pregnancy test had, and represented reassurance that things were go-ing well.

Now that her sons Erik and Ian are 3 and 1, Beth is back to her pre-pregnancy weight, but with a slightly looser belly and breasts whose sizes fluctuate according to how much milk she's producing. "Pregnancy didn't ruin my body, it just changed it," she says. "I still want to look nice and presentable, but I don't obsess any more."

Beth's tips for maintaining a healthy body image:

• *Focus not on what your body looks like, but what it's capable of.* "There's no such thing as a perfect body. Love your body for what it can do—growing a baby, giving birth, breastfeeding."

• *Exercise.* "When some women get pregnant, they treat it like an illness and become sedentary. It's better to adjust along with your new body shape by staying physical. I did prenatal aerobics classes twice a week. It was also a good place to bond with other moms."

• *Wear clothes that make you feel good.* "I had one outfit—a silky black tunic with palazzo pants—that I loved to wear and was a real pick-me-up."

• *Resign yourself to change.* "When you're pregnant, you have a whole different body. It was like going through puberty for 9 months."

• *Remember, your changing shape isn't flab—it's baby.* "People might look at me and say, 'Oh, she's fat.' But I looked at myself and said, 'I'm beautiful.' "

GOOD ADVICE: ON ADVICE GIVERS

Sometimes the voices of experience start to grate like an ominous Greek chorus, especially when perfect strangers chime in. How to cope with annoying advice givers or other invaders of your privacy?

- *Keep an open mind.* Lots of comments spring simply from affection or the excitement of your condition. And you might pick up a good tip or two.
- *Practice diplomacy.* If you argue, they'll just keep nagging. Better to smile, nod—and do your own thing.
- *Retain your right to privacy,* though. If the curious go too far—say, asking if you took fertility drugs if you're expecting twins—invoke your right to snap, "That's none of your business."
- *Learn to separate fact from folklore.* Just because they say it, that doesn't mean that it's so.
- *Blame your doctor,* as in "Sorry, but my doctor says I should do so-and-so."
- *Cut 'em off.* When the advice concerns some gruesome topic you'd rather not hear about (long, hard labors and births gone wrong are two stories that folks never tire of telling pregnant women), don't be shy about interrupting and saying, "Sorry, I've got to go," or "I don't want to talk about that, thanks."

IS IT TRUE...

That worrying can cause birthmarks or left-handedness? Fears and frets can incite indigestion, insomnia, and headaches. But rest assured that what's going on in your head won't affect what's going on in your uterus. Birthmarks are caused by irregular pigmentation. The cause of handedness isn't known, but maternal fretting is not one of the theories researchers are pursuing.

Checkups and Tests

Second-Trimester Exams

Checkups take place monthly during the second trimester of a normal pregnancy. At each visit, your weight, blood pressure, and urine will be checked, along with the size and position of your uterus. To check the baby's size, growth rate, and position, your belly will be measured on the outside from your pubic bone to the top of your uterus (called the *fundal height*); from about week 20 to week 36, the tape measurement (in centimeters) will roughly correspond to how many weeks pregnant you are. You probably won't get an internal exam unless a problem (such as preterm labor) is suspected.

Certain other routine and optional tests may be performed as well. These include:

- *Alpha-fetoprotein (AFP) test.* (routine) Offered between 15 and 20 weeks (with the surest results between 16 and 18 weeks), this maternal-serum blood test measures the levels of AFP (a protein produced by the fetus) in your blood. A higher-than-usual reading indicates the possibility of a neural tube defect such as spina bifida, which is a defect of the neural tube that results in a gap in the bone surrounding the spinal cord, or anencephaly, in which the brain does not develop properly. A low level of AFP can indicate that the fetus has Down's syndrome. This test only screens for the possibility of these abnormalities, however; it cannot pick up every Down's baby or every neural tube defect. This test also has a high rate of false-positives, the vast majority of which turn out to be normal babies.

An ultrasound typically follows a suspicious AFP reading to try to determine its cause. The spine can be checked, for example, or a due date can be verified, which is important because AFP levels vary with how far along you are. For the 50 percent of cases in which the ultrasound is inconclusive, amniocentesis is then offered.

• *Multiple-marker screening tests.* (routine) When the blood drawn for the AFP test is also used for other tests, it's called a multiple-marker screening. One common combination is the triple-screen, in which levels of the hormones estriol and hCG (human chorionic gonadotrophin) are also checked. The triple-screen offers the advantage of screening for Down's syndrome when amniocentesis is not performed and is a more accurate predictor of Down's than AFP alone. Estriol, produced in the placenta and fetal liver, tends to be lower than normal when the fetus has Down's. And hCG, a hormone produced by the placenta, tends to be higher when Down's occurs. The test cannot detect every Down's baby, however.

• *HBV screening.* (routine) This blood test checks for the presence of the hepatitis B virus (HBV), which can be transmitted to your baby, usually at birth. About 1 in 250 Americans is a chronic carrier, though a carrier may have no ill effects herself. If the test is positive, your baby will be treated immediately after birth with hepatitis B immune globulin and a vaccine to prevent infection. During pregnancy, an infected woman may also be given immune globulin, and prescribed bedrest and a special diet.

• *Glucose screen.* (routine) Around 24 to 28 weeks, sometimes later, you will be tested for gestational diabetes. (Or you may be tested earlier if you are overweight or have a family history of diabetes.) This condition is caused when hormones produced in the placenta alter the way a pregnant woman's insulin works. It shows up in about 3 percent of pregnancies, often (but not always) in those who are over 30, are overweight, or have a family history of diabetes. After delivery, it usually disappears. The risk of gestational diabetes is that you may have an unusually large baby (10 pounds or more), which could lead to a difficult delivery or related health problems in you or your newborn.

You'll be asked to fast overnight, with no food or drink except water before taking a *glucose screening test* (GST). For convenience, it's usually scheduled first thing in the morning. The test involves drinking a special sugar solution, which tastes like flat, thick soda pop. Some doctors use jelly beans instead to eliminate the nausea the drink causes some women. After 1 hour, a blood sample is drawn and your blood-sugar level is checked. If the reading is abnormal, as is the case about one-fifth of the time, you will be given a similar 3-hour *glucose tolerance test* (GTT) to definitively diagnose the disorder. The treatment for gestational diabetes involves controlling blood-sugar levels through special diet and exercise regimens, and occasionally insulin. (See "Gestational Diabetes," page 142.)

• **Ultrasound.** (optional) A second-trimester sonogram may be used to verify the due date or check for multiple births, and to check the progress of fetal growth. The sonologist will evaluate the anatomy of the fetus, look for birth defects, and check the location of the placenta. While not medically indicated for all pregnancies (or covered by all HMOs or insurance companies), the majority of women have an ultrasound at some time during their terms for one reason or another.

• **Amniocentesis.** (optional) This invasive, but information-loaded procedure is typically performed at 15 to 18 weeks, although it can be done earlier or later. Unlike tests that screen a mother's blood, this is a diagnostic test, which reveals information about the baby with a high degree of accuracy since it is based directly on fetal cells. An amnio may be recommended if you are 35 or older, if your family history shows a higher-than-usual risk of genetic disorders, or if your AFP or multiple-marker screen blood test results are suspicious. It's more than 99 percent accurate in diagnosing chromosomal problems; it can also reveal the gender of the fetus.

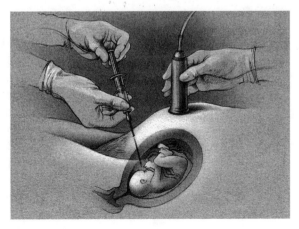

During amniocentesis, a small sample of amniotic fluid is withdrawn via an ultrasound-guided needle to test your baby for possible genetic disorders.

During the almost painless but nonetheless scary procedure, a doctor uses ultrasound to guide a thin needle through the woman's abdomen into the amniotic sac. A small amount (less than 1 ounce) of amniotic fluid is withdrawn through the needle. Discarded fetal cells in the fluid will be analyzed for chromosomal abnormalities and other genetic disorders, depending on your family history. Slight cramping or bleeding may follow. Amnio isn't routine in all pregnancies because the test itself causes one miscarriage for every 200 times it's performed. Note that the risk of miscarriage varies considerably with the experience of the physician and the point in the pregnancy at which the procedure is performed. (For a comparison with a similar test, chorionic villus sampling, see "CVS or Amnio?" page 46.)

• *Fetal fibronectin (fFN) test.* (optional) This new test, still being studied, may help predict whether preterm labor is likely. Performed in a doctor's office after 23 weeks, it's similar to a Pap smear. If the protein fFN is detected in the vagina, it may be a sign that the placenta and fetal sac are starting to separate and that early labor is likely. It's more helpful in cases where the woman is suspected of having preterm contractions than in a woman with no symptoms.

• *Percutaneous umbilical blood sampling, or PUBS.* (optional) Also called *cordocentesis*; this newer test detects blood disorders, genetic disorders, Rh-incompatibility, and infections (such as toxoplasmosis). It involves inserting a needle into the umbilical cord (guided by ultrasound) to remove fetal blood cells. The test is done after week 18 and carries a 1 to 2 percent miscarriage risk. It offers the advantage of rapid turnaround on test results (within a few days, as compared with 1 to 2 weeks for similar tests performed on amniotic fluid). It is not widely available, however.

WHAT IF...

My doctor's in a group practice—should I meet every doctor who might deliver my baby? Often in practices where your ob-gyn may not be on call the day you deliver, doctors begin rotating their patients in the second or third trimester, so you see a different physician at each checkup. This is done for *your* comfort, so that the face you see in the delivery room will be at least somewhat familiar. Rotating physicians should be strictly optional, though. Many women find it more comforting to see the same person (who really does get to know them) over the long haul every few weeks at regular checkups. And by the time you're ready to push the baby out, you're apt to care less how well you know the person who catches your newborn than whether he or she is capable and qualified—which all of your primary ob-gyn's colleagues will most likely be.

I can't bear to get weighed? If the pounds that begin packing on now unnerve you, let the nurse know that you'd rather not know the exact amount—just whether you're gaining at a healthy pace. Then look straight ahead when you step on the scale until the reading has been taken.

Mother to Mother:
"We Had a Prenatal Test Scare"

Lisa Kent, 30
Tucker, Georgia

At 14 weeks, Lisa gave a small sample of blood for an alpha-fetoprotein (AFP) screening test that her doctor described only as a routine check for abnormalities. She didn't think anything more of it until a few days later, when his office called to say that the reading on the test was "questionable" and she needed to come back for a sonogram. Meanwhile Lisa read up on the test. That's when she discovered that she'd had a screening for spinal diseases and Down's syndrome. Thinking of a cousin with Down's, she panicked.

"My doctor said not to worry or jump the gun because misleading readings happen all the time," she says. Also, only a very rare form of Down's is inherited. (More typically, it's caused when, for unknown reasons, an error in early cell division causes an extra chromosome to appear in the fertilized egg.) "But I was shocked. I never dreamed of something like this coming back wrong."

She was referred to a specialist for a thorough, hour-long sonogram, which revealed no signs of Down's syndrome (though ultrasound cannot conclusively diagnose Down's). The sonogram also showed her due date to be about 10 days earlier than previously thought, which may have skewed her AFP reading. Amniocentesis would boost the certainty of her baby's health from 95 percent to nearly 100 percent, she was told. The Kents elected not to do amnio because of the risk of miscarriage and because nothing would change the outcome of the child's health, other than that a specialist could be on hand at delivery. Still, she says, undue worry over the baby's health made for "a really scary time." Son Marshall was born with no defects right on Lisa's revised due date.

Lisa's tips for handling test anxiety:

• **Find out what every test is for and its possible outcomes.** "If you have questions about what you read on test consent forms, ask." You'll be better prepared to deal with results.

- *Question what will happen if suspicious results turn up.* "Learn about the tests' reputation for accuracy, and what the next steps are if there's a red flag."

- *Remember you have the right to refuse a test you really don't want.* This is especially useful to remember if the test can't conclusively diagnose a problem that you'd choose to live with anyway or that cannot be corrected before birth. "A test can be a needless worry."

- *Stay calm.* "It doesn't make sense to panic until you have something concrete to worry about."

What Should I Eat?

Nutrition Basics Now

As your appetite returns, constant hunger or peculiar cravings may kick in as well. Cravings that began in the first trimester may intensify or change. Eating lots of small meals will help regulate your ravenous pangs and ease digestion, too. You'll discover it helpful to keep snacks stashed in your desk at work or to have a box of raisins always at the ready in your purse. Resist the temptation to eat anything and everything, though. Your baby has a lot of growing ahead, and it's your job to supply him or her with the *best balance* of protein, vitamins, and minerals that you can.

What's ideal? The American College of Obstetricians and Gynecologists recommends a version, modified for pregnancy, of the Food Guide Pyramid developed by the U.S. Department of Agriculture. (See the illustration on page 119.) Those guidelines cover the average person's basic requirements. Adjusted for the added nutrients and calories needed in pregnancy, this means:

- *Grains (bread, cereal, rice, and pasta):* 9 to 11 servings (one serving equals 1 slice of bread, 1 large tortilla, 1 ounce of cold cereal, 1/2 cup of cooked pasta)
- *Fruits:* 3 to 4 servings (one serving equals 1 medium fruit such as an apple, an orange, or a banana; 3/4 cup juice; 1/2 cup chopped, cooked, or canned fruit)
- *Vegetables:* 4 to 5 servings (one serving equals 1 cup raw leafy vegetables, 1/2 cup cooked vegetables)
- *Meat, poultry, fish, dry beans, eggs, and nuts:* 3 servings (one serving equals 2 ounces meat, 1 egg, or 1/2 cup cooked beans)
- *Milk, yogurt, and cheese:* 3 servings (one serving equals 1 cup milk, 1 cup yogurt, 1 1/2 ounces cheese)
- *Fats, oils, and sweets:* Use sparingly.

More good-eating guidelines:

• *Keep a food diary.* For a week, write down everything you eat. Then assess it against the guidelines recommended above. Ask yourself: Do I drink enough milk? How many servings of fruits and vegetables do I really eat? How varied is my protein supply? Do I rely too much on fast-food meals? How can I make snacks and desserts work harder for me? (You don't have to cut them out entirely, but you can add nutrients by having sweet-potato chips rather than the regular kind, or by topping frozen yogurt with fresh berries or wheat germ.)

• *Get off to a good start.* Never skip breakfast. You'll be more tired and dizzy if you try to shave these calories off your daily intake. Some women are prone to fainting if they don't have breakfast, especially later in pregnancy. At minimum, consume some protein and carbohydrates—say, a glass of milk and peanut butter on half a bagel.

• *Think fresh and whole.* Generally, the less processed a food is, the better it is for you. Thus, an apple is more nutritious than applesauce; old-fashioned cooked oatmeal is better than oat cereal from a box; and 100 percent whole-grain breads are better than processed white ones.

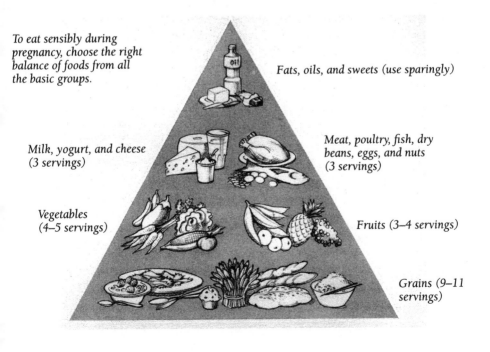

To eat sensibly during pregnancy, choose the right balance of foods from all the basic groups.

Fats, oils, and sweets (use sparingly)

Milk, yogurt, and cheese (3 servings)

Meat, poultry, fish, dry beans, eggs, and nuts (3 servings)

Vegetables (4–5 servings)

Fruits (3–4 servings)

Grains (9–11 servings)

• *Be a fruit and vegetable explorer.* Broaden your horizons. Tour a fruit stand or farmer's market. Vow to try something new each week. Remember that darker is better when it comes to green vegetables (pick spinach and romaine over iceberg lettuce).

• *Be broadminded about protein.* Especially from mid-pregnancy on, you'll need added protein to help produce the extra blood demanded by the tissue growth within, as well as to maintain your muscle tone and to fight disease. Don't overlook meatless sources, including eggs (the protein roosts in the whites), tofu and other soy products, beans, milk, cheese, wheat germ, peanut butter, rice, and grains.

• *Cook smart.* To retain nutrients, steam or microwave vegetables rather than boiling them. Remember that most of the good stuff is found in the peel or right below it. Broil or bake, rather than barbecue or fry. Roasting poultry (or meat) is one of the easiest ways to cook—all you do is pop it in the oven—and it's one of the most healthful, too, especially when you use a wire rack over a pan to catch the fatty juices. Add iron to foods, especially tomato-based sauces, by cooking in a cast-iron skillet.

• *Salt to your taste.* Don't eliminate it completely, since sodium helps regulate fluids. Especially in hot weather, loss of salt through perspiration can depress one's appetite. Adequate salt intake is also essential to the maintenance of your increased blood volume. On the other hand, excessive sodium can lead to hypertension and edema (water retention). Lightly salting your food is okay if you don't go overboard. Watch out for the hidden salt in ketchup, bacon, pickles, chips, pretzels, and fast food.

Are Nutrition Shortcuts Okay?

A relatively new issue for expectant mothers is whether or not the many artificial or nutritionally compressed foods available today are safe. Check the label first to be sure there is no contraindication for pregnant women. Many of these foods (such as Olestra and energy drinks) have not been tested on pregnant women specifically. When in doubt, ask your ob-gyn. Other guidelines:

• *Gatorade-type drinks.* If you're an athlete accustomed to these beverages, are continuing your workouts, and are eating an otherwise healthful diet, they may be an acceptable way to replenish liquids. Such drinks are high in salt, however. And because such drinks offer little in the way of actual nutrients, most pregnant women, even active ones, are better off with fruit juices and water.

• *Energy drinks.* Liquid nutritional drinks (such as Ensure, Boost, and Sustacal) were designed for seriously underweight people and those unable to eat solids. They contain 200 to 350 calories per 8 ounces and are made up of milk protein and vegetable oils. Pregnant women should consume them sparingly, and best under the supervision of a doctor. They're not substitutes for the fiber and nutrients offered by real whole foods.

• *Protein-packed–type concentrated snacks.* Snack bars can't harm you and can actually be helpful if you have severe morning sickness or other trouble consuming adequate protein. (Real foods are always the ideal, of course, as they offer more fiber and more natural nutrients.) But watch the vitamin content of such snacks. If you're already taking a prenatal supplement, you don't want to overdose on vitamins, which could harm your fetus.

• *Olestra.* Unfortunately, it's too early in this fat substitute's life to know much about its effects on pregnancy, so avoid Olestra-containing foods. Choose baked "low-fat" snacks as an alternative if you crave potato or corn chips.

TRY THESE RECIPES!

Mediterranean Couscous Casserole

Preparation time: about 15 minutes
Cooking time: about 30 minutes

This colorful casserole brims with the flavors of the Mediterranean—olives, leeks, tomatoes, fresh herbs, and roasted red peppers. Although it's mixed with bits of flavorful salami or turkey, you can omit these ingredients to make an entirely vegetarian dish. Serve this wholesome grain with crusty bread and a tossed salad.

2 tablespoons olive oil
1 medium leek (white part only), very thinly sliced
1/2 cup finely chopped roasted red pepper or pimiento
1/2 cup diced salami or turkey
1 1/2 tablespoons chopped fresh thyme, or 1 teaspoon dried
Salt and freshly ground black pepper
10-ounce box instant couscous

½ cup cherry tomatoes, quartered, or 1 small ripe tomato,
   cut into small cubes
⅓ cup Niçoise or good-quality black olives, pitted
1 6-ounce jar marinated artichoke hearts, drained and chopped
2 tablespoons chopped fresh dill

Preheat the oven to 350 degrees. In a medium casserole, heat 1 tablespoon of the oil over moderate heat. Add the leek and sauté 5 minutes, stirring frequently to prevent browning. Add the red pepper, salami or turkey, thyme, and salt and pepper, and cook another 3 minutes. Remove from the heat.

Meanwhile, in medium saucepan, bring 2⅓ cups of water to a boil. Add a pinch of salt and the remaining 1 tablespoon olive oil. Stir in the couscous, cover, and remove from the heat. Let sit for 5 minutes. Using a fork, fluff up the couscous to prevent clumping.

Add the cooked couscous to the casserole and gently stir in the tomatoes, olives, artichoke hearts, dill, and salt and pepper to taste. Cover the casserole. (The recipe can be made up to a day ahead of time up to this point. Keep covered and refrigerate until ready to use.)

Bake casserole for 15 to 17 minutes, or until hot throughout. Yield: 4 servings.

Healthy Tuna Pockets

Preparation time: 10 minutes

Chopped celery, bean sprouts and lettuce, plus a touch of mayo or yogurt, make this tuna salad nutritious but light. Serve it on pita bread or toasted rye.

1 6-ounce can tuna packed in water, drained
¼ cup finely chopped celery
¼ cup finely chopped black or green pitted olives, drained
2 tablespoons lemon juice
2 tablespoons low-fat mayonnaise or plain low-fat yogurt
1 large pita bread or 2 slices thinly sliced bread, such as rye
¼ cup shredded lettuce
¼ cup bean sprouts (optional)

In a small bowl, mix the tuna, celery, olives, lemon juice, and mayonnaise. Cut the pita bread in half or place the bread on a work surface and divide the mixture between the 2 halves, then top with the lettuce and sprouts. Yield: 1 to 2 servings.

Whole Wheat Pizza

Preparation time: about 15 minutes
Sitting time: about 1¹/₂ hours
Baking time: about 8 minutes

Think of this pizza dough as a canvas and the contents of your refrigerator as the paints that create an edible work of art. Anything goes with pizza: try leftover slices of chicken, beef, or lamb; combine various cheeses; add raw or cooked vegetables, or herbs. The dough can be made a day ahead, or frozen for up to a month. Double the recipe and freeze half for a hectic day.

Whole Wheat Pizza Crust
    1 tablespoon active dry yeast
    1¹/₂ cups warm water
    3 to 3¹/₂ cups whole wheat flour, or about 1¹/₂ cups all-purpose flour and
        1¹/₂ cups whole wheat flour
    ¹/₂ teaspoon salt
    2 tablespoons olive oil
    About 2 tablespoons cornmeal, for dusting

Toppings
    About 2¹/₂ cups chopped vegetables and/or meat
    About 1 to 1¹/₂ cups grated cheese
    About ¹/₂ cup tomato or other sauce

To make the pizza dough, mix the yeast with the water in a large bowl and place in a warm spot for 5 minutes, or until the yeast begins to bubble.

Sift 3 cups of the flour(s) and salt into the yeast and gradually mix to form a ball. Mix in the olive oil and enough additional flour to form a soft ball.

Transfer the dough to a lightly floured work surface and knead it until soft and elastic, 5 to 8 minutes. Shape the dough into a ball and place it in a lightly oiled bowl and cover with a clean tea towel. Place in a warm spot for about 1 hour, or until the dough has doubled in bulk. Punch down the dough and re-shape into a ball. Let sit another 20 minutes, or until the dough rises again. Divide the dough in half; you can freeze the other half or make 2 pizzas.

Roll out half the dough on a floured surface. Sprinkle a cookie or baking sheet with the cornmeal and place the dough on top.

Preheat the oven to 450 degrees.

Add your toppings of choice and bake for about 8 minutes, or until the crust begins to turn golden brown and the cheese is bubbling and melted. Yield: 2 to 3 servings for each pizza.

Minestrone Soup

Preparation time: about 20 minutes
Cooking time: about 1 hour

Don't let the long list of ingredients scare you: this soup is simple to put together and a great dish to make ahead of time. (It's ideal, too, in late pregnancy and early motherhood, when cooking is the last thing on your mind.) View this as a master recipe, and use virtually any combination of vegetables you like (depending on the season and whatever you happen to find in your refrigerator). Make it even heartier by adding chunks of ham or turkey.

1 tablespoon olive oil
3 leeks (white part only) or 1 onion, chopped
2 garlic cloves, finely chopped
6 carrots, chopped
4 celery stalks, chopped
2 large potatoes, peeled and cubed, or 4 new potatoes unpeeled and cubed
2 medium zucchini, cubed
1/2 head broccoli, cut into florets
3 scallions
1/2 cup chopped fresh parsley
4 ripe tomatoes, cored and cubed, or 3 cups canned whole tomatoes, chopped
Salt and freshly ground black pepper
1 bay leaf
2 pints chicken broth, homemade or low-sodium canned, or water
1 1/2 cups water
1/4 cup dry white wine (optional)
1 cup corn kernels, fresh shucked or canned (optional)
1 19-ounce can cooked white beans, drained (optional)
1 cup grated Parmesan cheese

In a large pot, heat the oil over moderate heat. Add the leeks and sauté about 4 minutes, until tender but not brown. Add the garlic, carrots, celery, and potatoes and sauté another 3 minutes. Add the zucchini, broccoli, scallions, and half the parsley and stir well. Add the tomatoes, salt and pepper, bay leaf, broth, water, and wine, if using, and raise the heat to high. Bring to a boil, reduce the heat to moderately low, cover partially, and let simmer 30 to 45 minutes, or until the potatoes and vegetables are tender.

Remove the bay leaf from the soup, and taste for seasoning. If the soup tastes weak, simmer vigorously for another 5 to 10 minutes to reduce slightly. Add the corn and beans, if using, and simmer another 2 minutes. Sprinkle the soup with the remaining parsley just before serving. Serve the grated cheese on the side. Yield: 8 servings.

Smart Swaps

Some foods are more nutrient-packed than other choices. Consider these easy dietary reforms.

INSTEAD OF THIS	SUBSTITUTE THIS
Whole milk	Fat-free or nonfat milk (formerly called skim milk)
Fried chicken	Broiled, baked, or roasted chicken
Boiled vegetables	Steamed vegetables
White rice	Brown rice
White bread	Whole wheat, pumpernickel
Orange juice	Orange juice fortified with calcium
Presweetened cereal	Hot, low-sugar cereal
Potato chips	Air-popped popcorn
Croissants	Bran or banana muffins
Creamy salad dressing	Oil and vinegar
Canned fruit in syrup	Fresh fruit
Cake	Cranberry-pumpkin bread
Ice cream	Fruit sorbet
Soda pop	Juice or juice sparkler

IS IT TRUE...

That craving pickles means my body needs salt? That might seem logical, but it's not true. (Just look at the totally inexplicable yens that some pregnant women have for fluffer-nutter sandwiches or Lucky Charms cereal.) In fact, the cause of cravings isn't known. Rather than being omens of nutritional shortfalls, it's more likely that we acquire preferences for certain foods because of changes in our taste buds and sense of smell. Pregnancy's yo-yo emotions play a role too, creating a basic yearning for comfort foods. As for why some women crave old favorites while others develop sudden new tastes for tuna, watermelon, or pickles, no one really knows. If it's good for you, indulge. If it's not, indulge in moderation.

One odd craving to avoid, which some women actually develop, is a lust for laundry starch, dirt, clay, or chalk. Called *pica*, this strange but not uncommon urge often arises from a serious dietary deficiency and should be reported to a doctor.

That I should avoid sugar? In a zeal to get their diets under control, some pregnant women try to cut out all sources of sugar in their diets. While trimming empty calories is a good idea, there's no need to banish the crystals completely. Sugar, after all, is glucose—and glucose is what your growing baby is using for fuel. A diet made up of 10 to 15 percent sweeteners won't make you a diabetic or overly fat. But do try switching to healthful sweets, like carrot cake, pumpkin bread, 100 percent juice popsicles, or milkshakes.

That organic produce is healthier? You'd think that fruits and veggies grown pesticide-free would be the purest things you could eat. The problem is that pollutants and toxins are everywhere, including the soil and water in which the organic produce is grown. And it's unproven whether some of the natural pesticides used in organic farming may be nonetheless toxic to a developing fetus. If you want to spend the extra money on such foods, that's fine. But there is no difference in the nutritional composition of organic and nonorganic produce. You're probably not losing any nutritional edge if you buy the regular stuff and wash it well or peel it before eating.

GOOD ADVICE: SNEAKING IN NUTRIENTS

Bored by eating basic foods? Having a hard time cramming in all the recommended servings of each food group? Consider these tasty ideas:

- Slice fresh fruit (berries, banana, kiwi, dates, peaches, apples) onto your breakfast cereal, or add dried fruit.
- Top pancakes with fruit yogurt, rather than syrup.
- Grate zucchini or carrots and add a cup to your favorite banana bread recipe.
- Layer your pizza with spinach and add Parmesan cheese to the crust recipe.
- Scramble eggs with cheese and tomatoes.
- Put sliced bananas on your peanut butter sandwich instead of jelly.

- Accent salads with peanuts, garbanzo beans, or tuna.
- Add sprouts, avocado, spinach leaves, tomatoes, thinly sliced cucumbers, or shredded cabbage to your sandwich.
- Slip applesauce into waffle batter.
- Make soups with milk instead of water.
- Swap wheat germ or oatmeal for a little of the flour in cookies, cakes, and breads.

WHAT IF ...

I still have morning sickness? If you're still feeling sick after the fourth month, you should work doubly hard to make sure that what you *can* stomach is packed with nutrition. As the fetus grows, it will take certain nutrients from your body stores if they're not being supplied, putting your health at risk. If appetite-stealing nausea persists into the fifth month, inform your doctor so you can get dietary advice and be monitored for possible related problems such as anemia and dehydration.

I forget to take a prenatal vitamin? One day's lapse won't do any harm if you're eating a generally balanced diet. *Don't* try to make up for the nutrient loss by taking two pills the next day; an overdose of vitamins is more harmful than a brief deficit. Taking your vitamin at the same time every day helps reinforce the habit. (If you used birth-control pills, make it the same time you used to take them.) Pop your vitamin with a glass of orange juice to improve iron absorption.

I'm lactose intolerant? Women who have difficulty digesting milk sugar because they lack the enzyme lactase run the risk of not getting enough calcium in pregnancy. Those of African-American, Asian, Hispanic, or Mediterranean heritage and older women are most commonly affected by the bloating and gastric distress that this incurable disorder brings on when certain dairy products are consumed. Doctors usually prescribe calcium supplements (different from prenatal vitamins). You can also buy lactase pills or drops (brand names Lactaid, Dairy Ease) that supply the missing enzyme needed to break milk sugar down. Other options are lactose-reduced milk and cheese (ask your grocer), buttermilk, acidophilus milk, and some yogurts. Sometimes the problem eases late in pregnancy, perhaps as the body's way of helping it get as much calcium as needed.

I hate milk? In addition to trying the suggestions above, make an effort to consume more of the calcium-rich foods you do like. Try yogurt (frozen or regular), cheese, dark-green vegetables (collards, spinach, bok choy), small-boned fish such as sardines, custards or puddings, tofu, calcium-fortified bread, and orange juice with added calcium. Work harder to sneak milk or nonfat dried milk powder into your soups, sauces, scrambled eggs, mashed potatoes, and baking mixes. Don't drink coffee or tea or eat salty foods when you do eat calcium-rich foods, because those things can slow calcium absorption.

Fit for Pregnancy

Exercising Caution

As you begin feeling more like your old self in this trimester, you'll probably take more pleasure in exercise routines. Clearly, though, you're not exactly the same. Work the following caveats into your workouts:

• ***Don't lie flat on your back.*** After the fourth or fifth month, the weight of the baby and uterus can restrict blood flow when you lie flat. Modify your stretches accordingly.

• ***Watch your step.*** As the hormone relaxin loosens up your ligaments and your center of gravity shifts, your surefootedness begins to fail you. Take extra care with—or eliminate altogether—activities that involve a lot of hopping or quick changes of direction, such as step aerobics, tennis, and jogging.

• ***Stand straight.*** Between your aching back and a chronic off-balance sensation, good posture gets harder to maintain. But keeping your back and shoulders straight during exercise will strengthen muscles and help prevent injury.

Relaxation

Relaxation soothes muscles after a workout and helps you maintain a mental even keel. It can lower your heart rate and blood pressure. Don't limit relaxation exercises to just workouts, however. Take mini-relaxation breaks throughout the day or at specific times, such as first thing in the morning and last thing at night. When you use basic relaxing techniques throughout pregnancy, you're also preparing yourself for labor, when the ability to fight the instinct to tense up can make you more comfortable. Begin to practice techniques now and they'll be second nature by the time you need to call on them in labor.

Some basic approaches:

• ***Progressive relaxation.*** You can do this by yourself. The idea is to relax each part of your body individually. Lie down on your side and breathe deeply. Isolate one muscle group, such as your shoulder. Tense the muscles, then release. Accompany the release with an exhale or an audible sigh. "Tour" your body so that you relax each major muscle group one by one. Don't forget your fingers, your toes, your jaw, and even the way your tongue rests in your mouth.

• **Imagery.** Start with slow, easy breaths. Picture a pleasant, reassuring scene—rocking your healthy new baby in your new nursery, for example, or lounging on a favorite beach. Use all your senses to focus on the details of the scene, such as the light on the water, the movement of the waves, how the sun feels on your skin. You might imagine this on your own, or develop a picture that your partner guides you through verbally. Some women tape-record a visualization so that they can more fully relax while listening to it.

• **Touch relaxation.** Like gentle massage, this approach uses gentle stroking or pressure over various parts of the body to relax them one by one. Your partner should start with the hands, then the arms, the shoulders, and so on.

• **Meditation.** The simplest form is to concentrate on a given object or image. Dim the lights and play soft music, if you like. Position yourself comfortably and breathe deeply. Focus on the image or, alternatively, close your eyes and focus on a phrase or affirmation that you repeat over and over, such as "I feel so healthy and I can't wait to meet my baby."

The Tip-Top Ten

Stretching should be part of any prenatal exercise routine. Easy enough for anyone to master, stretching limbers muscles that naturally shorten up in pregnancy, prevents muscles from tightening during other activity, enhances flexibility, and nicest of all, makes you feel great. Make these ten basic stretches part of your daily prenatal routine. Repeat each exercise four times in each direction unless otherwise instructed.

1. HEAD CIRCLES
Position: Sit or stand
How to do it: Lengthen your neck down and forward. Roll your head to the side; look up at a high angle while stretching your spine up and slightly back. (Don't drop your neck back or you may strain a muscle.) Now roll your head to the other side. End by dropping the head forward again. Repeat in the other direction.

Arm stretches.

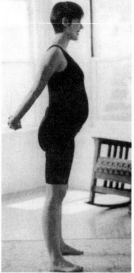

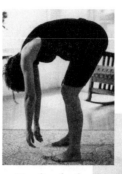

Standing back stretches.

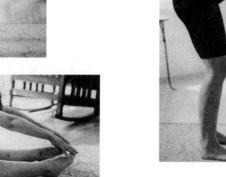

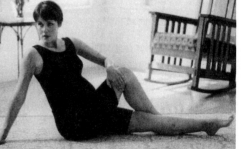

Sitting back stretch.

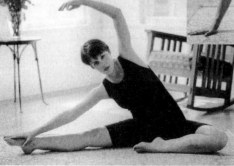

Thigh stretch.

Side stretch.

2. SHOULDER CIRCLES

Position: Sit or stand

How to do it: Circle your shoulders forward, up, back, and down in the largest circle you can make. The movement should be soft and easy-going. Repeat; reverse the motion.

3. ARM STRETCHES

Position: Sit or stand

How to do it: Clasp your hands behind your back. Stretch them back and down, then release. Repeat.

4. WAIST TWISTS

Position: Sit or stand

How to do it: Turn side to side slowly from the waist and look over one shoulder, then the other. Allow your arms to move freely. Repeat this a little faster so it becomes a swinging movement.

5. STANDING BACK STRETCHES

Position: Stand with your feet about 12 inches apart

How to do it: Roll your head and torso down toward the floor, bending your knees as you go. Return to standing straight by rolling up smoothly through your spine. Maintain the feeling of weight in both your feet. Repeat.

6. SITTING BACK STRETCH

Position: Sit on the floor with your legs stretched out parallel in front of you

How to do it: Slowly drop your head toward your knees and stretch your fingers along your legs as far as they will comfortably go. Straighten up slowly. Imagine that you're straightening up because your torso is filling with air, like a balloon, not because you are using your muscles to hoist yourself up. Repeat.

7. THIGH STRETCHES

Position: Sit on the floor with your legs outstretched

How to do it: Cross your right ankle over your left knee. Use your left hand to pull the right thigh toward the left, stretching the outside of the right leg. Increase the twist by looking over your right shoulder. Hold for a minute. Do once on each side.

8. SIDE STRETCH

Position: Sit on the floor with your left leg out to the side, your right one bent

How to do it: Raise your right arm over your head. Reach high and make a big arc as you lean over your left leg and try to touch your fingers to your toes. Reverse the arc to bring yourself upright. Repeat, then do the other side.

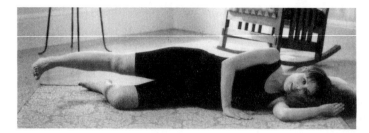

Leg stretch.

9. PELVIC TILT

Position: Kneel on all fours

How to do it: Start with the head and pelvis in a relatively straight line. Curve the center of your back upward, contracting your abdominals, then lower it until straight. Repeat.

10. LEG STRETCH

Position: Lie on your left side, your head on a pillow or folded towel. Bend your left leg at the knee and hip, and brace your right hand on the floor. Your right leg is straight.

How to do it: Stretch your right leg long as you lift it off the floor. Lower it to the floor. Repeat, then do the other side.

GOOD ADVICE: REMEMBER TO KEGEL

Thank one Dr. Arnold Kegel for creating a very private—but essential—little exercise that every pregnant woman and new mom should know. Called the Kegel, it dates back to the 1940s. The exercise is a way to strengthen the *pubococcygeus* (PC), the main muscle of the pelvic floor, which surrounds the urethral, vaginal, and rectal openings. Why is it important? In a word, support. The vagina and pelvic muscles undergo a lot of stretching and strain in pregnancy, supporting the uterus, baby, placenta, bowels, and bladder. Unless the PC muscle is kept in good shape, you could wind up, postpartum, with one or more of several unsavory conditions, including incontinence, a loose feeling during sex, or a prolapsed uterus (which occurs when the uterus drops down into the vagina).

Hence, doctors and childbirth educators continually harp about the importance of keeping up your Kegels (also called pelvic-floor squeezes) before and after pregnancy. To locate the muscle in question, try interrupting an imaginary urine flow. Now squeeze and hold for 10 seconds, 10 to 20 times in a row, ideally three or more times a day.

Some tips:
- Never actually do Kegels while you're urinating, as this may lead to urinary tract infections.
- But get in the habit of doing a series before you leave the bathroom.
- Do them while you're in the middle of a long telephone call or a boring meeting. (No one can tell.)
- Try holding the muscle during intercourse, which produces a pleasurable tightening sensation around the penis.
- See how many you can do as you drift off to sleep.
- Gradually increase the length of time you can hold the squeeze (without straining).
- Remember that it's much easier to condition the PC muscle while you're pregnant than once you've delivered—which, guaranteed, is when you'll wish you'd started sooner.

The Pregnant Look

Maternity Clothes: A Buyer's and Borrower's Guide

Your favorite skirt no longer zips up, your shirt buttons pucker, and you gave up your blue jeans weeks ago. Now you're ready to assemble your maternity wardrobe—the clothes you'll love to slip into and then, after a few months of repetitious wear, grow to hate the sight of.

Thankfully, the style and quality of maternity wear has improved since the early baby boomers began having babies. No modern mama-to-be need masquerade as a ruffly kewpie doll or a circus tent anymore. In fact, a maternity look can be attractive, fun, and yes, even chic. Resist the impulse to simply buy bigger sizes of regular clothes. Maternity garments are cut to fit your unique shape—with expanded waists, chests, and hips, but unchanged arms, shoulders, and legs, and also with hemlines that won't ride up as your stomach expands. Because of this attention to detail, they're actually more flattering than extra-large regular clothes would be. If you look around, you can find styles that range from classics to loungewear to looks that are downright hip.

First, chances are good that some pregnant relative, neighbor, friend, or coworker will have already gladly volunteered her maternity leftovers. Say yes to everything you're offered. Then weed out what doesn't work for you in the privacy of your own bedroom. Don't feel obligated to wear it all. (They'll never notice, and if they're rude enough to mention it, just sigh and say, "It just didn't fit me right.") Maternity wear is sized to your pre-pregnancy size, so if you've always worn a 10, that's what to look for on maternity tags. But don't judge solely

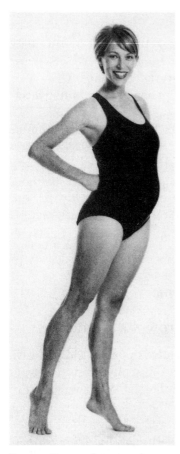

Because it expands as you do, a leotard is a maternity wardrobe essential.

by the labels: not only can "small" and "medium" be misleading, but sometimes what doesn't fit well at first looks great by 25 or 30 weeks, once you've plumped out more in front. The point is that by borrowing voraciously, you might unearth almost everything you need—or at least a few fresh pieces—and all for free.

Where else to look? Maternity specialty shops (Motherhood, Pea in the Pod, Japanese Weekend) are an obvious destination, especially for career wear and specialty items like nursing bras or bathing suits. Some department stores (Macy's, J.C. Penney's) and discount stores (Target, Kmart) have maternity departments—great for stocking up on inexpensive basics such as black stretch pants and underwear. Other fruitful sources are catalogs and mail-order houses, where the choices are often most fashion forward (Belly Basics, Garnet Hill), factory outlets (Dan Howard), secondhand and consignment shops, and rent-a-dress boutiques that specialize in formal occasions (most carry a small selection of maternity party frocks).

If you're handy with a sewing machine, you can find easy-to-make styles in every pattern book. Not least, raid your partner's closet. If he's a big guy, you're in luck for sportshirts, sweaters, or a bathrobe. Even if your builds are comparable, men tend to have broader shoulders and longer torsos, so his oxford shirts and denim jacket might work better now than yours, at least for a few months. Think sleek, though: team oversized pieces with slender bottoms—leggings or a straight dark skirt and tights—rather than his baggy sweatpants.

To construct a basic wardrobe, start with a set of solid-hued separates: pants, leggings, skirt, jumper, and matching long solid tunic. To these you can add a big white shirt and some coordinating tops with prints. A dress or two, overalls (shorts or long pants) or a jumpsuit, a sweater for the cold, and some exercise wear or a bathing suit are nice extras. The goal is to have enough variety without overbuying. Since maternity clothes have a finite lifespan, it doesn't make sense to stuff your closet with them. (Trust experience: these items will not be joining your permanent wardrobe and soon enough you will be gladly handing them off to the next pregnant woman you know.) But don't bore your reflection to tears. Toss in a wild-print shirt or a sock-it-to-me red sweater to cheer up the monotony—and make you feel cheerier.

When assemblying your maternity wardrobe, remember these tips:

• *Go natural.* Choose natural fibers whenever possible; cotton knits are cooler than rayon or polyester blends, important as your internal furnace stokes up. Lean to a layered look, for the same reason.

• *Pick quality over low-low prices.* True, you won't wear the stuff forever, but you will be washing it over and over. And if you think you'll have more than

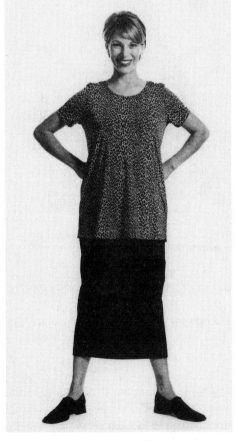

An oversized white shirt—his or yours— is a polished partner for a pair of leggings.

Feeling a bit too basic? An animal print top will give your outfits (and your spirits) a lift.

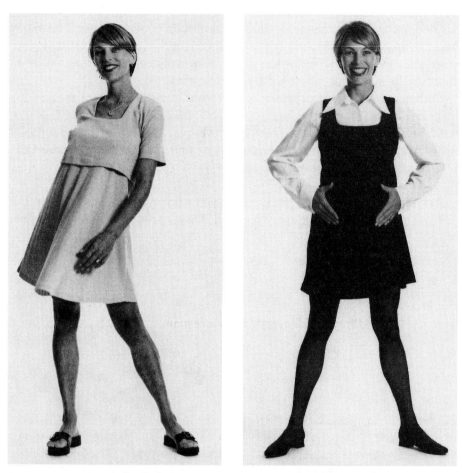

Extra-roomy nursing clothes do double duty as maternity wear.

Looking businesslike is literally a cinch with a dress that can be tied in the back or worn loose.

one child, splurge a little. Justify expenses by calculating the cost per wear.

• ***Look for built-in flexibility.*** Many styles feature tie-backs, decorative alligator clips, adjustable buttons, and drawstrings that let you cinch in—or let out— fabric as needed.

• ***Try everything on.*** Invest some fitting-room time to determine which kind of waists suit you best. Most pants and skirts feature either elastic waistbands, stretch panels, or special supportive bands that are designed to be worn *under* the belly. You might tolerate all three well or discover a comfy favorite. Check to be sure that bathing suits offer ample stretch in the rear as well as the belly.

• **Beware stirrup pants.** Some moms love their elongating look, but others find that the straps can interfere with circulation and exacerbate foot swelling. If you wear them, stick to loose-fit stirrups.

• **Consider a few nursing clothes now.** Tops and dresses that feature hidden openings for breastfeeding tend to be cut roomy, extending the usefulness of your pregnancy purchases. Likewise, look for maternity wear that buttons down the front so it'll do double duty postpartum while nursing. (Though you may wish to burn all your well-worn maternity clothes the day you get home from the hospital, rest assured that your old body won't be there yet, and you'll be grateful for maternity leggings for many weeks to come.)

• **Don't ignore the right lingerie.** It will make your clothes look and feel better. (See "GOOD ADVICE: Buying Comfortable Lingerie," page 73.)

IS IT TRUE...

That my hips will get wider with each pregnancy? Not inevitably. During pregnancy your pelvic supports do loosen to help accommodate birth. But within a few weeks of delivery, they return to their normal position. What many women experience as bigger postpartum hips is actually lingering fat—the last 5 to 10 stubborn pounds that cling to their figures, especially around the hips, waist, and rear.

That I'm more likely to get freckles if I'm carrying a girl? No. A freckle face is hereditary. Hormones can darken preexisting freckles during pregnancy, whether your baby is a boy or a girl.

GOOD ADVICE: A PROFESSIONAL LOOK

What if you can't wear any old sack to the office—but can't afford to buy out the designer racks at the local boutique? Try these tricks for adding polish to your pregnant look:

• Coordinate understated maternity basics—skirts, jumpers—with your best jackets and blazers, worn unbuttoned (the longer, the better).
• Buy the best you can afford but consider more than the price tag—evaluate workmanship and fabric carefully.
• Cliché but true: nothing communicates confidence as well as black, charcoal, and navy.

- Extend a lean line with dark opaque hosiery.
- Rely on good jewelry and silk scarves to finish a look.
- Don't give up heels, if you like the look. A slight lift is actually healthier for the leg, but avoid 2-inch and up stacks.
- Consider a shorter haircut or wear hair neatly pulled back. A trimmer head adds balance to a burgeoning body.
- Since hair tends to grow faster and thicker in pregnancy, be careful to maintain or step up your schedule of trims.

What About Sex?

What's Normal Now?

The range of what's normal about sexuality during pregnancy is widest during the second trimester. Many women who in the first trimester felt too nauseous to think about bed in any context beyond sleep suddenly find their libido awakening during the fourth or fifth month. Some find themselves more sexually oriented than ever in their lives. Feeling aroused several times a day, having multiple orgasms, or masturbating frequently are not uncommon. Some women achieve orgasm for the first time ever during pregnancy. Yet it's also common to have zero interest in sex.

What causes so many different responses? Sexual arousal is stoked by the same hormonal changes that fuel a pregnancy. By your second trimester, the manufacture of estrogen is in overdrive, producing as much in a single day as a nonpregnant woman's ovaries do in 3 years. But whereas erotic inclinations may have been masked in early pregnancy by nausea or fatigue, they now become more apparent as those impediments lift. What's more, a fuller belly and breasts, lustrous hair, and glowing skin give most women erotic "bloom." Dispensing

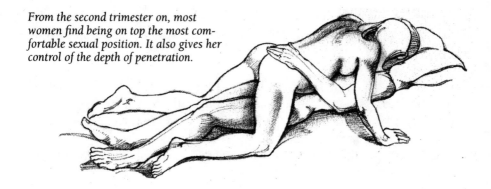

From the second trimester on, most women find being on top the most comfortable sexual position. It also gives her control of the depth of penetration.

with birth control often inspires new freedom. And some studies suggest that steadily increasing levels of oxytocin—the hormone that ultimately initiates and maintains labor—ignite lust, too. With the genitals already engorged and their nerve endings growing more sensitive as they stretch, the net result can be insatiability.

On the other hand, still other realities of pregnancy can nix these natural developments. They include ongoing sickness, physical discomfort, worries about a high-risk pregnancy, feeling fat, or perceiving that your partner finds you unattractive. All of these circumstances and feelings are understandable. In fact, your level of desire will probably change from day to day, depending on which factors have the upper hand. It's your prerogative to decide the level of sexuality that's comfortable during pregnancy, so long as you and your partner can communicate openly about your feelings and your overall intimacy isn't imperiled.

By mid- to late pregnancy, an expanding belly requires some physical accommodation. Positions that work well include side-by-side variations, the woman on top, and the man entering from behind with the woman on all fours.

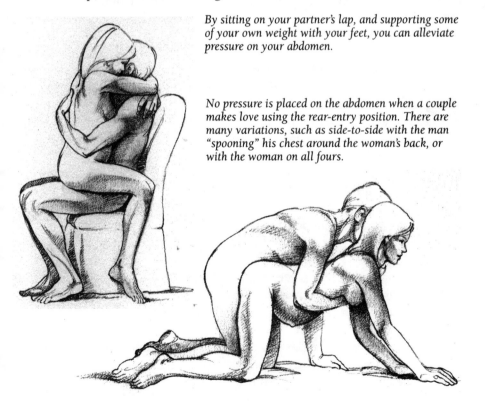

By sitting on your partner's lap, and supporting some of your own weight with your feet, you can alleviate pressure on your abdomen.

No pressure is placed on the abdomen when a couple makes love using the rear-entry position. There are many variations, such as side-to-side with the man "spooning" his chest around the woman's back, or with the woman on all fours.

Dad's Views

Fathers-to-be experience their own range of sexual feelings during pregnancy. Responses include:

• *Fear of hurting the baby.* Some men hold back sexually out of fears about the baby's safety, especially once the baby is showing or once they have felt it move. Some basic anatomical information can allay such concerns. The baby, safely bundled in the amniotic sac, won't be harmed by intercourse or orgasm.

• *Feeling left out.* At first he's slightly in awe of the tremendous changes taking place within his partner. He wants to be supportive of her sickness and fatigue. But in terms of a pecking order of attention in pregnancy, he's a distant third after mother and fetus in the eyes of well-wishers and, often, of the mother herself. Eventually he becomes impatient. The catch here is that many men are uncomfortable articulating feelings of being left out—especially when they don't want to appear self-serving during this special time. Try to anticipate *his* feelings even as you're absorbed with your own. Find ways to make him feel special and involved with the pregnancy. Be careful not to squelch all sexual expression even when you're not in the mood.

• *The three's-a-crowd phenomenon.* Just knowing that the baby's there is enough to dampen some guys' ardor. He still adores you, still finds you sexy, but seeing a kick in mid-passion or maneuvering clumsily around a beach-ball belly works like a cold shower on his ardor. In this case, he just has to confront the reality that sex during pregnancy, like sex after baby, is going to be different, period. Advice for him is to get used to it, and get over it.

• *He's just not attracted.* Some men have a hard time seeing their partners as both mothers and sex objects. Or they misread the swelling belly as fat and, in words or deeds, fail to support the mother's need to add pounds for the baby's benefit. Either way, the result is a turn-off for him and devastating to her. Painful though such a conversation may be, try to get him to articulate the possible "whys" behind such feelings. Is he afraid you'll never lose the weight? Is he worried about what life will be like with a baby in the house? Serious problems of this nature, while rare, may benefit from counseling.

• *He's very attracted.* The most common scenario, fortunately, is that dads-to-be *like* the changes they see in their mates. In fact, studies have shown that pregnant women notoriously underestimate how attractive their men find them, maybe because women are so programmed to be insecure about their looks even when they love being pregnant. Her alluring new endowments, her renewed arousal, his primitive masculine pride at having brought forth life, and their charged excitement about the forthcoming baby—all can combine to make sex as good as ever. If you're doubtful, just ask. He'll probably be glad to make it clear how he really feels.

MOTHER TO MOTHER:
"Pregnant Sex Was Great"

Wanda LaGrave, 32
Hobbs, New Mexico

In the first trimester of each of her three pregnancies, nausea left Wanda feeling like she was in a "daze." After it lifted, though, "everything you do is intense, just like at first you're too busy throwing up, but after that you enjoy eating everything," she says. Her attitude toward sex proved no exception.

Physical changes she felt in the second trimester—heightened responsiveness and a "primal urge" fueled by surging hormones—were accompanied by aroused emotions. "You are so proud that you're bearing life," she explains. "I'm normally overweight, but when I'm pregnant it doesn't matter. I feel like I'm full and bursting with life. Being naked and pregnant is very liberating."

Sex also proved relaxing. "The closeness and release of sexual tension is a natural high," she notes. Still, conflicting schedules (and, in her later pregnancies, the presence of older kids) meant that "how often I indulged was a lot less than I felt like." And by her third trimester, her bulky middle required a lot of creative positioning. Overall, though, she and her husband remember these months as a very erotic time: "Pregnancy makes you appreciate being a woman. That's what it's all about."

Wanda's tips for enjoying your sexuality in pregnancy:

• *Don't be afraid that your partner will find you unattractive.* "A pregnant woman is very sensuous. Really look at your body and see how beautiful it is. Beauty is found in its curves, dips, and valleys."

• *Buy French-cut maternity panties.* "They let you feel sexy because they make your legs look longer."

• *Take bubble baths.* "I took them all the time. It was very sensual."

• *Be creative.* "Sex doesn't have to be in the bed. If you're someplace else and it's private, why not?"

IS IT TRUE...

That orgasms are stronger during pregnancy? Sometimes. Increased blood flow to the breasts, vagina, and clitoris tend to cause pregnant women to achieve orgasm more quickly or intensely. On the other hand, this engorgement can also feel uncomfortable, inhibiting responsiveness or stranding a woman at a point where she's aroused but unable to climax.

That oral sex in pregnancy can kill you? Cunnilingus is perfectly safe now, with one exception. Care must be taken not to blow air into the vagina, which could cause a life-threatening air bubble in the bloodstream (called an *air embolism*).

Special Situations

Gestational Diabetes

Fewer than 3 percent of mothers-to-be develop a form of diabetes unique to pregnancy. In any kind of diabetes, the body fails to efficiently produce or process insulin, a hormone produced by the pancreas that lets the body turn glucose, or sugar, into usable fuel. During pregnancy, the mother must produce extra insulin to meet her fetus's growing energy needs (especially from mid-pregnancy on). At the same time, hormonal changes can interfere with the way she processes insulin, sometimes causing her blood-sugar levels to rise too high. Fortunately, this can be detected in a glucose screening test. Usually there are no warning symptoms, though you may experience extreme thirst or fatigue.

The risk to the baby is that it receives too much sugar and produces its own extra insulin to process the sugar, which is stored as fat. This can lead to a baby with a larger than normal birthweight (a condition called *macrosomia*). While most big babies can be delivered vaginally with no problems, there is an increased risk of a traumatic delivery or a Cesarean delivery.

If gestational diabetes is diagnosed, you'll probably be referred to a dietitian, who can screen your current eating habits and suggest changes based on your weight and your stage of pregnancy. Preapproved exercise can help further control blood-sugar levels. You'll also be checked once a week or more to verify that the levels are stabilizing. If not—which is the case about 10 percent of the time—they require insulin injections. The shots do not adversely affect the fetus. You'll be instructed how to do this (usually at least twice a day) and how to monitor your own blood-sugar levels throughout the day with a home glucose meter or strips. Your unborn baby's size and heart rate will be monitored as well. You'll also be checked postpartum. In most cases, gestational diabetes disappears after delivery, although your risk of developing diabetes later in life is increased.

Preterm Labor

Ten percent of all births in the United States occur earlier than the usual 37- to 42-week window. When labor begins after 20 weeks and before the 37th week, it's called *preterm*. Not all preterm labors lead to immediate delivery. The longer birth can be postponed, the better a baby's odds of good health, since growth is so critical from mid-pregnancy on. (A baby born preterm is called premature, hence the term "preemie.")

The cause of preterm labor isn't known, though getting good prenatal care and not smoking definitely reduce your odds. What happens is that the uterus begins to contract and the cervix starts to thin (*efface*) and open (*dilate*) in readiness for the fetal exit through the birth canal. Unlike a full-term delivery, though, this occurs before the baby is fully mature. It can happen to anyone. Common risk factors, though, include a history of preterm labor, carrying more than one fetus, uterine problems such as fibroids, second-trimester bleeding, placenta problems, excess amniotic fluid, and birth defects.

Early detection of the problem is critical, though the symptoms are not always obvious. Even more confusing, many of the symptoms of preterm labor can occur for other reasons. Nonetheless, warning signs to report to your doctor include:

- Unusual vaginal discharge (any changes in color, texture, or quantity)
- Mild cramping
- A constant backache
- Pelvic or abdominal pressure
- Regular contractions (not always painful)

Note: The uterus contracts mildly from the third month on. Later, using your hands, you will be able to feel your midsection firm up. It's usually painless, though you may feel a slight discomfort later in pregnancy. These "practice" contractions, called *Braxton-Hicks contractions*, ready your body for delivery and do not signal preterm labor. But if you begin to feel them in the second trimester, even without any other warning sign of preterm labor, monitor their length and frequency and inform your practitioner.

Your doctor will examine your cervix for any suspicious changes. If it's still tightly closed, you are probably not experiencing preterm labor. If your cervix is thinning or opening, you may be examined by ultrasound and your baby's heart rate will be monitored. If the diagnosis is made early and neither you nor your baby are in any immediate danger, your labor can be halted through a combination of bedrest, hydration (by drinking eight to ten or more glasses of water a day or via IV), and drugs called tocolytics, which are delivered by mouth, injection, or IV to stop uterine contractions.

Late Bleeding

Bleeding in mid- to late pregnancy is cause for concern because it is much less common than during the first trimester. Always contact your caregiver immediately. Often the cause is a minor inflammation of the cervix and not a sign of trouble.

Vaginal bleeding can also signal one rare, but dangerous form of miscarriage called *incompetent cervix*. What happens is that the cervix dilates very prematurely and with little advance warning, usually in the fourth month. This causes the entire amniotic sac with the fetus to pull down and rupture. The first sign is a leakage of amniotic fluid and discharge of the mucus plug, which sealed the cervix from infection. The woman may notice the plug itself, a mass of mucusy tissue tinged with blood, or there may simply be heavy bleeding. By the time this happens, though, miscarriage is inevitable. The root cause is unknown, although the condition has been associated with an earlier trauma to the cervix,

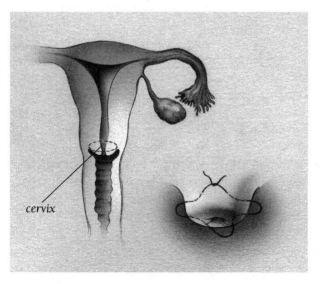

cervix

A cervical cerclage—surgical stitching to close the cervix—is used to prevent premature delivery.

such as after surgery, an abortion, or a complication in a previous delivery.

Losing a baby because of an incompetent cervix can be devastating, especially because it happens with little forewarning. The silver lining is that in future pregnancies, the cervix can be sutured closed until around 36 weeks, a procedure called *cervical cerclage*, almost always ensuring that the tragedy won't repeat itself. The stitching can be likened to pulling a drawstring tight around the opening of a pouch (the uterus). The cerclage is released when the pregnancy is full term, allowing labor to begin. Also, modified bedrest is frequently urged for future pregnancies.

Bedrest

As many as 20 percent of expectant mothers are given the vague prescription "bedrest" as a precaution against premature labor, preeclampsia, unexplained bleeding, or other complications of pregnancy. Whether your visit to "Club Bed" lasts a few days or a few months, get clarification on exactly what your physician expects. Since your partner is apt to do most of the household work and care for you, too, it's a good idea for him to accompany you to a doctor visit to discuss the treatment. Ask:

• *Should I rest in a special position?* You may be told to lie down periodically throughout the day or may be forbidden to get up at all. Though you should not lie flat on your back, you may be told to favor one side, or that it's okay to prop yourself upright with pillows.

• *How often can I use the bathroom, or get up to cook or eat? What about bathing or showers?* Restrictions can vary. The extreme is to be confined 24 hours a day, with bedpans. Most women are able to rise briefly to shower or use the bathroom. Keep a cooler stocked with water, juice, and refreshments at your bedside so you won't need to get up more than is absolutely necessary.

• *Can I work?* If so, for how long during the day? In bed only or not? Can I prop myself in front of a computer (or set it up at bedside)? If work is okay, rearrange the room to give you easy access to a phone and a workspace from bed; a lapdesk or bed tray are handy.

• *Can I exercise?* Sometimes stretches, relaxation techniques, Kegels, or pelvic tilts are permissible. Ask first! At the very least, wiggling your fingers and toes aids circulation.

• *How much can I take care of my children?* Remind your doctor about older kids when you discuss your case. You may be able to perform basic childcare, except for lifting them. Or you may need to bring in household help. Ask friends to wash or sort laundry, take the older child on outings or to school, bring food, or make library runs. Set up a special table in your bedroom where your child can eat with you and play.

MOTHER TO MOTHER:
"Sentenced to Bedrest"

Jennifer Davids, 29
Jersey City, New Jersey

At 27 weeks into her pregnancy with twins, Jennifer awoke with pain in her uterus and down her legs. When the sensation persisted, her doctor monitored her for contractions. She was having them every 3 or 4 minutes, though they were slight enough to feel more like menstrual cramps to Jennifer. After a week of medication and bedrest to quell the contractions, they eased except when she'd get up. The recommendation: back to bed for the duration.

"I cried when I heard that," Jennifer says. "I didn't want to be helpless and confined." First she went into denial, since she basically felt fine. *Maybe it's a mistake,* she reasoned. When reassured that it wasn't, adjustment took a while. "At first I just sat and watched the wall and completely brainless TV shows. I hadn't made any preparations for the babies yet and couldn't do the things I'd planned."

Finally it hit home that the twins' health was at stake. She resolved to make the best of the situation and dug out her long-postponed work on a graduate-school dissertation. She began to balance her checkbook and pay bills from bed, and her husband took over all the cooking, cleaning, and shopping. "He yelled at me if I tried to do anything like get a glass of water. It was nice to know I could rely on him," she says.

Jennifer's tips on making bedrest better:

• *Set a schedule because it offers a sense of control.* "I'd get up at 8 A.M., watch the *Today* show, shower, and eat breakfast. Then I'd work for 3 hours on my dissertation, eat lunch, and watch *Oprah.* I'd also go on the Internet for an hour, where I found other moms in the same situation."

• *Keep in contact with the outside world.* "Write letters, call people, go on-line. Shop for baby things by catalog."

• *Accept—without guilt—that you need help.* "My mom came to stay for a week and my friends brought me dinners."

• *Find out if you can exercise, and resist the temptation to gorge out of boredom.* "I'd move my feet in circles and do leg stretches, and was also allowed to move around the apartment a little bit every day."

• *Be easy on yourself.* "Don't feel pressured to accomplish some great tasks. People think, in this hectic life, it would be great to be put to bed to read *War and Peace*, but the main point, after all, is to rest. Do whatever you need to do to pass the time—even if it isn't intellectually stimulating."

Work Worries

Planning Childcare

You can hardly imagine birth yet, much less the end of your maternity leave several weeks or months later. Still, it's not too early to begin thinking about who will take care of your baby if you plan to return to your job. Ask neighbors and coworkers for recommendations and begin investigating the possibilities. (See "Which Type of Childcare?" page 148.)

Clearly, the pros and cons of each type of care are highly subjective. Your schedule, budget, work locale, and community options will all influence your plans. Before you decide, make at least two visits to a provider: one prearranged, so you can observe and also talk to the director, and one unannounced. Check out the toddler and preschool programs, too, as time will pass quickly. Additional considerations include:

• **Where is the care located?** A site near your home will make drop-off and pick-up convenient, but one near your workplace may enable you to visit more easily during the day and get there quickly in case of emergency. If you're considering an individual provider, will she come to your home or care for the child in hers? (In the latter event, do you need to provide extra equipment, such as a crib, high chair, or car seat?)

• **What is the caregiver like?** What is her experience and training? How does she handle crying, illness, or discipline? What do references say about her? Most of all, do you like her?

• **What is the child-caregiver ratio like?** In group situations, there should ideally be four or fewer infants per caregiver. While some age spread among the children can be stimulating for the kids, it might also be hard for one caregiver to adequately attend to a broad mix of infants, toddlers, and preschoolers. (Most centers segregate ages.)

• **What is the atmosphere like?** Are there interesting things to do? How would the caregiver entertain your child? Is there a schedule? A plan for sick children? Is the equipment safe, clean, and in good shape? Can the children go outdoors? Are meals provided?

Which Type of Childcare?

Try to let go of preconceived notions about different types of care, because wide variations exist within each. Your three basic options are these:

Group Care in a Childcare Center

Advantages: Open even when primary caregiver is sick; usually trained staff; usually wide range of activities and toys; must meet minimum safety standards. *Disadvantages:* Less individual attention; need backup care (or you must stay home) when child is ill; can be expensive; demand for quality programs exceeds supply. *Note:* Many centers have waiting lists for infant care, so it's not too early to apply; in some areas, you may want to get your name on several lists even before you've made a final decision. Centers meeting the highest standards are accredited by the National Association for the Education of Young Children.

Group Care in a Private Home (Family Daycare)

Advantages: Usually least expensive; hours may be more flexible than an institution's; may take sick children; typically homier atmosphere. *Disadvantages:* Caregiver usually has little formal training; turnover can be high; not always licensed or regulated; may lack backup care if caregiver is sick. *Note:* Amount of attention your child receives depends on the total number of kids and age mix; find out the anticipated enrollment when your baby will be there.

In-home Care (By a Nanny, Au Pair, or Relative)

Advantages: Inexpensive (if a relative); one-on-one attention; more flexibility in terms of hours and child illness; saves drop-off and pick-up time; exposure to fewer germs; nanny may do housework as well. *Disadvantages:* Expensive (if a nanny or au pair, unless more than one child); need backup care when caregiver is ill; high turnover—you may be in the lurch if caregiver quits suddenly; as employer, you must deal with salary and taxes; loss of some privacy if caregiver lives in; toddlers and preschoolers may lack group interaction. *Note:* You may not be able to line up a caregiver until after you've delivered, as few of them make plans so far in advance. You can register early with placement agencies, though.

For More Help: Childcare Resources

- Child Care Aware, 2116 Campus Drive SE, Rochester, MN 55904; 800-424-2246. Can direct you to referral agencies and help evaluate forms of care.
- American Council of Nanny Schools, Delta College, University Center, MI 48710; 517-686-9074. For a list of places that train nannies.
- National Association for the Education of Young Children, 1509 16th Street NW, Washington, DC 20036; 800-424-2460 or http://www.naeyc.org/naeyc. Publishes a booklet on choosing an early-childhood program.
- Child Care Aware Resource Referral Line. 2116 Campus Drive SE, Rochester, MN 55904; 800-424-2246.

Checklist: Smart Snacks to Stash at Your Desk

Snacking wards off hunger and is easier on your digestive system than three big squares a day. Pack yourself a workplace survival kit containing simple, nutritious noshes like these:

- ☐ Bottled water or juice boxes (if you don't have easy access to a dispenser)
- ☐ Pregnancy trail mix: almonds, unsalted pumpkin or sunflower seeds, peanuts, raisins, diced apricots
- ☐ Fresh apples, bananas, or grapes
- ☐ Crudités (carrot and celery sticks, raw broccoli)
- ☐ Cold cereal that can be munched without a spoon (like bite-size Shredded Wheat)
- ☐ Granola bars (but note that some brands contain much more sugar and fat than others)
- ☐ Saltines or graham crackers
- ☐ Peanut butter

I'm on my feet a lot? Standing still for long periods can cause circulatory problems and has been linked to preterm labor. Ask your employer about modifying the length of time you must stand, using a stool to sit on and taking frequent breaks, or even switching to a less taxing job. Get a doctor's note to verify your need. If your work interferes with your health, you may qualify for disability insurance. Jobs that keep you on your feet but walking aren't necessarily bad if you can incorporate rest periods or sit down once or twice an hour.

I'm being discriminated against because of my pregnancy? Numerous federal and state laws safeguard against firing, demoting, or failing to promote a worker just because she's pregnant; denying her normal sick leave, disability, or health insurance benefits; and refusing to reinstate her to her same job or a comparable one at equal pay if she has taken an allowable maternity leave. But infractions—both blatant and subtle—abound. It's smart to make copies of all your performance records and to document other positive feedback as well as discriminatory comments or actions you experience. The Civil Rights Act of 1991 ruled that pregnant women can sue for compensation for such discriminatory practices. Contact the Equal Employment Opportunity Commission (EEOC) at 800-669-4000 (you'll be connected to a local office) or see "FOR MORE HELP: Work/Family Resources," page 199.

Other Big Deals

Finding Out: Boy or Girl?

Thanks to the miracles of modern technology, "Do you know what it is?" has become the number-two question pregnant women are asked, after "When are you due?" But should you find out your baby's sex?

Here are reasons parents want to know:

- You can set up a gender-specific nursery.
- You can begin buying appropriate baby clothes.
- You only have to select one name.
- You have something else to talk about during your pregnancy.
- You can prepare older siblings.
- You can bond more concretely with the unborn baby.
- Why not? Learning the sex is no different from learning about the expected size or health problems.

Here are reasons parents *don't* want to know:

- It's like reading ahead to the last page of the novel.
- It's meddling in one of life's great mysteries.
- People will give you more functional shower gifts than boy's or girl's clothing.
- You get to pick two names.
- You have something else to muse and fantasize about during your pregnancy.
- In the event something goes wrong, knowing makes the unborn child seem *too* real.
- Ultrasound sex diagnosis can be wrong!

Whether you find out the gender now or on your baby's birthday, you may grapple with letdown if your imaginary or long-sought "he" proves to be a "she" (or vice-versa). A certain amount of regret, even grieving, is normal. But most parents get so caught up in their newborn's individuality that close-held fantasies about gender tend to fade away.

Choosing a Childbirth Class

It's best to start a childbirth-preparation class before the second trimester ends, since many classes meet over 6 to 12 weeks. Why take one at all? The purpose of a childbirth class is to better understand and prepare for what you'll be experiencing, so you can respond accordingly. Preparation won't provide a painless delivery. But it has been shown to ease pain, enhance relaxation, and lead to better overall feelings about birth. Even if your heart is set on painkilling medication, a class can help you be an active rather than passive or helpless participant, which can only improve the experience.

Not all instruction is alike, however. Different methods of pain management are taught, and instructors' experience, teaching styles, and general approaches to labor and delivery vary. Start by thinking about what kind of birth experience you want: Where do you plan to have the baby? How much control would you like? How fearful are you? Ask friends and your doctor for their input on educators. Hospitals and maternity centers, HMOs, and independent instructors all offer courses. Then consider interviewing several teachers the way you would a new doctor or a home contractor. Sit in on a class. One red flag: soft peddling. If the instructor refers to labor pain as "discomfort," look elsewhere. Another caveat is to consider hospital-run courses carefully; they tend to tout the procedures that are routine to that particular institution (so if continuous fetal monitoring is de rigueur there, you may never hear about other options).

The method you select depends on the amount of control you want and on

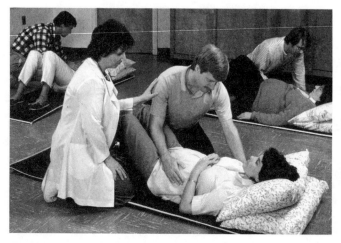

Childbirth classes give couples a chance to work toward a common goal—the birth of a healthy baby.

your philosophy about birth. Most cover the anatomy of birth, birthing positions, and a blend of relaxation techniques. Prenatal nutrition, breastfeeding, and postpartum care may also be discussed. Those classes that meet over a period of weeks (up to 10 or 12) may seem inconvenient, but they allow you to better practice and remember what you learn. All-day workshops cram a lot in and may overwhelm you, leaving you less well prepared. If you must go this route, schedule an all-day class for your late seventh or early eighth month. Six to eight couples is an ideal class size, providing you more individualized attention than larger groups can. The main methods taught include:

• **Lamaze.** The goal of the most widely used method is to avoid unnecessary medical or technological intervention during childbirth, though most courses include a thorough overview of anesthesia, pain relief, and hospital routines. A host of relaxation methods are introduced, including visualization, guided imagery, massage, and verbal coaching from partners. The centerpiece of Lamaze's mind-over-matter approach is patterned breathing exercises that, taught to become a conditioned response during the various stages of labor, help the mother feel a crucial sense of control over her contractions. Be aware that the term "Lamaze" is bandied about generically these days; for the real McCoy, look for a teacher who is certified by the American Society for Psychoprophylaxis in Obstetrics (ASPO/Lamaze) and who uses the initials ACCE (*ASPO-certified childbirth educator*) after her name.

• **The Bradley Method (husband-coached childbirth).** The aim here is to view birth as a natural process requiring no drugs, with the partner involved as coach. The emphasis is on both parents working together to actively ride through the pain (rather than control it). This is done through guided visualization, open-mouthed abdominal breathing, extensive coach training, and much outside reading. Unlike in most classes, you won't hear much about epidurals or painkillers. The classes, which meet over 12 weeks, are taught usually by couples who used the method. Bradley is a good option if you're sure you want to try natural childbirth, or if you're planning to deliver at a maternity center that provides no epidurals.

• *ICEA (International Childbirth Education Association).* Unlike Lamaze or Bradley, ICEA classes refer not to a single approach but to a host of them. The well-respected institute certifies its own instructors, but individual teaching methods and materials vary. Usually mothers-to-be are exposed to a range of strategies (medicated and nonmedicated) for working through the pain and avoiding panic.

Taking Other Classes

While you're checking out childbirth education, you may come across these other valuable options:

• *Hospital tours.* If this isn't a feature of your childbirth prep course, sign up for a tour of the facility where you'll deliver. Firsthand familiarity with where to park and check in, the labor/delivery rooms, nursery, and neonatal intensive-care unit will boost your comfort level on your labor day. Check-in procedures and policies on visitation and other matters are covered, too. Make a tour in your second trimester, if you haven't already. You want to be sure you're comfortable with the types of procedures standard there (such as whether you'll be monitored continuously or must have an IV) and have time to make a change if not.

• *Breastfeeding classes.* If you're planning on nursing, these courses (usually one session) provide invaluable advice about what to expect, common problems and solutions, equipment (pumps, pads, and so on), and other tips for successful breastfeeding. They're usually taught by lactation consultants or childbirth educators. You may also want to discuss preparation for breastfeeding with your obstetrician or pediatrician (if you've selected one).

• *Newborn care classes.* Not every new mom (or dad) comes with experience in diapering, bathing, dressing, and looking after a fresh-born baby. Practical skills and healthcare tips are usually reviewed. These classes are fun to take together in the last trimester.

• **Sibling preparation classes.** If you have a preschooler or older child, these can make the abstract baby-to-be seem more real. Usually run by hospitals, they incorporate stories and demonstrations with hands-on doll care and feature a visit to the nursery. (Some courses also target toddlers, but don't get your hopes up about how much a very young child will understand or retain.)

For More Help: Prepared Childbirth Resources

Each of the following can provide printed materials or referrals.

• American Society for Psychoprophylaxis in Obstetrics/Lamaze, 1200 Nineteenth Street NW, Suite 300, Washington, DC 20036; 800-368-4404 or http://www.lamaze-childbirth.com.
• The Bradley Method, Box 5224, Sherman Oaks, CA 91413-5224; 800-423-2397 or http://www.bradleybirth.com.
• International Childbirth Education Association, P.O. Box 20048, Minneapolis, MN 55420; 612-854-8660 or http://www.icea.org.

Going Out and About

Thinking about a last fling alone together? Wondering if a business trip will be okay? The second trimester is prime for traveling, since the rate of complications is lowest and your mood is highest. Unless you're in a high-risk pregnancy, have a chronic or pregnancy-caused illness, or have experienced problems (such as bleeding), you won't need your doctor's blessing to take off. However, do check before long trips and prior to all trips after 34 weeks to be sure there are no signs of labor. Most doctors prefer that their patients stick close to home by the eighth month. Jostling in a car, train, or subway may be less comfortable than usual but won't harm the baby.

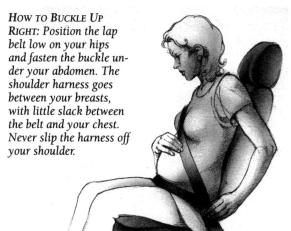

HOW TO BUCKLE UP RIGHT: Position the lap belt low on your hips and fasten the buckle under your abdomen. The shoulder harness goes between your breasts, with little slack between the belt and your chest. Never slip the harness off your shoulder.

For a better trip:

• *Keep moving.* Wherever you go, and however you get there, remember to take frequent walking and stretching breaks, including while you're in transit. Relieve leg cramps—and your bladder—every hour or two.

• *Practice care with airbags.* Statistics show that the risk of injury or death in an accident is vastly greater when an adult driver or passenger is *not* protected by an airbag, which is programmed to open at a sudden stop or collision. You can lessen the full impact of inflation by tilting the steering wheel up, away from your abdomen, and pushing the seat back as far as possible. (The gas in the airbags is harmless.)

• *Pack your papers.* If you're traveling far from home, bring a copy of your medical records, which your doctor can furnish. He or she may also be able to recommend reputable physicians or hospitals at your destination, just in case.

• *Take special care by air.* Most air travel is perfectly safe, including small unpressurized aircraft used by private flights or short-distance commuter airlines. (Some doctors warn that changes in oxygen levels in unpressurized cabins could compromise the fetus's health, but no studies confirm this.) In any aircraft, you should drink more than usual amounts of water—one glass per half hour—to ward off dehydration. Eat lightly so you won't get nauseous, but skip the salty peanuts and request low-salt meals when you book your flight. For convenience and comfort, go for an aisle bulkhead seat. *Note:* Check airline regulations regarding late-pregnancy travel; some won't let you board after the eighth or ninth month and may require a doctor's verification of how far along you are.

• *Cruise with caution.* Motion sickness aboard a ship may bring back memories of your just-finished morning sickness, so veteran cruisers tend to do better than first-timers. Ask your doctor in advance about over-the-counter remedies. (Most are recommended for only short-term use.) Lack of medical care is a potential hazard to cruising, though most ships have a doctor on board. Like airlines, many cruise lines prohibit passengers late in pregnancy (some as early as the sixth month).

Readying the Nursery

There's more to nursery planning than selecting a decorating theme. Here's how to furnish your baby's space with both flair and care:

• *Crib.* New cribs must meet federal safety requirements, but don't rule out family heirlooms and garage-sale finds. Just make sure that slats or bars are no more than 2³/₈ inches apart, and that there are no cutouts in the headboard or footboard or corner posts on which clothing could get snagged. If you're unsure whether the paint contains lead, as pre-1978 cribs may, have someone else strip and repaint it. Position the crib away from windows, heating elements, lamps, cords, and wall decorations. Invest in a firm mattress and snug-fitting crib bumpers (with ties shorter than 6 inches long). Don't use sheepskin coverlets, crib-size futons, waterbeds, thick comforters, or pillows, which can suffocate a baby.

• *Mobiles.* Choose the kind where the images face the baby (you'd be surprised how many look good to adults but not to the little fella lying on his back in the crib). Mobiles with replaceable toys or music add interest. Black and white or bright colors are best for newborns and young infants. Consider a second mobile for the changing table.

• *Changing table.* Whether you choose the type with drawers or open shelves, place all necessary toiletries (diapers, ointments) within immediate reach so you won't have to step away from the baby for a second. Put a diaper container (with a tight-fitting top) nearby, too. A terry-cloth–covered foam liner pad atop the table adds comfort and security (but don't cover the safety strap). High sides are another plus.

• *Dresser.* Select a model that can't tip over, ideally with rounded (not sharp) corners and gliding drawers that a preschooler will be able to open himself later.

• *Chair.* A comfy rocker will make middle-of-the-night feedings easier and provide a cozy spot for bedtime stories as your baby grows. Worth the splurge are glider styles, which are designed for nursing moms. A footstool lets you put up your feet, smart for breastfeeding.

• *Lighting.* Skip floor lamps, which could tip over. Smaller nursery lights provide soothing diffuse illumination; place on a high shelf or dresser with the cord out of reach. Consider a dimmer switch for overhead lights. A low-wattage crib light, which attaches to the crib or changing table, is helpful for the early weeks (but should be removed from a crib once the baby can pull up). Install electrical outlet safety plugs now and you won't have to remember to do it in a few months, when your baby starts to crawl.

• **Windows.** Choose blinds, shutters, short curtains, or valances instead of long drapes, which could be pulled down. Avoid window treatments with cords, which pose a strangulation risk, or encase the cords in childproof cord wraps. Window screens should lock. If you use blinds, note that many plastic and vinyl types made before 1997 contain lead, which can be dangerous to a child under 6 if the blind or even dust on it is mouthed. Look for blinds cartons labeled "nonleaded formula" or "no lead added."

• **Flooring.** Your call. Wall-to-wall carpeting is cozy, though you should be aware that some new carpets are treated with high levels of chemicals. Some synthetic carpeting has been linked to seizures in infants and children, who typically spend more time in close contact with carpets than adults. Natural fibers (such as woven wool) are safer, particularly without glued-on backings. Wood or vinyl floors are easy to clean. Be sure throw rugs have nonslip backing.

IS IT TRUE...

That you can teach your baby in utero? It's true that the fetus can hear, taste, smell, and even sense light in utero. What's more, memory may be at work—in one famous study, women read Dr. Seuss's *The Cat in the Hat* repeatedly to their unborn children, who showed a preference for that story over another within hours of birth. How long these impressions are retained, however, is another matter.

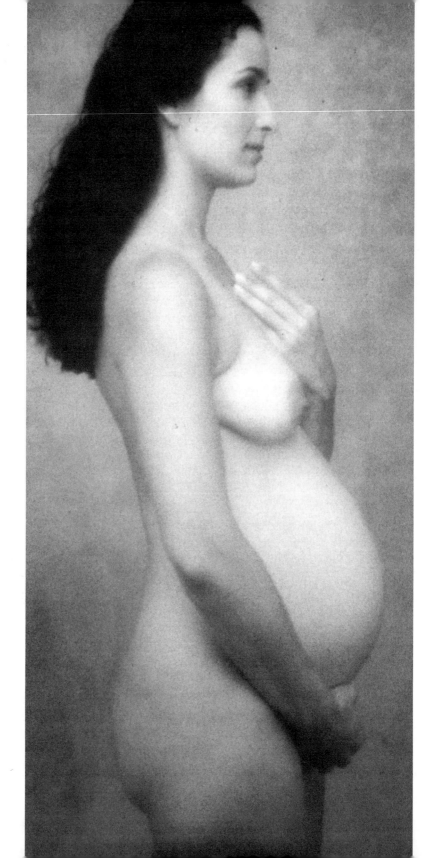

CHAPTER 3

YOUR THIRD TRIMESTER

TWENTY-NINE TO FORTY WEEKS

A strange mix of revved-up excitement and plodding fatigue marks the final span of pregnancy. Time seems to pass both very quickly and unbearably slowly. As your midsection grows ever bulkier, daily activities become more challenging. It takes careful maneuvering to rise from your chair, squeeze behind the steering wheel, or even roll over in your sleep. You find yourself bumping into doorways or other people, unaware of your body's new boundaries. And thanks to that new silhouette—along with stretch marks, wider feet, and a wide-open navel—your old, pre-pregnancy body can seem like a fond, fuzzy memory. You're getting tired of your maternity clothes, tired of everyone asking how you're doing. You feel like you've been pregnant forever.

At the same time, your undeniable size serves as a delicious reminder that your baby will be here sooner, rather than later. You may suddenly feel like you haven't got *enough* weeks left for baby-readying tasks like finding a pediatrician, selecting birth announcements, attending showers (and writing thank-you notes), and folding the tiny pieces of your new layette and placing them in their freshly lined drawers. Labor looms nearer, the final hurdle between you and new motherhood. You worry, *How will I know when it's really time? What will it be like?*

The last-trimester homestretch is a time of wondering, waiting—and waiting some more.

Week-by-Week Highlights

From now on, growth in both the mother and the baby is less predictable and more variable than in the early months. Here's what's ahead in the third trimester:

Week 29: The fetus is not quite 12 inches long and weighs between 2 and 3 pounds—and will double or triple in size between now and birth. As space gets

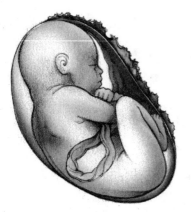

Month 7: Growth is rapid this month. The eyes can now open and shut. The bones begin to harden, and the fetus kicks and stretches to exercise its limbs.

Size: *15 inches long*
Weight: *3 pounds*

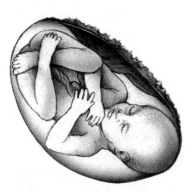

Month 8: The uterus is becoming crowded, and there's little room to move around. But you will still feel plenty of kicks. Soon the fetus should settle into a head-down position in preparation for birth.

Size: *18 inches long*
Weight: *5 pounds*

tighter in its amniotic waterbed, less acrobatic tumbling takes place, though you'll still feel plenty of stretching and kicking.

Week 30: The fetus has eyelashes and the head of hair he or she will be born with (if any). This hair may fall out a few months after delivery, however, and grow back in an entirely different texture or color.

Week 31: Though the scenery in the womb sure isn't Paris or the Grand Canyon, the fetus can see in utero—discerning light and dark, and blinking or shutting the eyes. Take care of pre-baby decisions while you can: write your birth plan (an outline of what you would ideally like to take place during your delivery), interview pediatricians, and preregister at the hospital if you haven't yet.

Week 32: A layer of fatty padding is being laid down beneath the thin, wrinkly fetal skin. Review your childbirth class notes and don't forget to keep practicing breathing and relaxation exercises. A glucose screen may be repeated around 32 to 34 weeks.

Week 33: The fetus is exercising its lungs by practicing breathing—inhaling amniotic fluid. You're gaining a pound a week now; roughly half of that goes right to the fetus. In fact, the baby gains more than half its birthweight during the next 7 weeks, fattening up for survival outside the womb. Thanks to these fatty deposits, the skin grows plumper and pinker.

Week 34: Most babies settle into the head-down position, although it may not be final. The skull bones are still quite pliable and not completely joined, to ease the exit through the relatively narrow birth canal. Pack your hospital bag now—better to be early than to be sorry to have forgotten something in a last-minute scramble.

Week 35: Your doctor will probably check you weekly until you deliver. You'll be tested for Group B *Streptococcus* bacteria between weeks 35 and 37. Ninety-nine percent of babies born now survive, the overwhelming majority with no major problems. Not only are the lungs more developed but, thanks to advances in neonatal care, respiratory problems—once a leading killer in preemies before 35 weeks—are much more readily overcome.

Week 36: Your uterus has expanded to 1,000 times its original volume, and now reaches up to the base of your rib cage. The baby may drop lower in your abdomen, the head engaging with the circle of pelvic bones at the birth canal. Don't let your friends hold your shower too late; you're almost in the due-date zone.

Week 37: By the end of this week, your pregnancy has come full term; the baby could be born any day now. More good news: your weight gain will probably hit its zenith.

Week 38: Most of the fetus's downy coating of hair (lanugo) and cheeselike skin coating (vernix) have disappeared. (Some may remain at birth.) They get swallowed by the fetus along with other secretions and lodge in the baby's bowels—where they'll become the child's first BM, a tarry waste called *meconium*.

Week 39: The average full-term newborn weighs 7 to 7 1/2 pounds. On average, boys tend to be slightly heavier than girls. Take it very easy now; if you aren't inclined to do much, don't.

Week 40: Can't be long now! Don't fret if your baby isn't born by your due date—just 5 percent hit the mark exactly. Most doctors wait another 2 weeks before considering a pregnancy overdue.

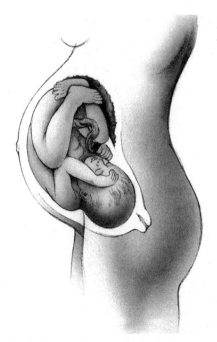

Month 9: In the last month, the fetus gains about half a pound a week. By the last week of pregnancy, it is fully mature and completely fills the inside of your uterus.

Size: *20 inches long*
Weight: *6 to 9 pounds*

What's Going on in Your Body

Preparing for the Big Day

By now you may have detected a pattern to your baby's movements, as he or she settles into a predictable sleep-wake cycle. Sharp jabs and slow grinding rolls replace gentle flutters. Any movement is reassuring, of course. Another way to check on your baby's well-being as your due date approaches is to do a *fetal kick test*. At the same time every day—first thing in the morning, after a meal, or right before bedtime work well—count the number of movements you notice over a given time period. Then compare the movements from day to day. Your doctor may suggest how many minutes to monitor (usually 5); call if you have any doubts or questions about your baby's movement. (If at any point you feel fewer than ten movements in an hour, call your healthcare provider.)

Toward the end of the last trimester, your body gradually gears up for its dramatic denouement, labor. You may notice *Braxton-Hicks contractions*, a tightening of the uterus that can last from 30 seconds to 2 minutes, as the uterine muscles rehearse the squeezes that they will eventually use to push the baby out. Though generally painless, they can be slightly uncomfortable. Shifting your position often makes them disappear. Unlike real labor, these involuntary practice contractions are not strong enough to do anything more than help thin your cervix. Some women notice them for weeks; others not until labor is about to begin or not at all.

Sometime in the last month (usually between 36 and 38 weeks for first-

How Does Your Baby Lie?
The position of the baby in the womb is called its "lie." To determine it, your doctor or midwife will use one or more methods, including observation of your shape; how the baby feels from the outside; where the fetal activity and heart tones are located; and ultrasound. Possible presentation include:

Vertex (head down): By the time they engage in the birth canal, more than 95 percent of babies have assumed this position because the head, which is the heaviest part of the fetus's body, naturally shifts downward. It's the best lie for a vaginal delivery because the widest part of the baby, the head, is to be born first. Almost always, the crown of the head is nearest the cervix (and therefore delivered first). But sometimes the presenting part can be a forehead, chin, or part of the face. In those cases, the baby may be turned manually or delivered by Cesarean, as such labor can be slow. This also minimizes bruising and swelling of the baby's face.

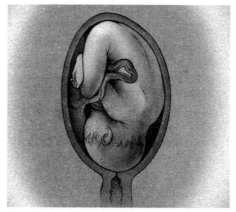

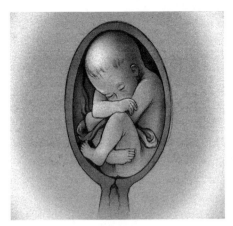

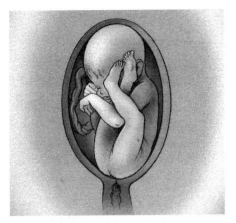

Complete breech: Breech babies are sitting head up with the feet facing down. Unless the body can be turned externally by a doctor, the baby is usually delivered by C-section.

Frank breech: When the body is folded into a V-shape, the buttocks would greet the world first. The legs are straight up with the toes up near the face. Such babies tend to be delivered by C-section.

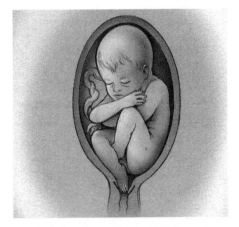

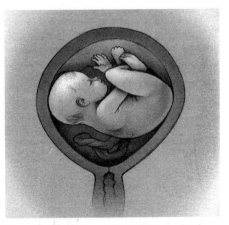

Footling breech: The baby is head up, like a complete breech, but one leg is bent and the other leg, or just a foot, dangles next to the cervix. If delivered vaginally, the foot would appear first and doesn't provide as strong a wedge to lead the rest of the body out (as the head does in a vertex lie), prolonging labor. Footling breeches are delivered by C-section.

Transverse (horizontal): A baby in this lie must be delivered by Cesarean if the body can't be manually turned by a doctor before labor has begun.

timers), the baby will drop noticeably lower in the abdomen, as he or she settles into position for birth, an event called *lightening* or *engagement.* As a result, you'll suddenly find it easier to breathe and eat—but walking around may feel less comfortable as the weight of the baby bumps against your cervix. Your outward profile changes, too, and people may comment that you're "carrying lower." But don't worry if you never detect the baby drop; this sometimes doesn't happen until labor has begun, especially in second-time mothers.

Just before labor starts, your cervix will soften and thin, or *efface*. Your cervix may also begin to open, or *dilate*. It will open to a width of 10 centimeters, or about 4 inches, before the baby is delivered. Sometimes the thick protective mucus plug that has been blocking the cervix for the past 9 months is expelled through your vagina, and the bag of waters, or amniotic sac, breaks before you're actually in labor. Because the risk of infection is increased after the sac ruptures, you should call your doctor immediately. (For more details, see "Is This It?" page 221.)

Common Aches and Pains

The rapid growth of the fetus in the last 3 months means less space for everything else within you—causing a host of less-than-pleasant reactions:

• **Backaches.** Back pain tends to worsen as the pregnancy progresses. That's because your natural posture has become more sway-backed to accommodate your big belly, as the musculature that normally supports a straight back loosens. Aches are generally located low along the spine, almost to the tailbone. Good posture (see page 185) and the pelvic tilt (see page 132) are the best remedies. Tucking a firm pillow behind your back when you sit helps, too. Especially in a woman at term, a persistent dull backache (often accompanied by cramps) may be a signal that labor is imminent.

• **Fatigue—and insomnia, too.** It's one of the irksome paradoxes of the third trimester that just when you need more rest than ever, you have a harder time getting it. Most women need 10 or more hours of sleep at night now, thanks to the sheer physical stresses of carrying a fetus. But you might find it hard to rest comfortably, and shifting positions can be a pain. So is getting up frequently to empty your bladder. Late in pregnancy, some women find it helpful to sleep in a recliner rather than a bed. It also helps now, more than ever, to cushion your belly and back with pillows. Catnap by day, if you can.

A commonly overlooked cause of fatigue is lack of exercise. Many women forgo their exercise routines in the last trimester as their size overwhelms them. But this is a mistake, since activity can actually make you feel better mentally and physically. The oxygen pumping through your bloodstream benefits the baby, too. Simplify workouts if you feel the need, but don't skip them.

• **Gastric reflux.** There's less room in your stomach than there used to be, since the uterus has pushed it from its customary position. As a result, stomach contents may back up your esophagus, leaving a bad taste in your mouth. The simplest solution is to eat less at each sitting, while grazing more frequently. In addition to being more generally healthful, lighter foods are less apt to irritate your stomach than richly sauced, creamed, or fried ones. Drinking a lot of water helps flush your system and can help prevent preterm contractions, too. If gastric reflux strikes most often at night (when lying flat further slows your digestive tract), avoid late snacks or meals. Try propping your head with extra pillows.

• **Frequent urination/stress incontinence.** As the weight of your uterus presses on your bladder, the need to frequently use the bathroom returns. A trick to emptying your bladder as completely as possible: tilt your pelvis back a bit as you sit on the toilet to ease some of the weight of your uterus off the bladder. Alternatively, you can gently lift your belly with your hands as you sit to help release all the urine.

You may also discover, to your dismay, some urine leaking when you sneeze, cough, laugh, or do certain kinds of physical activity. Called *stress incontinence*, it can occur anytime in pregnancy but is most common in the third trimester when the uterus exerts greatest pressure on the bladder. Your best defense: dutifully practice your Kegel exercises (see "GOOD ADVICE: Remember to Kegel," page 132), which strengthen the pelvic floor. Nearly two-thirds of pregnant women who try Kegels experience marked improvement in this condition, according to one study, and one-fifth are cured completely. In most women, mild urinary incontinence disappears within 6 months after delivery, as hormones return to normal and muscle tone improves. But left unchecked, the condition can worsen after pregnancy. In that event, your doctor may prescribe special pelvic inserts (to strengthen muscles), medication, or as a last resort, surgery. Don't be too embarrassed to bring up the problem with your doctor; the majority of cases are treated successfully.

• **Shortness of breath (dyspnea).** As your lungs and diaphragm are squeezed in the great organ shift taking place within you, you may find it more taxing to climb a flight of stairs or to walk a few blocks. Most women must modify their exercise routines to accommodate this change and take more frequent breaks. There's nothing else you can do about this side effect of late pregnancy than to live with it until the baby drops (which gives your lungs more room) or you deliver.

• *Round ligament pain.* Don't panic if you feel an occasional sharp pang across your abdomen that you're certain is neither a fetal kick nor a cramp. The muscles that support your uterus sometimes overstretch, usually when you're changing position, such as getting out of bed or a chair, producing a searing jab. The pain can last a few minutes or longer, but disappears within a day. Try rubbing the spot and resting. Call your doctor if you're worried or if the pain persists. Called round ligament pains, the name comes from the large muscles, called round ligaments, that connect your uterus and pelvis.

• *Swelling (edema).* Don't feel bad if you need to remove your wedding ring this trimester. Fluid retention increases now, including in the face and fingers but especially around the ankles and feet. (Some women transfer their rings to neck chains.) The problem can be worse in warm weather and late in the day. Part of the reason for swelling is the sheer amount of fluid circulating in your body in the form of added blood, amniotic fluid, and water. Your body and your baby need this fluid. It's why pregnant women are often thirsty. So don't allow yourself to become parched in a misguided effort to reduce swelling. The best remedy is moving around. Don't sit or stand for long periods. When you do sit, place your feet higher than your hips and don't cross your legs. If marked puffiness seems to appear overnight, alert your doctor—it may be a sign of preeclampsia.

• *Leaky breasts.* Some pregnant women release *colostrum,* a thick yellowish fluid that will nourish the newborn after delivery for a few days before the milk comes in. It can leak when your breasts are stimulated, or for no apparent reason. If this is a problem, tuck circular nursing pads in your bra to soak up the excess liquid. (Available at maternity stores and pharmacies, the pads come in disposable or washable types. Or cut up old T-shirts for the same purpose.)

IS IT TRUE...

That I should avoid baths in the last weeks? There's no medical reason to forgo the relaxation of the tub. Since you're less steady on your feet, though, be extra careful about slips and falls. And avoid extremely hot water. Exception: Don't bathe once your water has broken.

That boys are more active in the womb? Don't stereotype your baby before it's born! Both boys and girls kick and squirm with equal vigor in utero. You can't tell the baby's gender this way.

Checklist: When to Call Your Doctor

Alert your physician or midwife immediately if you:

☐ Notice a marked decrease in the baby's activity
☐ Have any bleeding or a discharge that's pink, red, or brown
☐ Leak fluid from the vagina
☐ Experience contractions every 5 to 10 minutes that are regular and rhythmic

MOTHER TO MOTHER:
"False Alarm!"

Laura Patyk, 29
Indian Trail, North Carolina

Laura's due date was January 10, which meant plenty of jokes in December about the possibility of a nick-of-time income tax deduction. Sure enough, on New Year's Eve, she began to have contractions. They seemed to increase in strength as the afternoon wore on, and by evening were 7 to 8 minutes apart. "They weren't painful, really," Laura recalls. "More of a tight pinching or stretching." At 11:00 P.M., when the contractions were 6 minutes apart, she called the doctor. "He told me to ring in the New Year and come on in."

At the hospital, Laura was hooked up to an electronic fetal monitor. The pace of her contractions slowed to every 10 minutes. By 2:30 A.M., the pains settled in at 15 minutes apart. "As they began to slow down and I realized that I could take an interest in everything going on, I began to get the feeling this wasn't the real thing," she says. "I thought I was in pain, but I also wondered if this was as easy as it was going to get."

At 4:00 A.M., she and her husband, Paul, were sent home. "I felt exhausted, and a little bit disappointed," she says. "I also felt relief, because my parents weren't there and I wanted them to be. And the house wasn't clean and the sheets weren't on the cradle yet!"

Ten days later—right on schedule—Laura's contractions started again, this time at an unmistakably steady pace and strong enough that she couldn't talk through them. Son Bryson Robert was born exactly on his due date.

Laura's tips for moms who think they're in labor:

- **When in doubt, ask.** "It doesn't hurt to call your doctor and get checked. It could be the real thing. Never hesitate to get reassurance."

- **Be ready.** "Pack your hospital bags a month in advance."

- **Relax.** "You have shortness of breath and your heart is racing because you're excited. Slowing down and doing breathing exercises helped me to calm myself even before the contractions were painful."

- **Remember there's no such thing as a waste-of-time contraction.** "False labor contractions, and even the Braxton-Hicks contractions you feel long before labor, help prepare your body for the baby to come out. It may not seem like it, but they're all productive."

- **Don't berate yourself if it's a false alarm.** "Sure, it's disappointing, but don't feel stupid. Consider it a dry run. When the real thing came, we knew where to go in the hospital. The false alarm was not a waste of time."

What's Going on in Your Head

The Fog

First, you misplace your car keys. Then, while transferring wet clothes to the dryer, you get distracted by the telephone and discover 3 days later that you never finished the laundry, which now smells like mildew. Next thing you know, you're forgetting appointments and missing your usual exit on the drive home from work. You've entered the last-trimester fog.

As your due date approaches, your subconscious begins to focus on the Big Event, crowding out everyday life. Hormonal shifts, interrupted sleep, a preoccupation with the many changes in your body and the preparations at hand, all contribute to the space-case syndrome. There also may be a deeper purpose to absentmindedness: it's thought to be a subconscious way of tuning into the baby and the life changes ahead, a gentle reminder that there's more to life than the 1,001 mundane tasks that ordinarily clog your brain.

So if you feel not quite yourself, remember, you're not—you're yourself *and* your baby. Try to embrace the amazing reality of what's happening within. Accentuating the mental positives helps counter all the physical negatives you're feeling. Give in to your probable desire to be alone. Turn down dinner invitations and resist working overtime. Make time for solitary walks and self-indulgences like leisurely shopping outings. Consider a meditative visit to a day spa or a bed-and-breakfast getaway.

Nesting

You may look more like a penguin than a sparrow, but the instinct is the same: to feather a nest for your hatchling-to-be. The nesting instinct may manifest itself as a sudden drive to finish every detail of the nursery or as a compulsive urge to refold everything in the linen closet. Nesting is a practical outlet for the pregnancy fog: it diverts your attention away from increasing anxiety about labor and the changes ahead and instead focuses your attention on the baby. Nesting provides a measure of self-confidence and control, too, as if you're telling yourself, *If I can do this, I can do anything.* Washing and folding hooded towels help make the baby seem more real. There's probably a practical reason behind this burst of baby-focused energy, as well; once lightening occurs, your organs loosen up a bit after their recent, tightly packed weeks, making you feel livelier.

Above all, have fun. But take care not to get overwhelmed. Pace yourself. You probably can't endure a shopping marathon or an afternoon shoving furniture around, anyway. Be aware of psychic overload, too. Modern American nesting involves a lot of consumerism, and simply making all the necessary decisions can feed anxiety: Cloth or disposable diapers? Naturally shaped plastic nipples or the traditional kind? Diaper pail or Diaper Genie? It's easy to get flustered by the variety, or to harbor silly—but nonetheless very real—embarrassment about what your choices reveal to the world about your readiness for the job of Mom. Self-doubt and panic can creep in when you least expect them. Do your best and rely on the advice of experienced friends. Don't worry about what your mother-in-law or the saleswoman may think about your purchases and plans. And don't try to do everything before the baby's born.

Fears of the Unknown

Anxieties about the coming weeks are bound to surface. Maybe you lie awake fretting quietly in bed after your 3 A.M. trek to the bathroom. Maybe you dissolve in tears when your husband asks a simple question. Though prenatal worries take many shapes, what they all have in common is Fear of the Unknown. Fear is the dark side of the excitement and thrill of having a baby. And even though it's distressing, it's perfectly normal. The best defense is to acknowledge your fears. Every mom-to-be has them. Then you can arm yourself with reassurances to the contrary. Distraction also helps to shake off persistent fears, so use relaxation exercises such as deep breathing or visualization, or take a walk. Common worries include:

• *Fear of labor.* Will I make it through all right? How much will it hurt? Will I do or say something embarrassing? Will I somehow fail to achieve my vision of the perfect birth? Fear of labor is probably the number-one worry expectant mothers have. You can't know what it's really like until you're there, and you can't control everything about it. (This is equally true for second-time moms, who have some idea what to expect, since every labor evolves differently.)

Don't play ostrich and bury your worries. *Do* learn as much as you can about the mechanics of labor, take a childbirth class if you haven't already, or review your notes. A must do: read ahead to the next chapter in this book about labor and delivery. Be sure to tour the place where you'll deliver, too. That way your imaginary fears won't be compounded by the shock of the new or by complete surprise when you're actually in labor. You may also find it reassuring to hear others' birth stories. (Just be sure to talk to a broad range of women; some people take a perverse pleasure in retelling horror stories, which can provide a skewed portrait of labor.) But if hearing friends' tales upsets you—especially accounts of atypical birth experiences—politely decline to listen. Remind yourself that millions of women go through labor every year, and that your body was designed for the task. There's no "right" way to have a baby.

• *Fear for the baby's health.* No matter how many tests you've taken or how often you've heard the fetal heartbeat, it's hard to rest easy about your unborn child's well-being until you've had a chance to count fingers and toes and have received a pediatrician's blessing. If you've been diligent about receiving prenatal care and following your doctor's instructions, there's nothing more you can do. Articulate your worries to your doctor or midwife during your prenatal visits to receive added reassurances. Remind yourself that the overwhelming majority of infants are born healthy. Even if you're at risk for a particular problem, the odds are in your favor; a genetic counselor can equip you with added information.

• *Fear you'll be a bad mother.* Maybe you've never felt maternal stirrings. Maybe you had a poor role model and don't want history to repeat itself. Or—most common—you simply doubt your ability to be a loving, patient, knows-just-what-to-do kind of mother. Anxiety about how well you'll do in your new persona of mother is not much different from any kind of performance anxiety. Think of your first day on a new job or the hours before you got married. Give yourself some credit: tote up all the other things you do well in life. Why wouldn't you make a great mom, too? Give your standards a reality check: remind yourself that you don't need to know about toilet training and handling adolescent angst right off the bat; tiny newborns come with pretty basic, easy-to-master needs, and you'll grow into the rest of the job as your child grows. And rest assured that the Perfect Mother is a big myth. You're going to make mistakes, probably lots of them, but good days will outnumber the bad ones. Talking to other mothers really helps—everyone has had lapses in confidence that they've overcome through trial and error.

• *Fear of the baby.* Some women are more afraid of the baby than the delivery. Typical worries: How will I know what she wants? What if I don't fall in love? What do I do with a baby all day long? Infant phobia is especially common among women who haven't spent much time around young children. It can help to take special classes in newborn care or to hang around friends or neighbors who have recently delivered. Some pregnant women find themselves gravitating to babies, while others shy away. Both responses are perfectly normal, so don't feel forlorn if diapering and dressing your friend's drooling, pooping babe leaves you unmoved. Nothing prepares you for the responsibility of a baby like being responsible for one of your own. While a small percentage of new moms don't feel instant attachment to their newborns (particularly if they've had a long, difficult delivery), most find that their prenatal jitters evaporate once they're faced with the real thing.

• *Fear you won't love a second baby as much as the first.* It's hard enough to picture another little personality in your life, let alone to imagine feeling as love-blind about it as you do your firstborn. And why not? You've had a lot longer to get to know that child, and the intense mother bond you feel with him or her is like no other relationship you've ever had. You might even feel a twinge of betrayal, since an only child tends to be blissfully ignorant of the demands a newborn will make on your time and your body in a few short weeks. You might feel guilty about all this, for the oblivious unborn baby's sake. Well, you know what? As soon as you lay eyes on that child for the first time, your heart will swell three sizes. You'll find yourself capable of plenty of love to go around for all, and you'll somehow love each child equally. It's corny, but true. Wait and see.

Pregnant Dreams

Often the worries rattling around in an expectant mother's brain haunt her when she's most vulnerable—at night. Thanks to more frequent trips to the bathroom and shifting often in search of a comfy position, pregnant women are more likely to awaken during REM (rapid eye movement) sleep, the stage when dreams take place. Thus, their dreams are remembered more vividly than those of nonpregnant folks. And the later in pregnancy, the more bizarre these dreams tend to become.

Fear not, though. Most pregnant dreams are actually reassuring—the mind's way of helping you understand your fears and work through them. Common themes include:

• **Neglecting the baby.** You dream you oversleep and miss night feedings, or forget about the baby for so long that you discover a teenager lying in the crib in a filthy, long-outgrown diaper. Though frightening, such visions reflect a normal ambivalence about becoming a mother and natural anxiety about the enormity of the job and what it will be like.

• **Losing the baby.** Sometimes women dream that the baby dies—or that they wake up to discover their pregnancy was "just a dream." This is not wishful thinking. Rather, dreams of loss usually represent thoughts about leaving behind your old childless lifestyle, or thoughts about labor, when the fetus to whom you've grown so attached will physically leave your body. Every woman wants the best for her child, so such nightmarish visions may also be a way of exorcising what-if-the-worst-happens fears and mentally preparing yourself, just in case.

• **Checking the oven.** Many women report dreams in which they—or their doctors or partners—remove the fetus to check its health or size, then pop it right back in, like a pan of cookies that need to bake a bit longer. Here, the mind is offering a chance to act out reassurances about worries over the baby's health.

• **Baby as frog.** Perhaps because during waking hours the baby is so often envisioned as a small creature (not clearly a human being), animal images persist in sleep. It's common in early pregnancy to envision the baby as a tadpole or a fish, and later as a larger mammal such as a puppy, a kitten—even a pig or a cow! Such images don't mean you'd rather have a pet than a child. They reflect efforts to imagine the life within you, which can sometimes seem rather abstract.

• **Marriage disruption.** Dreams of war involving you and your partner, whether or not the baby pops up as a character, can signal fears about what the baby will mean to your relationship. These are normal fears about stresses that, to some extent, inevitably await even the closest couples.

GOOD ADVICE: PAMPER YOURSELF IN THE HOMESTRETCH

Who deserves R&R more than you right now? Try to indulge in three or more of the following every day:

- Put your feet up and commune with your baby.
- Take a nap.
- Skip vacuuming (and definitely ditch the dustrag).
- Soak in the tub, using scented oils and soaps.
- Flop on the sofa and listen to a CD that you haven't played in ages.
- Go out for lunch instead of brown-bagging it.
- Drop everything and take a walk.
- Make a milkshake.
- Record your thoughts or dreams in a diary.
- Have your hair trimmed.

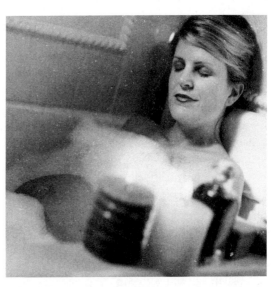

Take time to pamper yourself now. Once your baby arrives, leisure moments will be few and far between.

- Gently massage your midsection with an extravagant moisturizing lotion.
- Buy fresh flowers.
- Rent a corny movie, like an old musical. (But nothing with babies or dark scenes.)
- Order yourself a present from a catalog. If your budget allows, sign up for a gift-of-the-month club that will send a shipment of fresh fruit, bath products, flowers, books—even gourmet pizzas—to you once a month for the next year.

IS IT TRUE...

That it's a girl if you carry low? Or a boy if your skin darkens? Or a girl if you gain weight in the face? Or a boy if a needle on a string that's held over your stomach doesn't move? Or ... It's almost cruel to burst these favorite shower-game and wise-granny tales, but none of them is scientifically valid—or, if you ask enough women, even anecdotally true. Examining the fetus's chromosomes (such as by CVS or amniocentesis) or its genitals (by ultrasound) are the only ways to be certain about the baby's gender before birth. And even ultrasound can be wrong, as many a shocked parent's face in the delivery room will attest.

FATHER TO FATHER:
"We're Pregnant"

Joe Mockler, 28
Richland, Washington

Soon after Joe learned his wife of 2 years, Ann, was expecting their first child, he bought a stack of books about fatherhood. "I didn't know my role anymore. Ultimately, I learned I had to work things out on my own and that whatever I was feeling was okay."

His main priority, he says, was to make life easier for Ann. So he gave up alcohol and caffeine along with her. He attended every checkup but one. He helped pick their childbirth instructor and type of class—the Bradley Method, a husband-coached approach. Worried about hurting the baby, they also curtailed sex at first. "It never did pick up to its full strength, but it can still be enjoyed and you can still have closeness," he says.

Playing an active role in the pregnancy helped Joe deal with worries about how well he'd manage the emotional and financial responsibilities of fatherhood, as well as anxiety over Ann's and the baby's health. Even their baby shower was unisex. He empathized right along with her—to the tune of gaining 80 pounds to her 35 pounds. "It was how I handled stress," he explains. (The father-to-be's development of physical responses to his partner's pregnancy—weight gain, backaches, food cravings, mood swings—is known as *couvade syndrome*. Some 20 to 80 percent of dads are thought to be affected, especially in the very first and last months.)

Son Dylan was born after a 22-hour labor. "It's tough," says the proud papa about the pregnancy and birth. "I don't know how women made it through history without more help."

Joe's tips for expectant dads:

• ***Spend a lot of time with your partner.*** "We would wake up on weekends and I'd go get the paper, then we'd stay in bed together reading and talking. I miss those times now."

• ***Put yourself in her too-tight shoes.*** "If after a long day you come home and your wife asks for a massage and you don't really want to, realize she may have had a terrible day."

• *Respect her mood swings—and keep communicating through them.* "Not everything she does makes sense. Even something like watching her decide on clothes tested my patience. I'd think something looked nice, but she'd have tears in her eyes because she thought it didn't. Don't take things personally. You have to talk to see what she needs."

• *Be involved—but remember you're the third star on this stage.* "I tried to let Ann have the center light. As long as she was happy, I was happy."

Checkups and Tests

Last-Trimester Visits

Sometime in month 7 or 8, you'll begin having checkups every 2 weeks. In the ninth month, your pace advances to once a week. At each visit, you'll continue to have your blood pressure, weight, and urine checked. Your baby's growth, heartbeat, and position will be monitored as well. Toward the very end, you may be examined internally to see whether there are any changes in your cervix—is it effacing (thinning), ripening (softening), or dilating (opening)? Although these changes may begin to occur in the last weeks, they are not a predictor of when your labor will start. It's possible to walk around 1 to 3 centimeters dilated for several weeks, for example. Or the condition of your cervix may show no changes at an exam during the day, then you go into labor that very night. These measures provide a comparison from checkup to checkup and for when labor does begin.

By 38 or 39 weeks, you'll hit your highest weight and probably gain little more; it's not uncommon to lose a pound or two at the very end. You may also have one of several routine or optional tests:

• *Group B strep.* (routine) This new test, in which sample cells are taken from the rectum, vagina, or cervix (or all three) and then cultured, screens for Group B streptococcal (GBS) bacteria. GBS is present in up to 30 percent of all healthy women, where it's usually harmless to them. But it's the leading cause of life-threatening infections in newborns, who can be exposed to it during delivery. GBS can result in mental retardation, impaired vision, and hearing loss in newborns. The screening, which has greatly reduced the prevalence of the infection, is done between 35 and 37 weeks. Those who test positive are treated with antibiotics during delivery, protecting the baby.

• *Ultrasound.* (optional) A sonogram can determine fetal position if the doctor can't tell manually. If a doctor is concerned about the baby's well-being, ultrasound may also be used at this point in pregnancy to see if the baby is growing properly, is moving and breathing adequately, and is surrounded by adequate amniotic fluid. Called a *biophysical profile*, this thorough workup is reserved for overdue babies and cases where the baby does not seem to be moving much or when growth problems are suspected. An external electronic fetal monitor (which is strapped around the mother's belly to detect the baby's heartbeat) and other tools are used.

• **Nonstress test.** (optional) A fetal monitor is used to determine whether the fetal heart rate increases as the fetus moves, which is a good sign. It's typically used for overdue babies.

• **Stress test.** (optional) Again, a fetal monitor evaluates the baby's heart rate, this time in response to contractions that are stimulated either by a small intravenous dose of *Pitocin* (a synthetic version of the hormone oxytocin) or by having the woman rub her nipples to trigger the release of natural oxytocin. It's also called a contraction stress test.

Planning for Birth

During your last trimester you should have a conversation with your doctor about your delivery. He or she will let you know what to do when labor begins: What are the signs to watch for? How far apart should contractions be before you call the doctor or midwife? Do you go directly to the hospital if the doctor's office is closed for the day? What do you do if your water breaks? (See "Is This It?" page 221.)

This is also the time to review your birth preferences. Be sure your doctor knows your feelings regarding pain relief, episiotomy, having the newborn brought to you immediately after birth, and other issues where choices are involved. These should be written in your patient record or attached to it in the form of a written *birth plan* that you provide and go over together. (See CHECKLIST: "Your Birth Plan," page 177.)

Caution: Birth plans articulate your ideal vision of delivery. But having a baby isn't like building a house—your plans cannot be regarded as absolutes. That's because labor and delivery are fraught with unknowns. You can't control the duration or intensity of labor, the baby's size or position, or possible complications. A birth plan can't be too rigid or filled with unrealistic absolutes. But if you have a doctor or midwife whom you trust and who has a clear understanding of your preferences—and if you've checked in advance that the facility where you will deliver is open to your plans—you'll feel much more confident about your birth experience than if you leave everything to chance.

Checklist: Your Birth Plan

Setting your thoughts about labor on paper, or discussing them with your healthcare provider, can help crystallize your preferences. You'll find it helpful to read up on labor and delivery, and to take a child-birth education class, before solidifying your opinions. Consider your stances on such topics as:

Labor

1. *During labor, do you want to:*
   - ☐ Move around
   - ☐ Stay in one place
   - ☐ Be able to take a bath or shower
2. *For refreshment, would you prefer to:*
   - ☐ Eat
   - ☐ Drink
   - ☐ Have ice chips or popsicles
   - ☐ Use an IV (if you wish to avoid a routine IV, say so explicitly)
3. *Do you want the baby's heartbeat to be monitored:*
   - ☐ With an internal electronic fetal monitor
   - ☐ With a portable telemetry unit (so you can walk)
   - ☐ With an external monitor
   - ☐ With a fetal or Doppler stethoscope
   - ☐ Intermittently, if at all possible
4. *How do you feel about pain medications?*
   (Note that once you begin to receive pain relief, you're confined to bed.)
   - ☐ I want to use all appropriate pain-relief options.
   - ☐ I would like to take them if the pain is too intense (and if so, do you prefer narcotics or an epidural?).
   - ☐ They should be avoided if possible. (Do you want the staff to refrain from asking if you want drugs until you ask first?)
5. *What nonmedical pain-relief methods would you like to try?*
   - ☐ Breathing exercises
   - ☐ Acupressure
   - ☐ Massage

☐ Visualization
☐ Hypnosis
☐ Water (warm bath, shower)
☐ Other: _____

6. *Whom do you want to be present during labor? (If you want more than one person, is this okay with the hospital, and do you need to sign them in ahead of time? If you don't want medical trainees present, say so.)*
   ☐ My partner
   ☐ Another birth coach
   ☐ A doula (professional labor assistant)
   ☐ Friends or family members
   ☐ Older children

Delivery

1. *What positions would you like to try for pushing?*
   ☐ Reclining in bed
   ☐ Squatting
   ☐ All fours
   ☐ Other: _____

2. *How do you feel about an episiotomy?*
   ☐ I would like one if the doctor thinks I will tear.
   ☐ I would prefer that the birth attendants massage and stretch my perineum in order to avoid an episiotomy.

3. *Would you like your partner to cut the cord?*
   ☐ Yes
   ☐ No

4. *In the event of a Cesarean delivery, do you want to:*
   ☐ Be conscious
   ☐ Watch the procedure
   ☐ See and touch the baby after the operation
   ☐ Have your partner present at all times

After Delivery

1. *Do you want to postpone noncrucial procedures until after you've had a chance to hold your baby?*
   ☐ Yes
   ☐ No

2. *Do you want to try to nurse the baby immediately?*
   ☐ Yes
   ☐ No
3. *When do you want to have the baby with you? (Note that hospitals may have specific policies on this.)*
   ☐ All the time
   ☐ Whenever I'm awake
   ☐ Whenever the baby is awake
   ☐ At scheduled feeding times or when baby is hungry
4. *Is it okay for the hospital staff to give your baby:*
   ☐ A pacifier?
   ☐ Sugared or plain water? (not generally advised if breastfeeding)
   ☐ Formula? (not generally advised if breastfeeding)
5. *If you have a son, do you want him circumcised?*
   ☐ Yes
   ☐ No
6. *Barring complications, how long do you want to stay in the hospital?*
   ☐ I want to rest and recover as long as I can.
   ☐ I want to go home as soon as possible.

IS IT TRUE...

That first babies are usually late? Not really. Every baby follows his or her own schedule. Just over half of all babies are born after their projected due dates; 35 percent arrive early, and just 5 percent arrive on the very day they're expected. If your first child was especially early, you can generally expect the same for subsequent births.

That you can predict the baby's size? Some grandmas swear by a formula that involves averaging the parents' birthweights. While it's true that a very small maternal birthweight increases her baby's odds of being small also, that's not a very reliable predictor. Experienced doctors can make an educated guess based on the measurement of the fundus and how the baby feels externally. An ultrasound is another way to tell a baby's size before birth, but even this high-tech method has an error margin of 10 to 15 percent.

That I'll need a C-section if I'm narrow-hipped? No. Many a petite woman has delivered a 9-pound whopper vaginally. It's the size and position of your baby relative to your pelvis that are the key determinants. Usually a woman must begin labor before it's clear whether the baby will fit through her birth canal.

What Should I Eat?

Do a Diet Check

Nutritionally, the third trimester proceeds pretty much like the second. You're still gaining as much as 1 to 1½ pounds a week as your baby edges toward its birthweight. It's as important as ever to consume a broad variety of foods, especially protein and B vitamins (found in animal proteins, dark leafy vegetables, bananas, and legumes), to fuel brain development. Keep up your intake of fluids, too, to assist the production of blood, to keep you and the baby well hydrated, and to ward off premature contractions and such common late-pregnancy side effects as constipation. The biggest change now may be an inability to comfortably eat very much at one sitting without experiencing heartburn or getting the bad taste in your mouth known as gastric reflux.

As the pregnancy advances, however, many women backslide on good nutrition. It's understandable, but not advisable. As the novelty of the experience wears off, old habits resurface. Or you're so big and so tired that you feel you deserve to cut some corners and eat more treats. Well, some old habits and some treats are fine—but your baby still needs optimal nutrients in order to build strong bones, develop brain cells, and generally complete its growth.

Check your progress with this quiz:

- Are you still taking your prenatal vitamin every day? (Don't neglect to refill the prescription once the first bottle runs out.)
- Do you take your vitamin with orange juice or some other source of vitamin C (such as grapefruit, melon, or strawberries) for better iron absorption?
- Do you eat breakfast every day? (If you skip even one day a week, the answer is no.)
- Do you drink eight to ten 8-ounce glasses of water a day?
- Do you eat fish, beans, or a potato to make sure you get enough iron every day?
- Does your protein come from a variety of sources?
- Do you serve yourself two different vegetables at lunch *and* at dinner?
- Do you drink 2 to 4 glasses of milk a day—or the calcium-rich equivalent from foods such as yogurt, small-boned fish, or dark-green leafy vegetables?
- Are you still cutting back on caffeine?
- Are you avoiding alcohol?
- Are your snacks adding nutrition to your diet, as opposed to purely empty calories—in other words, are you snacking on fruits, nuts, raisins, oatmeal cookies, blender shakes?
- Are you gaining about a pound per week?

To score:

- If you answered yes to ten or more questions, keep it up!
- If you answered yes to six to nine questions, you're in the Homestretch Lag and need to redouble your efforts.
- If you answered yes to fewer than five questions, ask yourself how you can improve your eating habits. It's not too late to make changes that will help protect your baby's health. You may want to seek the advice of a nutritionist to shore up your weak spots.

TRY THESE RECIPES!

The following recipes have just the right ingredients for the last trimester: they're packed with nutrition and quick to prepare.

Corn Chowder

Preparation time: 10 minutes
Cooking time: about 35 minutes

This easy soup makes a meal by itself. It's full of calcium and fiber.

1½ tablespoons vegetable oil
1 medium onion, diced
3 medium potatoes, peeled and cubed
2 cups water
1 bay leaf
Salt and pepper
3 cups milk, heated
4 cups fresh or frozen corn kernels (use a small, sharp knife
    to cut kernels from ears)
2 tablespoons flour
Sweet Hungarian paprika

Heat the oil in a large soup pot. Sauté the onion for 5 minutes, until softened but not brown. Add the potatoes, water, bay leaf, and salt and pepper to taste. Bring to a boil, then reduce the heat and simmer, uncovered, for about 25 minutes or until the potatoes are just tender.

Add the warm milk and corn, and stir well. Place the flour in a small bowl. Take 3 tablespoons of the hot chowder and whisk into the flour to form a paste.

Slowly add the flour mixture back to the pot, stirring to create a smooth soup. Let simmer 3 to 5 minutes, until thickened. Season to taste and serve with a sprinkling of paprika. Yield: 6 servings.

White Beans Provençal

Preparation time: 10 minutes
Cooking time: 10 minutes

These protein-packed beans—which conveniently start with canned beans—can be eaten straight from the pot or used in a wide variety of ways. Drain the beans and then sauté with onions, garlic, and tomatoes, or add the beans to soups and stews.

1 tablespoon olive oil
1 medium onion, finely chopped
1 garlic clove, finely chopped (optional)
2 cups cooked canned white beans, rinsed and drained
1 ripe medium tomato, cut into small cubes (optional)
1 teaspoon dried thyme, or 1 tablespoon fresh
1/2 teaspoon dried crumbled rosemary, or 1/2 tablespoon fresh
Salt and freshly ground black pepper
2 tablespoons dry white wine or water
1/3 cup finely chopped parsley (optional)

In a large skillet, heat the olive oil over moderate heat. Add the onion and garlic, if using, and sauté for 5 minutes, stirring frequently to prevent browning. Add the beans, tomato if using, thyme, rosemary, salt, pepper, and wine or water; simmer for another 5 minutes. Sprinkle with the parsley, if desired, and serve hot. Yield: 4 servings.

Salmon Cakes

Preparation time: 15 minutes
Cooking time: about 4 minutes per cake

Made easily with canned salmon, these cakes are light, flavorful, and a good source of protein, which promotes fetal brain development. Serve them on a large platter surrounded by lemon and lime wedges, or alongside a bowl of tartar sauce or green sauce. To make a quick green sauce, mix a cup of mayonnaise with 1/4 cup finely chopped pickles, ¹/₄ cup capers, ¹/₄ cup finely chopped parsley, a squirt of lemon juice, and freshly ground black pepper to taste.

1 tablespoon olive oil
¹/₄ cup finely chopped onion
1 small red bell pepper, finely chopped
Salt and freshly ground black pepper
1 14³/₄-ounce can salmon, drained
¹/₄ cup finely chopped parsley
3 tablespoons finely chopped fresh dill
Juice from 1 large lemon
¹/₂ to ³/₄ cup bread crumbs
Dash of hot pepper sauce
1 to 2 tablespoons vegetable oil

Garnishes:
Fresh dill sprigs
Lemon and lime wedges

In a large skillet, heat the olive oil over moderately low heat. Add the onion and sauté for 3 minutes. Add the red pepper, salt, and pepper, and sauté another 7 minutes, stirring frequently to prevent browning.

In a large bowl, separate the salmon into flakes using a fork. Add the parsley, dill, and lemon juice. Add the sautéed vegetables and stir to mix. Add enough bread crumbs to hold the mixture together. Taste for seasoning and add additional salt, pepper, or hot pepper sauce. (The mixture can be made only about an hour or two before cooking.)

Preheat the oven to 250 degrees.

In a large skillet, heat 1 tablespoon of the vegetable oil over moderately high heat. Using your hands, form 2¹/₂- to 3-inch cakes. Add a few salmon cakes to the skillet, being careful not to crowd the pan, and press them down with a spatula to flatten. Let cook 2 minutes, flip the cakes, and flatten again; cook another 2 minutes. Remove the salmon cakes to an ovenproof plate and keep warm in the oven. Repeat with the remaining mixture, adding more oil as needed. Serve hot or warm on a large platter and top each cake with a sprig of fresh dill; surround with the lemon and lime wedges. Yield: About 14 salmon cakes.

Quick Apple Crumble

Preparation time: 15 minutes
Cooking time: 30 to 35 minutes

Treat yourself. This is a great last-minute dessert because it takes under an hour from start to finish. Serve with vanilla yogurt or ice cream.

4 tablespoons unsalted butter, plus 1 teaspoon
5 large apples, peeled, cored, and cut into thick slices
1 teaspoon ground allspice
$1/2$ teaspoon ground cloves
$1/2$ cup all-purpose flour
$1/2$ cup granola
$1/3$ cup sugar
$1/3$ cup apple cider

Preheat the oven to 350 degrees. Grease the bottom of a large ovenproof skillet or baking dish with the 1 teaspoon butter. Place the apples in the dish and toss with half the allspice and cloves.

In a medium bowl, mix the flour, granola, sugar, and remaining allspice and cloves. Cut the butter into small cubes and, working with your hands, a pastry blender, or 2 flat knives, mix it into the flour mixture until it resembles small peas. Spoon the topping over the apples and pour in the cider. Bake for 30 to 35 minutes, or until the apples are tender and the topping is golden brown. Yield: 6 servings.

WHAT IF...

I'm gaining weight too fast? A steady advance on the scale goes with the territory after 24 weeks; *don't* begin to diet or cut back. *Do* be sure to keep exercising; a short session is better than none. Water retention can also make it seem like you're gaining fast, especially in summer. Even if your weight jumps from one checkup to the next, there may not be cause for alarm; your doctor will be monitoring your vital signs to rule out problems such as high blood pressure or sugar imbalance. *Important:* If you gain more than a pound or two in a single day, and also notice sudden puffiness in your ankles or face, alert your doctor, as this can be a warning sign of preeclampsia.

I'm gaining weight too slowly? Every woman wears a pregnancy differently. Your doctor checks your weight at each visit to verify that you're gaining adequately. If the numbers seem too low, he or she may review your diet and suggest more calorically dense foods (such as peanut butter, nuts, avocado, vegetable oils for cooking). Review your activity level, too; your lifestyle or workout routine may be expending more calories than is optimal right now.

Is It True...

That eating spicy foods close to your due date can trigger labor? Tabasco sauce and onions may trigger heartburn—especially in the third trimester—but not labor.

That eating strawberries causes strawberry birthmarks? At face value, it seems logical. The fruit's size and color are comparable to strawberry hemangiomas (a type of birthmark that affects one in ten newborns and tends to disappear in early childhood). But berries do not cause these marks. They're a good source of vitamin C and fiber, though, so enjoy.

Fit for Pregnancy

Posture Basics

Who would expect that you'd need to learn to stand and sit up all over again just because you're pregnant? But in a way, that's the case. Good posture and careful movement are especially important now to counter loose joints, unsteady balance, and an overstressed back. You'll feel better and be less injury-prone. Some basics:

• *Standing.* Imagine the top of your head being pulled toward the ceiling. Automatically, you'll tuck in your chin, lift your shoulders, and tuck in your stomach and buttocks. Take care to distribute your weight evenly on both legs.

• *Getting out of bed.* Rise slowly to prevent dizziness. While still lying flat, swing your legs over to the side of the bed. Then use your arm to push up your body and slide to your feet. Never bolt straight up from the waist, jackknife style.

• *Lifting.* If you must lift a heavy object, always bend at the knees, not the hips, and keep the object close to your body. It can be difficult to hold large objects closely with a big belly, though, so be careful and get help if you're at all in doubt about straining yourself.

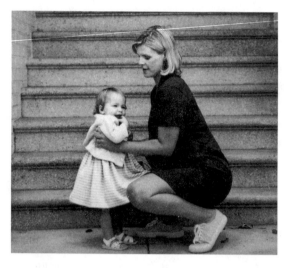

An alternate way to lift your child without causing back strain: hold her close and bend at the knees—not the waist.

• **Carrying children.** To prevent back strain, avoid carrying an older child on your hip. When lifting a child, try having her stand on a stool or chair so you won't have to bend so far down.

WHAT IF...

I don't feel like doing *anything*? By the eighth or ninth month, your sheer size can make getting out of bed seem like an athletic event—let alone putting yourself through the paces of a workout. But it's worth the effort to try. While you probably won't be able to maintain exactly the same routine as you followed earlier in pregnancy, you ought to be able to keep up basic exercises such as stretches and Kegels, along with easy aerobic activities such as walking or swimming. Try cutting back to just three times a week instead of five or seven, taking more frequent breaks, or reducing your overall exercise time or distance. By continuing to do *something*, however, you'll improve your mood as well as your strength for labor. *Exception:* You're excused from all of the above for the last couple of weeks before your due date. No one feels like doing much then—nor should you!

I fell—how do I know the baby's okay? Wobbliness goes hand in hand with waddling, thanks to your shifting center of gravity. But falls rarely cause injury to mother or baby. Don't forget that your child is securely trundled in the womb—and your own softened ligaments make you less likely to sprain. After a tumble, sit down and wait to feel the baby move, a sign that he or she is just fine. If you're still not convinced, your doctor can monitor the fetal heartbeat or do a sonogram. If you have severe abdominal pain, vaginal bleeding, or other fluid releases from your vagina, alert your doctor immediately.

IS IT TRUE...

That vigorous exercise will get my labor going once I reach my due date?
Sorry, there's no proven way to initiate labor on your own.

The Pregnant Look

Skin Changes

Count on the extra blood and hormones circulating within you to make themselves visible in one or more ways. The best, most common result is a healthy flush and a less oily complexion. Or you may experience one of the following, less glamorous changes:

• *The mask of pregnancy (chloasma).* Pigmentation tends to deepen in pregnancy, such as on freckles and breast areolae, because of the hormone MSH (*melanocyte-stimulating hormone*). On the nose, cheeks, and forehead, however, brownish patches (or, in some dark-skinned women, light patches) called chloasma may appear. If you were prone to such marks when taking birth-control pills, you're more likely to get them now, too. Exposure to sunlight can worsen the problem. Don't attempt to bleach these marks; stick to cosmetic concealers if you feel they're needed. Chloasma usually disappears after delivery.

• *Linea nigra.* One day in the seventh month or so, you may discover a dark, vertical stripe running down the middle of your abdomen, along the path where the muscles part slightly to accommodate the uterus. It may look odd with your bikini—if you're bold enough to still be wearing one—but never fear, the line fades after pregnancy.

• *Varicose veins.* Caused by blood pooling in overstretched blood vessels, they're unsightly but no cause for alarm.

• *Spider veins.* Smaller than varicose veins and usually limited to the face, neck, arms, and upper chest, these thin branches are tiny broken blood vessels, which have become more sensitive in pregnancy owing to hormones and your magnified blood volume. Fair-skinned, fair-haired women are most vulnerable. They usually disappear within a few weeks of birth.

• **Stretch marks.** Up to 50 percent of pregnant women develop these pink to deep red or purple streaks, sometimes indented, which can appear virtually anywhere on the lower body. Think of them as the membership badges of motherhood, since there's nothing you can do to avoid them, short of being born with highly elastic skin. They're caused by chemical changes in the skin's connective tissue. Many stretch marks fade to silvery white, or disappear, within 6 months of delivery. When they persist postpartum, they can be minimized through topical treatments that use prescription formulations such as glycolic acid or by postpartum laser treatments. Both of these fairly new options must be done by a dermatologist. Though not an option for nursing moms, a recent study found that Retonoic acid reduced the length of stretch marks by 14 percent and the width by 8 percent.

• **Mole changes.** Along with the other pigmentation changes of pregnancy, moles tend to darken. But if one changes shape, size, or color, point it out to your doctor.

• **Red palms** (palmar erythema). It looks like you've just given a long, hard, standing ovation. This very common condition, affecting nearly two-thirds of pregnant women, will eventually disappear. It's believed to be caused by the normal increase in estrogen.

• **Skin tags.** These tiny flaps of skin can worsen during pregnancy or develop for the first time, especially on the breasts, neck, or underarms. If they're located in a place where they hurt because they rub against clothing, they can be removed postpartum. Again, hormones are the culprit.

• **Dry skin, itchiness.** The main reason for these common maladies is that your skin is stretching, especially across the abdomen where itching bothers most. Soothe with lotion rather than scratching. Try avoiding soap, too, which removes natural oils, as well as highly perfumed products that may only aggravate skin more. Slather on moisturizer or baby oil immediately after a tub soak to seal in hydration.

• **Wide-open navel.** One of pregnancy's little surprises is how an "innie" unfolds or an "outie" may flatten as your abdomen stretches to the brink. It doesn't mean anything. The navel can't open up—but it is an amusing development (and a good excuse to give your belly button a thorough cleaning).

GOOD ADVICE: WHEN YOU'RE SICK OF MATERNITY CLOTHES

On the one hand, dressing your voluptuousness probably takes little thought by the eighth or ninth month, now that you've got your maternity look down pat. On the other hand, it probably feels boring. What to do when buying ever-larger bras is not your idea of a fun way to freshen your wardrobe? Try these ideas for adding zip:

- *Buy one new item.* Sure, you won't wear it long, but if you scout resale shops, discount stores, or sales you can probably find a bargain. Pick a top with a zip-front or front buttons, so you can wear it the first month or two postpartum for nursing.
- *Buy some new shoes.* Not only may your feet have grown larger, but a slip-on style will make your life much easier than struggling to bend over to lace ties or fasten buckles. (Lace-ups generally provide greatest support, but a slip-on like a loafer can be a good choice if it's well-constructed and not too strappy.)
- *Trade with a pregnant friend.* Chances are, she's sick of her maternity clothes, too.
- *Check your mate's closet again.* Those big denim shirts or droopy cardigans that looked impossibly huge back in your fourth month might be just the thing now.
- *Switch to a smaller handbag.* It will make your overall line appear less bulky.
- *Have a makeover.* Visit a department store cosmetic counter for a free consultation. As well as lifting your spirits, you may glean useful tips on disguising the marks or puffiness that pregnancy has wrought. At the very least, cheer yourself up with a new lipstick.

IS IT TRUE...

That vitamin E lotion or cocoa butter will prevent stretch marks? Sorry, there's no known way to avoid stretch marks, though lotions can make a big taut belly feel better.

That scratching your belly can cause stretch marks? No. The red marks caused by scratches will fade in a day or two, whereas the damage that results in a stretch mark takes place deep within the skin and lasts throughout your pregnancy. But scratching *can* exacerbate itchiness—which is good enough reason to avoid the impulse.

What About Sex?

Homestretch Intimacy

Anything may happen now in terms of a couple's attitude toward sex: total disinterest in sexual activity (too big, too uncomfortable, too preoccupied by baby plans); sustained interest (less frequent maybe, but still active); or increased interest (those pregnancy hormones at work, the novelty and adventure of her new shape).

Medically, it's safe to enjoy sex until your water breaks. Nevertheless, the practical impediments are, well, growing. It's no wonder that the majority of couples gradually taper off or give up on sex by the ninth month. The only caveat: Neglect isn't always benign. To avoid sex without discussing it together can strain a relationship unnecessarily. Besides, the ability to be frank about your sexuality says a lot about how well you'll be able to communicate with one another once you're parents. Finally, remember that intimacy needn't equal intercourse. In addition to oral sex and masturbation, consider gentle massage, backrubs, and foot rubs—all of which feel blissful to the pregnant body and can have an erotic edge. By late pregnancy, many women feel a deep need simply to be cuddled. You might find yourselves feeling particularly close doing such ordinary activities as attending childbirth classes or assembling the baby's crib. Make it a point to go out to dinner or the movies as much as you can; getting away together won't be so easy in a few months. Cherish your couple time—remember that the days of just the two of you are soon coming to an end.

IS IT TRUE...

That sex can cause labor? Labor is a complicated event caused by many factors, and there's no evidence that sex is one of them. Stimulation of the breasts does promote the natural release of the hormone oxytocin, which can produce contractions in a woman near term, although contractions don't necessarily spell labor. Nevertheless, this may explain the oft-heard advice about having sex to jump-start an overdue labor.

Special Situations

Preeclampsia

A potentially dangerous condition called pregnancy-induced high blood pressure, or *preeclampsia*, develops in about 7 percent of expectant mothers, typically after 35 weeks, although it can occur earlier. First-time mothers are more at risk. (It used to be called *toxemia*, but that term has fallen out of use since it's now clear that no toxins are involved.) What happens is that normal blood flow to the uterus and, in turn, the placenta is restricted. The mother could develop kidney failure or *eclampsia*, a potentially fatal disorder characterized by convulsions, cerebral hemorrhage, and coma. The risk to the fetus includes early separation of the placenta (placenta abruptio) and possibly fetal death if the delivery doesn't take place in time.

Bedrest is the usual prescription to lower blood pressure. In the most severe cases, however, the onset of preeclampsia is sudden, and the baby must be delivered immediately to save both mother's and baby's lives.

The threat of preeclampsia is why the doctor monitors your blood pressure at each visit. But because problems can develop swiftly, get checked immediately if you notice:

- Swelling of the face and hands
- Blurred vision or seeing spots
- Severe or constant headaches
- Sudden weight gain (more than 1 pound per day)
- Severe pain in the upper abdomen

Preeclampsia's cause is unknown. Researchers have discounted the theory that sodium consumption is a factor (as it is in ordinary hypertension). Theories being investigated include a calcium deficiency, inadequate protein intake, and a glitch in the immune system.

Placenta Problems

The following conditions affect only a small fraction of mothers-to-be.

• *Placenta previa (low-lying placenta).* This is the most common cause of third-trimester bleeding. The placenta, the blood-lush organ that nourishes the fetus, is attached to the uterine wall where the fertilized egg first implanted itself. Normally the placenta is fastened high in the uterus. If it's positioned low, it can partly or completely cover the cervix, blocking the baby's exit from the womb. When the cervix starts to open in labor, the woman suddenly bleeds painlessly and profusely. Bleeding may also occur off and on in late pregnancy because of placenta previa; always inform your caregiver promptly about any bleeding.

An ultrasound, which shows the positioning of the baby and the placenta,

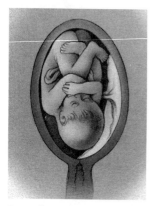

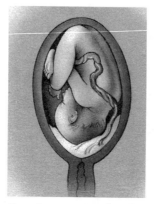

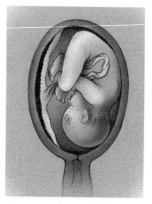

Partial previa: A partial previa occurs when a portion of the placenta obstructs the cervical opening.

Complete previa: When the placenta completely blocks the cervical opening, the condition is known as a complete previa.

Placenta abruptio: In placenta abruptio, the placenta prematurely separates from the uterine wall.

can verify the problem. Hospitalization generally follows to monitor the situation; labor is forestalled as long as possible to allow the baby to mature. The baby is delivered by Cesarean; in some emergencies, a preterm C-section is done immediately to save the mother's life, regardless of the fetal age. *Note:* Before the third trimester, as many as one in four or five placentas is low lying, but moves upward to a normal position later in pregnancy. Total placenta previa requiring a Cesarean delivery occurs in about 1 to 2 percent of pregnancies. The risk increases with each subsequent birth.

• *Marginal previa.* Sometimes the placenta is located next to or near the cervix, but does not touch or cover it. In those cases, a vaginal delivery may be attempted. Again, ultrasound is used to show the position of the baby and the placenta.

• *Placenta abruptio (premature separation of the placenta).* In about 1 in 150 first pregnancies, the placenta tears away from its moorings on the uterine wall. Symptoms include mild to heavy bleeding that may contain clots (though sometimes there's no bleeding at all), abdominal pain, and sometimes contractions. Treatment depends on how much of the placenta has torn and how late it is in pregnancy. Placenta abruptio most typically occurs in the third trimester. If a quarter or more of the placenta has come loose, mother and baby are in grave danger; the baby is quickly delivered by C-section. Placenta abruptio is most common in women with high blood pressure.

The Overdue Baby

Eighty percent of babies are born within 2 weeks before or after their due dates. About 10 percent are premature (born more than 2 weeks early) and another 10 percent haven't arrived 2 weeks after their due dates. These are called *post-date* or *postterm pregnancies*. Some physicians schedule inductions or C-sections if 14 days pass since the due date. They can't be sure if the baby is overdue because of a miscalculated due date or because a physical problem is preventing the onset of labor. If you're leery of those options, however, discuss the possibility of waiting a bit longer—more than 90 percent of babies born between 42 and 44 weeks suffer no problems as a result of their extended stay in the womb, according to the American College of Obstetricians and Gynecologists.

By the 40th or 41st week, an overdue expectant mother is carefully monitored with ultrasound, electronic fetal monitoring, and other tests for signs of a malfunctioning placenta or signs of fetal distress. The risks of a postdate pregnancy include a larger-than-normal baby; the possibility of the fetus inhaling *meconium*, or fetal wastes; and an abnormal heart rate. No matter at which point the baby is delivered, an overdue mother will also be carefully monitored in labor.

MOTHER TO MOTHER:
"My Baby Was Born Early"

Mitzi Clark, 31
San Antonio, Texas

In her seventh month, Mitzi noticed her hands and feet beginning to swell more than usual. She figured it was just part of being pregnant, worsened by her long hours on her feet as a pharmacist. Then one day her feet were so puffy she could barely put on her shoes. At a regular doctor's appointment, it was found that her blood pressure had risen and there was protein in her urine. She had also gained 12 pounds in one month and mentioned that she had been experiencing headaches and fatigue. "I thought the doctor would suggest cutting back on my hours, or bedrest," Mitzi says.

Instead, she was told she had severe preeclampsia and that the baby needed to be delivered immediately, 8 weeks early. "I was so in shock I couldn't even panic," she says. "I was scared to have a preemie because I wanted the baby to be okay." At the hospital, tests showed no signs of fetal distress. When Mitzi wondered what would happen if she didn't have an emergency C-section, her doctor explained the risk of the mother having seizures or a stroke, or of the placenta separating early (placenta abruptio), putting the baby at risk. "I said,

'Okay then, let's do it,' " she says. "My husband and I suddenly switched from shock to a let's-take-care-of-this attitude."

Son Christopher weighed 4 pounds, 1/2 ounce, and was taken immediately to the neonatal intensive care unit. He had respiratory distress syndrome (in which the lungs aren't mature enough to breathe properly on their own), and problems eating because his sucking reflex had not developed. "The first time I saw him, he was hooked to an IV and I was scared. I worried that he was going to die," she says. Mitzi was discharged 3 days after her Cesarean, while Christopher remained hospitalized for 4 weeks. "It was rough not taking him home right away. I cried the whole day—it was the first time I had let myself give in to my emotions."

Mitzi and her husband visited their son twice a day. When he was 2 weeks old, she picked him up for the first time. When he finally came home 33 days later, weighing 5 pounds, "I didn't really have many worries because we were used to him," she says. "He began walking at 9 months and talking at 18 months. We are very blessed."

Mitzi's tips for other mothers who have premature deliveries:

• **Get support.** "Don't hesitate asking for help taking care of the house or running errands. It's essential just having someone to talk to—family, friends, our church, and the Internet helped us. My hospital also had a Parents of Preemies support group."

• **Ask how you can be involved in your child's care while he or she is hospitalized.** "All the doctors and nurses encouraged us to do things with the baby—stroking his arms and legs or talking to him. If your doctor doesn't, ask."

• **Look past the medical tubes and your own panic.** "Remember that he's still the same baby, just a little smaller. Panic doesn't help you or the baby. Preemies are a lot more resilient than you may think."

MOTHER TO MOTHER:
"My 10-Month Pregnancy"

Mary Bailey, 33
Nashville, Tennessee

The nursery was ready. Her bags were packed. Her parents arrived from Florida to help out with the baby. Then Mary's long-anticipated due date came and went—uneventfully.

"I had already dropped. I had already effaced. I was having Braxton-Hicks contractions," Mary recalls. "I was definitely ready." Every day after her due date was "agonizing," she says. "My parents, my husband [Steve], and I went mall walking, ate pizza, did everything we'd heard about to stimulate labor. Every night I went to bed thinking, *This is it.*"

She stopped calling friends because she got tired of fielding their eager questions. She had already quit work, but after her due date passed, she pulled out a few projects again just to pass the time. "I never got nervous about the baby's well-being because I felt fine and she was moving the whole time. I started swelling a lot at the end, though, and often slept on the couch where I was more comfortable," she says. "I did worry that she would be too big and I'd need a C-section."

Ten days after her due date, a healthy Ruth Ellen finally arrived, by vaginal delivery, at 9 pounds, 3 ounces.

Mary's tips for other moms waiting it out:

• *Get on-line.* "I found parenting message boards where I could talk about things I was interested in—without having to dwell on my being late, which would always be the focus of conversations with friends."

• *Make constructive use of these bonus days.* "It was a good time to read books about newborn care, because I hadn't had much inclination to do that earlier in pregnancy and didn't have time after she was born. I also got thank-you notes out of the way to people who had already sent gifts, and started filling in parts of the baby book, like the family tree and the description of the nursery. I even cooked and froze some meals."

• *Rest.* "I was anxious to get labor going, so I expended a lot of energy I could have better used just napping and relaxing—or going to see movies, which I can't do now."

IS IT TRUE...

That I'll need a C-section if the baby is breech? Not necessarily. After months of free-floating about the womb, most babies dive head-first into the birth canal around 37 weeks, the most comfortable position for them once they reach a mature size for birth. Fewer than 5 percent of babies are still breech after 37 weeks. Some of these will still turn around on their own before labor begins. Breech babies can also be turned manually by a doctor (called *external version*). Such manipulations, usually done with the assistance of ultrasound in a hospital (in case an emergency delivery is warranted), work about half the time for first-time mothers and 90 percent of the time for women who have delivered vaginally before. It's usually clear within 5 to 10 minutes if version will be successful. If the baby is still breech once labor has started, a Cesarean birth is generally prudent, though some breech babies have been delivered vaginally by experienced doctors or midwives.

That I should arrange to store some of my baby's umbilical cord blood in a blood bank? A relatively new concept, the idea is that the blood could be used for a bone-marrow transplant for the child (or a sibling) if the child should develop such a need later in life (as for leukemia). The blood is otherwise discarded with the placenta. While a family with a history of a problem such as leukemia may want to consider such a plan, for most people there are plenty of reasons to think twice. For one thing, odds are slim—one in 200,000—that your child would ever need such a transplant. It's also unknown how long cord blood can be stored. What's more, private storage and upkeep of your child's cord blood can run into the thousands of dollars. Public cord-blood banks are run by some medical centers. If you'd like to donate the blood to a public bank to help others, ask your doctor if one exists in your area. Be sure to make arrangements before delivery.

Work Worries

Preparing Your Exit

Count on winding down your work days in a surreal atmosphere. As you begin to tire more easily and think more about birth, you may find it harder to concentrate, even as you feel an impending panic about finishing up everything before your leave begins. At the same time, your boss and coworkers may be in deep denial about your impending absence. They continue to count on you for work that you can't possibly finish on time, or drag their heels about discussing your transition plan.

Take the initiative in preparing everyone for your leave. If you haven't done so already, put down on paper just how all your responsibilities will be covered. Be specific. Consider charting in calendar form what's expected to happen when. Schedule individual time with your boss, your coworkers, anyone who reports to you, and your replacements, and make sure everyone is on track about your plans. If you intend to leave on a designated date, periodically remind everyone of it.

Psyche yourself for one surprise if you plan to work until your labor begins:

especially if your baby is overdue, you may be so well prepared for leave that there's virtually nothing left to do. One woman found that by the time she worked ahead and trained her temporary replacement, the days at the office crept by so slowly that she wished she had just arranged to take the time off to handle baby plans. Conversely, you may wind up having to quit sooner—and more suddenly—than intended if your baby comes early or if bedrest is ordered.

Nor should you shortchange your health now. Use your breaks to rest, not rush around. Drink water throughout the day. Take mini-breaks for stretching, walking, and relaxation. Prop up your feet on a box or stack of telephone books when seated.

Seeking Work-Family Balance

If you plan to join the ranks of working mothers, you're likely to encounter the dilemma of how to strike a balance between work needs and family ones. In fact, that was the number-one concern of working women in a major U.S. Labor Department survey. To be sure, progressive, family-friendly companies are still far from the norm. But as more and more women struggle to carve out new work situations that afford them balance, the tide is beginning to turn. Though it's hard to envision an ideal schedule before the baby arrives, it's not too early to mull the possibilities.

Look around your workplace (or the competition's) to see what kind of arrangements working moms have negotiated. Firms that are open to flexibility find it a good way to retain valued employees, and many save on benefits or overhead as well. Employees, of course, appreciate the acknowledgment that they have family responsibilities outside the office and the extra time or sanity such arrangements provide.

Options include:

• *Flex-time.* Flexible working hours usually mean working a full number of hours, typically around a core set by the company, with fluid stop-and-start times. *Pluses:* You generally keep full pay and benefits, but get to spend more time with your baby during the day. *Pitfalls:* Even 40 flexible hours a week may not give you as much time with your child as you'd like.

• *Part-time work.* This is the most popular choice for working mothers who seek alternative schedules. The possibilities are endless: half time; quarter time; full time except summers; or just certain days of the week or month. *Pluses:* You get the best of both worlds. Working just 10 fewer hours per week adds up to 2 fewer hours per day of childcare for your child. You can also keep current in your field. *Pitfalls:* Compensation plummets accordingly. Some women sense promotion stagnation as a result. Health benefits will probably be reduced.

• **Job sharing.** Two workers team up to split a single job. Some duos divvy their responsibilities equally, whereas others function as mini workteams, bringing respective strengths. *Pluses:* You work half the time. Since two heads are typically better than one, employers often find that the job is performed better than if by one person alone, though the company is paying for the equivalent of just one head. *Pitfalls:* It doesn't work for every job. It can also be hard to find an ideal partner with whom you can cooperate and get past petty competition. Benefits can be tricky to negotiate, as can part-time childcare.

• **Telecommuting.** Some 13 million workers now work at home, linked to central offices by computer, fax, and phone. Most put in a day or two per week of "face time" at headquarters; some companies have satellite offices where telecommuters can hold meetings, meet clients, do photocopying, and so on. *Pluses:* Depending on the job and how you structure it, you can earn full pay and benefits. Telecommuting saves companies office space and overhead. *Pitfalls:* You'll still need childcare from infancy through the preschool years. (You may, however, be able to work a reduced number of hours by day, and pick up again at night after the child's bedtime.) Some home workers feel isolated and strapped by the lack of a handy support staff.

• **Temping.** You can get temporary work assignments through a placement agency or, if you have a special skill or knowledge, negotiate such contracts with your current or former employers. *Pluses:* Temp work can be a stepping-stone to either full-time or part-time work. You choose when you want to work. *Pitfalls:* You'll need very flexible childcare, and pay can be sporadic.

• **Home-based business.** This option is ideal if you have skills you can market on your own. Examples are consulting, some sales, computer consulting, training, childcare, interior design, hairstyling, desktop publishing, graphic design. You'll need a separate area of your home that's strictly for business (both for tax purposes and for productivity's sake). *Pluses:* A home-based worker can be more available to a child, and you save on costs like commuting and dry-cleaning. *Pitfalls:* You'll need at least part-time childcare. Home-based businesses can require a huge investment of time (and sometimes cash) to launch.

For More Help: Work/Family Resources

- Families and Work Institute, 330 Seventh Avenue, New York, NY 10001; 212-465-2044 or http://www.familiesandwork.org. Publishes numerous handbooks.
- New Ways to Work, 785 Market Street, Suite 950, San Francisco, CA 94103; 415-995-9860. Advises companies, but also publishes career-specific resource guides.
- The Women's Bureau, US Department of Labor, 200 Constitution Avenue NW, Room S-3311, Washington, DC 20210; 800-827-5335. Offers a free "Work and Family Resource Kit."

Other Big Deals

Decisions, Decisions

Picking a nursery theme may seem taxing enough just now, but several important decisions await you that have greater consequences than Winnie the Pooh versus Peter Rabbit. Questions to resolve before you go into labor include the following:

• *Who will be your childbirth coach?* In recent years, the burden of labor support has fallen on fathers-to-be, and their presence has become expected in the delivery room. But dads aren't necessarily the best coaches. Not all men are cut out to provide the constant, capable, upbeat support that a laboring woman needs. And it can be hard for a husband to stay cheerful and objective while watching the woman he loves in pain. If you or your man can't see him as the labor-coach type—and in one survey, more than half the dads proved less than ideal for the task—neither of you should feel bad about it. The full burden of support needn't fall on his shoulders. Some clues that you might want additional labor support are: If he's not interested in childbirth classes or in helping you practice what you've learned; if the classes have raised his doubts about his ability to handle the job; if he's particularly squeamish; or if he thinks he'll find it difficult to see you in tremendous pain. That's not to say he shouldn't be at your side: Partners have an irreplaceable role in the delivery room as a soothing, supportive presence. (In fact, the word *coach* is falling out of favor in some circles since it connotes male-oriented sports analogies and is not an accurate image of what giving support involves; "labor assistant" or "support person" are now the preferred terms.)

For labor support, many women turn to a female friend or their mother. Or you may want to consider a newer option, a professional labor assistant, or *doula*. The word originates from Greek and means a woman who mothers the mother. Growing rapidly in popularity, a doula is a woman experienced in labor and delivery who provides support but not medical aid (unlike a nurse-midwife or a doctor). She focuses exclusively on the mother's needs and can help advocate the parents' preferences to the hospital staff. Use of an experienced doula is associated with fewer medical interventions, shorter labors, and a 50 percent reduction in the likelihood of a C-section. Ask your doctor for recommendations or contact a local birthing center. Most doulas charge a flat fee. Some insurance companies now cover their services, too.

• **Will you breast- or bottle-feed?** You don't need to make a hard-and-fast decision now, though it's wise to think through the options so you can best make preparations. Breast milk is considered by health experts to be best. In fact, the American Academy of Pediatrics suggests that new moms breastfeed for 6 months to 1 year or more for the optimal infant nutrition. Formula is a nutritionally sound alternative, although it lacks some of the infection-fighting properties that breast milk passes on to a newborn in the first weeks. You needn't stick to an either/or choice. Many mothers do both: they exclusively breastfeed at first (for anywhere from 6 weeks to 6 months), then switch to a bottle of expressed breast milk or formula. Others breastfeed with occasional bottle supplements or interchange breast milk and formula throughout the day.

Nursing provides impressive benefits for both mother and baby. Designed by nature to be the perfect nutrition for infants, breast milk passes along protective antibodies from the mother that guard the child against many diseases, including otitis media (ear infection) and diarrhea. The nutrients in mother's milk have been linked with higher IQ scores and a reduced likelihood of childhood asthma. And for you, producing the milk helps shrink the uterus to its pre-pregnancy size while burning extra calories, providing an edge in the battle to regain your pre-pregnancy figure. What's more, breastfeeding helps suppress ovulation and menstruation— aside from the birth-control assist this provides, having fewer ovulatory cycles has been associated with a decreased risk of cancer of the reproductive system and breasts. Women who nurse also have a reduced incidence of developing urinary tract infections and osteoporosis. A recent study even shows that breastfeeding an infant girl reduces her risk of breast cancer in later life.

Breastfeeding is also convenient in that you don't have to mess with bottles (mixing them, filling them, warming them, cleaning them). It's always ready, and free to boot. True, some women have trouble getting started nursing—like any new skill, it requires practice and patience—but once you and your baby have the hang of it, nursing is also very easy. Not least, breastfeeding is a lovely natural extension of pregnancy and childbirth, another amazing feat that your body was designed to do. For all these reasons, it's well worth planning on breastfeeding at the start. Then you can make a better informed decision about its longer-term suitability for both you and your baby.

You'll want to have on hand the phone number of a lactation consultant just in case you need advice. To find one, call your local La Leche League or ask your doctor, midwife, or childbirth educator. Taking a class or reading up on the subject can further prepare you. Stock up on nursing bras (at least three, to cover you when one is in the wash and another gets wet from leakage) and, to absorb leaks, breast pads (buy them at any drugstore or make your own from cotton fabric). Useful extras include nursing clothes with discreet openings, a comfortable rocker with a footstool, and a manual or electric pump for expressing milk, either to relieve fullness or to fill a bottle so someone else can take over an occasional feeding. To prepare your nipples for breastfeeding, stop using soap or perfumed lotion on them, because these products are drying; clean with plain warm water alone. If you have flat or inverted nipples, the last trimester is a good time to begin to stretch them manually or to use a breast shell that helps them protrude. Ask your doctor or childbirth educator to show you how. (See also "Breastfeeding Basics," page 303.)

If you plan to bottle-feed (either formula or pumped breast milk), you'll need a supply of bottles and nipples. Don't buy too many in advance, though. There are several different kinds and your choice may depend on your baby's preference. A bottle brush, a nipple brush, and a plastic cage for washing nipples and rings in the dishwasher are also useful. Ask your pediatrician which type of formula to buy, but, again, don't overstock until you see how well your baby accepts a particular brand. (See "Bottle-Feeding Basics," page 313.)

• **Will you circumcise your son?** Circumcision is the removal of a boy's foreskin, a layer of tissue that covers the head of the penis. The operation is usually performed within 48 hours of birth by an obstetrician in the hospital. In the Jewish tradition, it's done in a special ceremony on the eighth day after birth. Once routine in the United States, circumcision rates are declining. Some 62 percent of American boys are circumcised today; worldwide, however, 80 percent are not. (U.S. rates vary widely by region: the circumcision rate is 80 percent in the Midwest, 68 percent in the Northeast, 64 percent in the South, and 34 percent in the West.)

The decision is mostly a religious or cultural one, rather than a medical one. Research linking uncircumcised males to a greater incidence of urinary tract in-

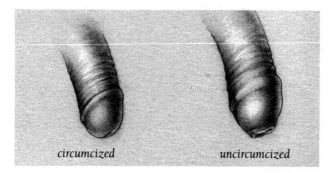

The majority of American boys—62 percent—are circumcised (left) *at birth. Worldwide, however, 80 percent of males are uncircumcised* (right).

circumcized   uncircumcized

fections and penile cancer is controversial, and both conditions are extremely rare. It's not true that it's harder to clean an uncircumcised penis. As for the argument that it can be traumatizing or upsetting for a boy not to look like his father, most psychologists now downplay this. The American Academy of Pediatrics has not recommended routine circumcision since 1989.

It's unclear how much pain the newborn feels during the procedure. While it's known that newborns not only do feel pain but also have a lower threshold for it than do adults, many doctors feel the event is forgotten as quickly as a pin-prick for a blood test. Anesthetic is increasingly used, though there is some concern whether this is safe for the baby; ask your doctor his or her advice. Some doctors reduce pain through acetaminophen or sugar-coated pacifiers, which have been shown to result in less crying afterward.

Your doctor will probably ask your preference before you deliver.

• **Who will be your baby's caregiver?** Strange as it may feel to scout a baby doctor before you have a baby, it's an essential job: you'll see this care provider a minimum of eight times in the first year alone—and that's just for well-child checkups. First you need to decide whether you will use (1) a pediatrician, a medical doctor with an additional 3 years specialized training in the care of children from newborn through adolescent; (2) a family physician, a medical doctor with an additional 3 years training in family medicine, including in-depth work on both children and adults; (3) a pediatric nurse practitioner, a registered nurse with added training in pediatric care who typically works in a pediatric medical group providing well-child care. This is a newer choice; in some states a pediatric nurse practitioner can work independently, with a referral relationship to a pediatrician.

Your friends with children are the best source of referrals. If you're new in town or the first in your crowd to procreate, ask around at your workplace or in your neighborhood. "Which doctor do you use?" is a good ice-breaker for meeting other moms, too. Your obstetrician or midwife may also make recommendations.

Factors to consider when choosing a pediatric caregiver include:

- **Location.** You won't want to spend any more time in transit than necessary with a sick child.
- **Size of practice.** If your doctor belongs to a large group practice, that tends to translate to expanded hours and prompt service. On the other hand, in groups you may not always get to see the doctor of your choice, whereas small offices ensure personal care. Find out if, and how, patients are rotated in a group practice.
- **Waiting time.** Can you get same-day appointments if your child is ill? Once you're in the office, will you be seen quickly? (Ask veteran parents for candid appraisals.) Larger group practices generally move patients more efficiently than one- or two-doc operations.
- **Office hours.** If you work, you may find evening and weekend hours a plus.
- **Atmosphere.** Are sick and well children segregated in different waiting rooms or seen at different hours? Does the place look child-friendly?
- **What happens when you have a nonemergency question?** Many practices set up a special free phone line staffed by nurses to handle nonemergency medical calls; at other offices, you can leave a message for your doctor, who returns calls at a certain point in the day. These conveniences can save the time and expense of an office visit, because you're bound to have plenty of tiny questions in the years ahead.
- **What happens in the event of an emergency?** Does another doctor respond if yours is unavailable? At which hospital does your doctor have privileges? If you live in a city with a children's hospital, it's best to have a doctor who's affiliated there because the staff has greater expertise in treating children and the equipment is scaled to smaller sizes. At the same time, you don't want to have to drive 45 minutes in an emergency, if you can avoid it, to reach your doctor's hospital. You'll also want to be sure the doctor you select has privileges at the hospital where you deliver, so he or she can perform the newborn and discharge exams on your baby.
- **Payment.** Check that your choice is covered by your health plan. Find out whether you're expected to pay at visits or if the office bills your insurance company directly. Note: Many health plans don't cover well-child checkups, which can mean a considerable outlay of cash for you; ask if the doctor offers installment pay plans.

It helps to interview more than one doctor for comparison's sake. Most do not charge for this prenatal visit. As you did when choosing an obstetric caregiver, get a sense of how well you like the doctor's manner, as well as his credentials, practices, and philosophies. Does he support breastfeeding? How does he feel about working mothers? Does he give written or verbal instructions? Does he give thorough, personalized answers or detached, rote ones? Find out the doctor's recommended schedule of well-baby visits so that you're clear when to bring your newborn in.

Checklist: Before You Deliver

Ready for baby? Take care of these details before the third trimester runs out on you:

☐ *Pack your bags.* Consult the checklist on page 211. Keep the suitcase near the door. To help you remember items you may still be using now (slippers, your glasses, a journal), keep a list of them on the top of the suitcase. That way you—or someone else in an emergency—can gather the last-minute items without forgetting anything.

☐ *Buy an infant car seat.* Start with the lightweight rear-facing kind designed for infants under 20 pounds. (Convertible seats made for infants and toddlers are usually too large to be entirely safe or comfortable for newborns and they're less portable; if you do use one, be sure to install it facing the rear.) Some brands of infant seats are made to snap out of a base; others can be easily unbuckled and carried out, a handy feature given how much young babies sleep, especially in cars. An optional insert pad designed to support the head will keep a tiny head from rolling around in the seat. Be sure you read the installment instructions provided with the car seat and use a locking clip if one is recommended. Always install a car seat in the back seat where there is no air bag; the middle of the car is safest.

☐ *Marshal your birth plan.* Put your preferences on paper or discuss them with your doctor. Copies of a written birth plan belong in your obstetrical records as well as in your suitcase (so you'll have a copy on hand in the delivery room just in case).

☐ *Preregister at the hospital.* You won't want to have to linger behind a desk once the contractions start.

☐ *Think through who will attend your birth.* It's becoming trendy for couples to invite their parents, older children, friends, and neighbors into the labor room. Think hard before you give all interested parties the green light, however. Birth is an intensely personal, inward time—you won't feel like playing hostess. Will, say, your dad's presence inhibit your ability to surrender to the primal urges of labor? How will you feel about the added noise, or about everyone watching if you need an episiotomy? A feeling of being watched has been shown to slow labor.

Kids under age 8 are too young to understand the pain of labor or to fully appreciate the magic of the event. They can be an unnecessary distraction. Most experts advise against young children's presence (though seeing the baby soon after it's born and cleaned up can be a wonderful way to bond and learn about birth). Even older children need careful preparation to attend a birth, as well as an adult (other than your partner) in charge of looking after them.

☐ *Rehearse your trip to the hospital.* Who will drive you? How will you alert your labor partner? Consider renting a cellular phone or pager to keep in touch. Enlist alternate drivers (such as a neighbor or taxi service) in case your partner can't be reached, and keep their phone numbers handy. Be sure you know the way, including options for rush hour and what you'll do in case of problems such as snow. Make sure there's enough gas in the car at all times. Also be sure you know exactly where to enter the hospital. If you have an older child, have several backup plans for childcare. If you're a city dweller, don't attempt to hail a cab yourself because drivers might not stop, fearing they'll wind up delivering the baby themselves.

☐ *Pick out birth announcements.* You may not have all the data yet, but the more work you can do on this task in advance, the better. Your options basically are (1) printed announcements (you select the design in advance at a stationery shop and phone in the name, birth date, and vital statistics; they're ready 24 hours to 2 weeks from when you place your final order); (2) preprinted announcements with blanks that you fill in by hand (which are less expensive but more labor-intensive); and (3) do-it-yourself announcements (the most personal but also the most time-consuming; best left to creative types or those who won't feel strange or guilty if all recipients have already met the baby by the time they get the announcement).

Whichever you choose, pick up and address the envelopes now. Computer-friendly parents can send announcements via electronic mail to connected friends and relatives, but since it's not likely that every interested party is on-line, you'll still want some of the traditional paper variety.

Some innovative announcement ideas: Draw one yourself or let an older child do the decorating (leave a space for the baby's snapshot) and color-Xerox it; design it by computer; or handpaint a onesie or bib with the key info and photograph your newborn wearing it. Some stationers can also print candy-bar wrappers that herald the news.

☐ *Stock up on items you'll need after delivery.* The most frequently forgotten: maximum-size sanitary pads (to absorb postpartum discharge, which will be considerable); breast pads; lanolin (to soothe cracked nipples); rubbing alcohol (to clean the umbilical stump); prepackaged snacks and drinks (crackers, granola bars, juice, for convenience); thank-you notes and stamps; a reliable infant-care guide; a week's worth of newborn diapers (count on using 8 to 10 a day; some brands are shaped to leave the umbilical stump uncovered, which is handy for the first week or so).

Nice extras: A cordless phone (or an answering machine set to a minimal number of rings so you can catch calls at your convenience), a breakfast tray (for holding the phone, food, books, and the TV remote—freeing both your hands for holding the baby), and extra nightgowns (between breast milk and spit up, you'll feel like changing *your* clothes almost as often as your baby's).

☐ *Line up postpartum help.* Count on living a zombie's life for the first few weeks. It's imperative to have 24-hour, live-in help when you return from the hospital, whether it's your spouse, your mom, or someone else. If you can afford it, professional postpartum doulas assist with lactation advice, baby care, and recovery; like doulas who act as labor companions, their job is essentially to "mother the mother." Cook ahead and freeze meals, while you have the energy, and welcome all offers to bring you hot meals after the baby's birth.

Checklist: Best Shower Gifts to Ask For

You'll be inundated with tiny undershirts and sleepers—few well-wishers can resist them. And if you know you're expecting a girl, you can count on receiving your fair share of sweet, beribboned dresses. But here's what your baby *really* can use:

☐ *A monitor.* It transmits sounds (some more expensive types can also transmit a video image) short distances from the nursery. A must if your home has two stories, but even in an apartment, you may not trust your ears.

☐ *A wearable soft carrier.* Many babies find these soothing for the first few months. Some sling designs cradle the baby and make nursing convenient; others allow the baby to snuggle against your chest, facing you or facing outward. Hip-slung models let you comfortably carry a baby into toddlerdom, but they aren't really suitable until the baby sits up. Some parents like metal-frame backpacks once a baby can sit up.

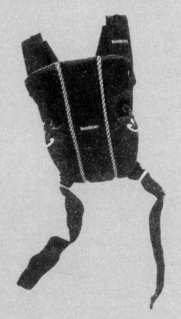

☐ *An infant seat.* The best models for young infants recline slightly and allow the baby to rock or bounce (hence the name "bouncy seat"). A removable bar of toys can be set in the baby's line of vision for entertainment.

☐ *Toiletry essentials.* Baby-size washcloths, hooded towels, mild baby shampoo and soap, infant nail clippers and scissors, diaper rash ointment, a soft hairbrush.

A wearable soft front carrier allows you to go about your daily activities without leaving your baby behind.

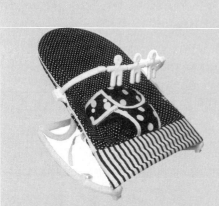

An infant seat is an ideal spot for your baby to eat, sleep, or just soak up the sights.

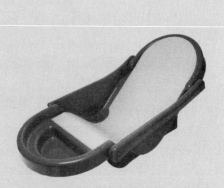

A baby can't go into a big tub until he can sit up on his own. In the meantime, you can keep your newborn squeaky clean in a baby bathtub.

☐ *A humidifier.* Pediatricians recommend these devices to moisten the air when your child has a cold. Humidifiers release cool air and are safer to leave in the room with an older child than the old-fashioned vaporizers, which heat water to create steam, because they can't cause burns if touched or tipped.

☐ *A tympanic (ear) thermometer.* Though not always reliable for use under 6 months, they give quick readings in an infinitely easier way than thermometers used rectally, orally, or by armpit on children of all other ages. Expensive but worth asking for now.

☐ *A baby bathtub and a tub seat.* A molded-plastic tub, large sponge, or bathinette will be used during the first 6 months or so for sponge baths; these tubs hold or prop baby securely. Once the child sits up solo, he or she graduates to the big tub, but a special seat makes the job easier. Most tub seats are circular, with suction cups that secure the seat to the tub and a rail to keep baby safe.

☐ *A baby swing.* Some feature carriage beds that allow even a newborn to swing gently while lying down. At the least, you want a reclining seat that's comfortable for a young baby and that can be positioned upright later.

□ *A play yard.* You may remember them as play *pens* (they've been re-named to soften some parents' concerns that they're too confining). An ideal, safe play space for babies while you dash to the bathroom or try to get something done, they also make a handy extra bed when traveling. Best are newer mesh-sided play yards that fold down in seconds. If you buy a used or older model, check to make sure that there are no tears in the mesh on which a baby could get snagged (a strangulation hazard) and that any wooden slats are spaced no more than 2³/₈ inches apart.

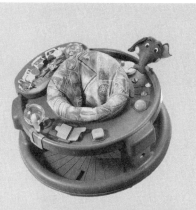

Stationary walkers—far safer than the walkers that can be moved around the room—let a baby entertain herself.

□ *A toy bar.* This is a freestanding bar of dangling toys that a small baby can see while lying down on the floor. Some models include a mat and can be folded up. Sometimes the toys are removable, which means you can change them periodically to add interest. Other great "toys" for young babies include a large unbreakable mirror and a play mat that features different textures and colors.

□ *A stroller.* The handiest type is a convertible model that folds flat to carriage position (for newborns and for sleeping older babies) as well as upright to a seat. It's even better if it has a hood and an adjustable handle that allows you to push from either side, which helps shield sun from the baby's eyes. If you or your partner are tall, check for stroller handles that are a comfortable height; some models can be fitted with handle extenders. Though you can't use a lightweight umbrella stroller until the baby is sitting up well, they're worth asking for. Many moms keep a spare stashed in the car trunk at all times.

□ *A high chair.* No, your baby won't need it for months. But he or she will eventually, making it a gift worth asking for. Plastic models are easiest to clean; some adjust to different heights or convert to a regular chair as the child grows.

☐ *A crib light.* These small, low-wattage lights attach to a crib or changing table, providing you with just enough illumination to check on a sleeping baby or change a nighttime diaper. (Not for use in cribs once the baby can sit or pull up.)

☐ *Clothing in larger sizes.* The darling zero to 3-month sizes will be ready for storage in weeks, and you'll welcome having replacements on hand. If you're expecting a girl, pass the word that she can use playclothes and sweats, so you don't receive only dressy dresses.

☐ *A diaper-disposal method.* Whether you use a diaper pail or the newer systems that compact and individually wrap dirty disposables (and reduce—but don't entirely eliminate—odors), you'll want one for each diaper-changing post. The best pails have a locking handle so they can't be opened by a curious baby.

☐ *Diapers.* The ideal gift because duplicates are no problem; you can never have too many. Count on going through 80 to 100 disposables in the first week. For cloth diapers, three to four dozen is a good startup supply (plus four to six diaper covers). Even if you use disposables, cloth diapers makes great burp rags for catching spit up.

What you don't *need:* A baby walker. In 1993 alone, 25,000 babies suffered walker-related injuries, particularly when the walker tumbled downstairs. There's no evidence that these devices actually promote walking, either. A better bet is an exercise/activity center that lets older babies use their legs to spin, bounce, and move—while remaining safely in place. Cheaper still is to spread a blanket on the floor along with a few brightly colored toys, which will promote scooting and pre-crawling motions.

IS IT TRUE...

That it's considered bad taste to list gift wishes on a shower invitation? Formally speaking, yes. That's because, even though everyone knows the purpose of a shower is to flood an expectant mom with baby gifts, issuing a list of wants to every guest with a party invitation smacks of blatant greed and extortion. Better to pass the word through the grapevine about what you really want. Furnish your hostess with a list, or let her tell invitees if you're registered at a department or specialty store. One other shower etiquette no-no, at least according to most manners mavens: never throw yourself a shower or let a member of your immediate family (such as your mom) host the event, for the same reason—it just looks greedy.

Checklist: What to Pack for Delivery

For the Mother

- ☐ Washable nightgown or T-shirt to labor in (better still, wear the hospital-issue gown, since it could get bloodstained)
- ☐ Nightgown for after delivery (you'll feel fresher in your own; splurge on one with special nursing openings)
- ☐ Slippers with nonslip soles
- ☐ Thick socks (to wear in labor; your feet will get cold)
- ☐ Robe (so you can walk the maternity floor)
- ☐ Toiletries (including shampoo, toothbrush and paste, and cosmetics)
- ☐ Two bras (nursing bras if you plan to breastfeed) and several pairs of panties you won't mind getting stained (in your pregnancy size)
- ☐ Sanitary napkins of the heaviest absorbency (*not* tampons); even if the hospital provides napkins, they may be the old-fashioned belted kind
- ☐ Eyeglasses (you'll want to remove contact lenses)
- ☐ Hair ties or combs (if you have long hair)
- ☐ Extra pillows
- ☐ Lip balm
- ☐ Hard candies (to keep your mouth moist)
- ☐ A favorite photo or object to use as a focal point in labor (some women can focus on a spot on the wallpaper, others use their partner's eyes)
- ☐ Baby book (for getting hand- or footprints and recording immediate thoughts)
- ☐ Light diversions (magazines, books, birth announcements to fill out)

- ☐ Comfort objects for you (a favorite sweater, a stuffed animal, a picture of an older child)
- ☐ Clothes to wear home (a loose maternity dress or a big shirt and maternity pants; you'll probably still be about your seventh-month size)

For Your Labor Support Partner

- ☐ Labor assists: massage oil, music (cassette player and tapes), labor handbook or notes
- ☐ Address book and long-distance calling card (shortcut: prepare a must-call list of names and numbers, in order of priority)
- ☐ Video or still camera, with tape or film (don't forget spare batteries)
- ☐ Snacks (the hospital cafeteria may be closed at night, or you may not want your partner to disappear in search of sustenance if your labor is long)
- ☐ Coins for phones and vending machines
- ☐ Health insurance and hospital preregistration information
- ☐ Change of clothes and toiletries if you're planning on staying overnight
- ☐ Swimsuit (in case your partner joins you in the shower or tub during labor)

For Your Baby

- ☐ Clothes for the trip home, including undershirt, spare diapers, sleeper, socks, hat, outer clothes, and receiving blanket (if you're expecting a large baby or are overdue, bring a few different outfits—some newborn-size garments may be too small)
- ☐ Rear-facing infant car seat (it's the law in all 50 states; most hospitals won't discharge you unless they see you've got one)

For More Help: Resources to Help You Prepare

- National Organization of Circumcision Information Resource Centers, P.O. Box 2512, San Anselmo, CA 94979; 415-488-9883 or http://www.naric.org. Anti-circumcision educational pamphlets.
- American Academy of Pediatrics, P.O. Box 927, Elk Grove Village, IL 60009; 847-228-5005 or http://www.aap.org. Educational brochures and fact sheets on children's health and psychosocial issues.
- La Leche League International, 1400 North Meacham Road, Schaumburg, IL 60173-4048; 800-LALECHE (800-525-3243). Check your phone book for local listings. Also, http://www.lalecheleague.org. Worldwide support, education, and information for breastfeeding women. For recorded advice, call the breastfeedling helpline at 900-448-7475, ext. 55 (there is a charge). Check your phone book for local listings.
- Doulas of North America, 1100 23rd Avenue E., Seattle, WA 98112; 206-324-5440 or http://www.dona.com. Provides doula referrals and informational brochures.

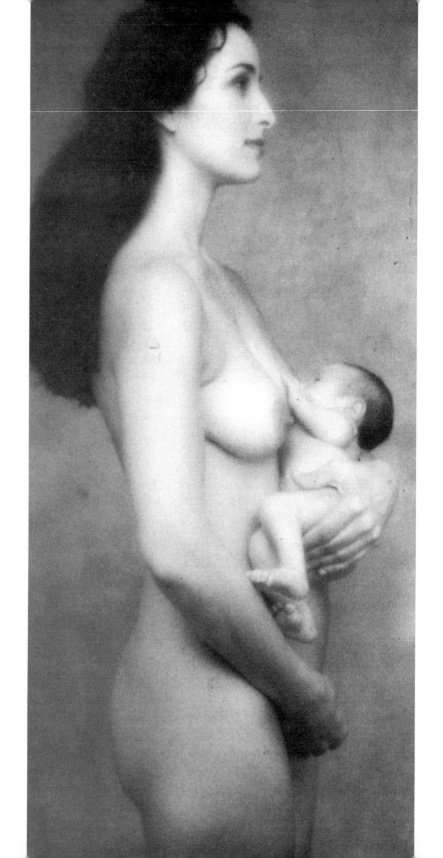

CHAPTER 4

YOUR BABY'S BIRTH

LABOR AND DELIVERY

By the time you've reached the brink of motherhood, you're uniquely positioned to appreciate just what a miracle birth is. First, a mother's egg and a father's sperm must dodge an obstacle course of structural, biochemical, and timing barriers in order to unite. To develop properly, the new, life-bearing cluster of cells that they form must sidestep countless perils, both within (genetic misfires, uterine problems) and without (poisons, bacteria). Continuing to thrive depends on just-right conditions and constant care.

Then, after nine months' cocooning, the fetus's mind and body mature to full readiness. For reasons that remain a mystery to researchers, something clicks in the fetal brain's hypothalamus. It's time to be born. Hormonal messages are dispatched more urgently than at any time since conception. The uterine muscles are cued to contract, the cervix widens, the baby heads down the birth canal—and emerges to take his or her first breath on earth. Or at least, that's what's supposed to happen. As was true throughout pregnancy, dozens of tiny variations in this scheme—from the fetus's position to the mother's health—must be navigated en route to a safe birth.

Awesome? Daunting? More thrilling than a James Bond escape? You bet.

But rest assured, millions of healthy babies trump the odds to burst into the human race every year. As was true of pregnancy, no two labors are exactly alike. By preparing yourself for what's ahead, you can boost your confidence, ease lingering fears, and smooth your way to the happy ending: cradling your newborn for the first time.

Once your baby's head crowns, the action usually proceeds quickly. It may only be a matter of minutes before you and your newborn will start to get acquainted. Your partner (and in some cases you) may even have the opportunity to cut the umbilical cord.

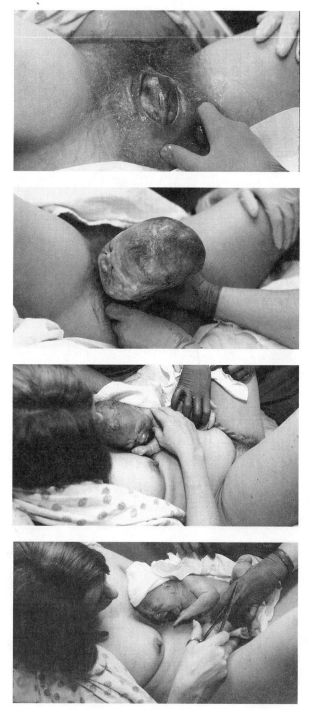

The Right Attitude

Common Worries About Labor

There comes a time late in every woman's pregnancy when she realizes that not only must the baby come out soon, but that the only routes are through her vagina or (in a Cesarean delivery) through her abdomen. Ouch! No wonder nervousness about labor tempers the excitement most first-time expectant mothers feel as their due date approaches.

Not only is apprehension perfectly natural but you're the exception if you don't experience a certain degree of it. Common anxieties include:

• *Fear of pain.* "How much will it hurt?" That's the million-dollar question everyone wants the answer to. While it's virtually impossible to go through a dress rehearsal for labor pain, confronting the idea—rather than ignoring it—puts you ahead of the game. (See "All About Pain," page 249.)

• *Fear of hospital procedures.* "What will they do to me?" Each individual tolerates medical procedures differently; some simply fear the loss of a certain amount of autonomy, privacy, and modesty that goes with the turf. (See "At the Hospital," page 224.)

• *Fear of loss of control.* "Will I swear at my husband in front of my doctor?" "Will I need an emergency Cesarean?" Not knowing what to expect in labor opens up the possibility that, well, anything may happen. That can be especially unnerving for control freaks who like plans or who pride themselves on being composed and in command.

• *Fear of failure.* "Will my labor be less than perfect, somehow?" "Will I let down my husband/midwife/mother?" The standard set by such worriers is usually self-imposed and unrealistic. It's often the result of comparisons to a friend who had a mere 2-hour labor, or a sister who went 24 hours with no medications, regardless of all the extenuating circumstances that shaped that individual's experience. Or the woman may be a perfectionist who's reluctant to fall short of the ideal birth experience that she learned about in a childbirth class.

• *Fear of a crisis.* "Will my baby be all right?" Even if the baby is kicking away in the ready-to-go, head-down position, most pregnant mothers worry that all's not well till it ends well. The specter of "what if" lurks until the healthy baby is safely in her arms.

• **Fear of death.** "Will I make it?" It's the ultimate fear of the unknown. Husbands share this worry, knowing their partners will be facing a physical feat they can barely imagine. Indeed, childbirth used to be a life-or-death experience in the days before anyone knew about proper hygiene or how to handle common complications. But this is the last thing you need to worry about today. Maternal deaths are exceedingly rare (8 per 100,000 births), and such cases are nearly always extremely high-risk pregnancies.

Easing Fears

Aside from reassuring yourself that everyone worries (at least a little) about labor, how can you deal with such feelings? First, surrender to the reality that you can't stage-manage completely what nature has in store for you. The size and shape of your pelvis, the size of the baby, and the pace at which your labor progresses are beyond your control.

Research has shown, however, that certain common denominators seem to strongly shape a woman's attitude toward her birth experience. The following factors can help you approach birth more optimistically—and wind up with more positive feelings about the experience afterward:

• **Expect pain—but don't be intimidated by it.** Labor hurts. Period. It's a truth that can't be ignored. (Okay, a small fraction of women report little or no intense pain, though they are far and away the exception. You *might* be lucky enough to be among them, but since you won't know for sure until showtime, you're better off preparing yourself to feel some significant amount of pain.) Surprisingly, however, research has found that lack of knowledge about the painfulness of labor is precisely what ends up terrifying women most. Sometimes the mother-to-be's own mother or friends downplay the reality so as not to scare her. Some women consciously choose to ignore all thoughts of labor (the "Oh, I'll just have them knock me out so what does it matter" school). But such blindness puts women at a disadvantage. Surprised by the intensity of their contractions, they mistakenly believe something must be amiss, escalating their anxiety and, in turn, their perception of pain. It's a vicious cycle.

There's an old saying that women get what they expect in labor. No one can predict the unique ups and downs of a particular delivery, of course. But if you go into labor expecting it to hurt—probably worse than anything you've ever experienced before—you'll be in the most receptive state of mind to confront that pain and deal with it.

• **Be prepared.** Whether you go natural or choose pain-relieving medication, a childbirth education class will help you understand the basics of birth and the options you face. You'll also get valuable reassurance about the likelihood of a safe, healthy delivery. Frightening as it may seem to contemplate less than ideal labors, it does help to know what *might* go wrong and how such possibilities would be handled. Preparation for birth has been shown to ease pain, enhance relaxation, and lead to better overall feelings about birth.

• *Exert control but be open-minded.* There are actually two types of control that give laboring women a sense of mastery: personal self-control (the kind you get through pain-management techniques) and situational control (having a degree of autonomy about everything from your body's positioning to whether you get to wear your glasses to watch the delivery). Situational control depends a lot on your choice of healthcare provider and birth setting and on your ability to make your wishes known. That's where a written birth plan comes in handy, along with a partner who shares your goals and can advocate them on your behalf.

At the same time, you must be flexible enough to alter your plans as conditions require. Such an attitude is also freeing: you can spare yourself from destructive self-recriminations that you've failed should anything not go according to plan. Your goal, after all, is not to be a superstar in labor—it's to be a mother.

• *Have support you trust.* It's no wonder that women harbor strong memories of their doctors and nurses 20 years or more after giving birth. Research has shown that the kind of support received in labor is one of the most critical factors in a woman's degree of satisfaction with the experience—more indelible than such factors as how long or hard the labor was. Whether your support comes from your mate, a friend, a professional labor assistant (such as a doula), or a labor-delivery nurse—or some combination thereof—your ability to completely surrender to the moment and be yourself can actually speed labor. Birth is a primal event. Especially in an unfamiliar hospital setting, feeling comfortable enough to let go is important.

Have confidence in your doctor or midwife, too. Not a blind trust, so that you automatically go along with every decision even if you don't understand it or agree with it; that kind of attitude backfires into fear. Rather, develop the sort of confidence that comes from being informed and treated with respect, making you better able to trust in a more experienced judgment should push come to shove.

• *Trust yourself.* Your labor-support team's job is to make you as relaxed and comfortable as possible. But a final measure of confidence comes only from within: your faith in yourself. Giving birth is a bit like attempting to scale a mountain or write a novel or piece together a quilt. Before you start, the task seems monumental, intimidating. But something inside you thinks you can do it, so you take a step, write a word, sew a stitch, or power through your first contraction. And you believe in your ability to keep going.

The Fashion Factor

No, we're not talking maternity clothes here. Like every other social convention, childbirth is subject to the ever-changing whims of culture, history, technology, and herd mentality. That means that the prevailing beliefs about birth today aren't carved in stone. Birth fashions change from decade to decade, from place to place—and from woman to woman.

One hundred years ago, home births attended by other women were standard in the United States. Fifty years ago, moms-to-be were routinely knocked out with powerful drugs known as "twilight sleep" while their husbands paced in hospital waiting rooms down the hall. Twenty-five years ago, an enema, a pubic shave, and strapped-down limbs were as much a part of labor as contractions. Ten years later, the pendulum swung in the direction of drug-free, even pain-free deliveries as the ideal (if not the reality), with fathers-to-be fully expected to be at their partners' sides.

Today, childbirth is characterized by choices. Epidural anesthesia is used by the majority of laboring women in the United States, but those who prefer natural childbirth rarely need to fight for the privilege anymore. C-section rates hover at 20 to 25 percent, but at the same time, more second-time moms than ever try VBACs (vaginal births after Cesareans). Midwives and homey maternity centers have gone mainstream. Depending on how vocal and persistent you are, as well as on your health and your baby's, the factors up for grabs include where you deliver, who attends you, what you eat and wear, how you cope with pain, what kinds of interventions you have, what positions you labor in, and what you'd like your first hours with your baby to be like.

This abundance of choice means that this is the best time to be giving birth in America ever. Medical advances are on your side—but so, thankfully, is the recognition that birth is a natural event over which women deserve to have control and be treated with respect. To be sure, not every doctor or every hospital will be as enlightened as the next. And it can't be stressed enough how much individual labors differ. Nevertheless, you *can* psyche yourself up with the confident knowledge that this is an experience to face with as much excitement and faith as healthy apprehension.

That I'll have a shorter labor if my mother did? Alas, a quick-opening cervix is not something you inherit. In general, first labors last about 14 hours, although it's not uncommon for them to go on for 24 or even 36 hours. Subsequent labors tend to be shorter because the cervix dilates more readily and the pelvic wall is already stretched a bit; also, experienced moms tend not to arrive as early at the hospital (where labor can slow if you're lying in bed or have an epidural too soon) and they know better how to push. Exception: if your second birth is vaginal, after a prior C-section, the labor will be more like a first labor.

That my doctor can't predict when I'll go into labor? As convenient as that information would be, physicians and midwives have only your physical clues such as the baby's position and the thinning, softening, and opening of the cervix to go by—but no conclusive proof pointing to a specific week, day, or hour. Everyone experiences both the onset of labor and the pace of labor itself differently. A medical specialist—no matter how experienced—who makes promises about when you'll deliver (unless, of course, it's a scheduled C-section) isn't doing you any favors.

That fewer babies are born on Sundays? Yes. According to the National Center for Health Statistics, one-fifth fewer deliveries take place on weekends, while Tuesdays and Fridays are boom days for births. How to explain the low ebb on Sundays? Simple: fewer C-sections and induced labors scheduled for weekends, when doctors, like the rest of us, like to have time off from work.

That more babies are born in summer? Statistically, births peak in August. Experts suspect that couples tend to be more amorous during the holidays—some 9 months earlier. Or maybe Thanksgiving turkey is an aphrodisiac.

Is This It?

Signs of Labor

In the movies, labor starts dramatically and unmistakably. The mom-to-be clutches her middle, announces "It's time!" and ignites her mate to a comic frenzy of activity. More typical in real life, however, especially for first-time mothers, is a scene that unfolds much more slowly. How will you recognize the onset of labor if you've never experienced it before? Happily, your body provides you with several warm-up clues. For most first-timers, these events occur so gradually that you may wonder whether you're really in labor or not. But they may also happen precipitously, almost all at once.

The signs of labor include:

• **The baby drops (*lightening*).** The baby's head settles into the birth canal anywhere from a few weeks to a few hours before labor begins.

• **The mucus plug dislodges (*the bloody show*).** The mucus plug is a thick seal that has protected your cervix against infection throughout pregnancy. As the cervix begins to widen, usually a few hours to a few days before labor begins, the plug dislodges. It may come out as a thick, slightly bloodied mass of mucus, or if the plug has been pushed into the vagina, you may just see increased vaginal discharge that can range in color from clear to pink to brown (also called "show"). Or a thicker-than-usual, mucusy discharge may be seen over a period of several days. You may not notice your mucus plug at all if it dislodges after your contractions have begun.

• **Contractions begin.** Picture your uterus as a wine bottle whose spout is the cervix. In order for your baby to be born, the neck must widen so that the bottle changes its shape to resemble a wide-mouth mayonnaise jar. A contraction is simply the involuntary tightening and relaxing of the long muscles that wrap around the uterus. As these muscles contract, they shorten, pulling up the muscles at the bottommost part of the uterus, around the cervix, causing them to gradually open. In this manner, the cervix widens enough for the baby to work his or her way out.

At first, you may feel the contractions as painlessly as any other muscle movement in your body. They then build in intensity. Depending on the phase of labor, each contraction lasts between 30 and 90 seconds. They come at fairly regular intervals that are usually widely spaced at first (anywhere from 10 to 20 minutes apart), then at closer and closer intervals.

Your doctor will have briefed you on when to call, usually when contractions are a specific distance apart (about 5 to 7 minutes, though the recommendation will vary, depending on your distance from the hospital, the time of day, or your history). *Always* let your doctor know when your water breaks (see page 223). If you have a high-risk pregnancy or if you have labor symptoms prior to 37 weeks, alert your doctor as soon as you think you're in labor. (Labor before 37 weeks is considered preterm labor, which places the fetus at increased risk.) When in doubt, call anyway. An internal exam can verify that your cervix is dilating. If you're deemed not to be in labor, or only in its earliest stages, you can return home to await more vivid signs as restfully as possible.

• *The membranes rupture (water breaks).* In the womb, the fetus floats in a sac of amniotic fluid. When the membranes that form the sac rupture—which can occur a few hours before labor or anytime during it—you may hear a pop, like a champagne cork. Warm liquid may gush profusely or, if the baby's head is blocking the flow, dribble out only slightly. As much as a quart of liquid may be released, and you continue to produce new fluid until delivery. (This means you're going to feel thirsty and should drink plenty of water or clear juices to replace your fluid stores.) If you're at home, place a clean towel between your legs to absorb the flow. Use a towel or thick sanitary pad when you walk. Some women prefer to place a plastic cover on their mattresses in the last month of pregnancy, just in case.

Take a look at the fluid that's released. It should be pale to clear. If you can see traces of green or brown, the amniotic fluid contains meconium, or fetal wastes. This can be a sign of fetal stress, so be sure to inform your doctor when you call to report that your water has broken.

If you're not certain your water has broken, the doctor can do one of two tests. In one, a sample of the fluid is placed on a special paper; if it changes color, it is indeed amniotic fluid. Alternatively, dried fluid is examined under a microscope; amniotic fluid will form a distinctive fernlike pattern.

Despite women's obsession with this dramatic sign of labor, in most cases water doesn't break until late in active labor. Often it must be done by the doctor with a special hooked tool in a painless procedure called an *amniotomy.* Only in about 1 in 10 women do the membranes rupture before the onset of significant, recognizable contractions (which is called *premature rupture of membranes,* or PROM). A combination of factors cause PROM, including contractions, the strength of the membranes, and inflammation of the membranes. Expect contractions to escalate in their intensity once the amniotic sac has ruptured.

What happens next depends on your caregiver. When membranes rupture at or near term, 90 percent of women go into labor on their own within 12 to 24 hours. But because studies indicate an increased risk of infection in the amniotic sac if the baby is not born within that length of time, many doctors will induce labor if it doesn't start spontaneously within a certain number of hours (often 4 to 6) after the water breaks. Other doctors feel there is little risk of infection if precautions are taken (no vaginal exams, no baths, no intercourse—all of which could introduce bacteria into the sterile uterine environment) and allow a woman more time to await spontaneous labor, up to 2 days. Current research indicates that the rates of infections among newborns whose mothers experience PROM are the same whether labor is induced or nature is allowed to take its course.

Your doctor needs to know when your water breaks. Depending on your stage of labor and whether the baby's head has engaged into the birth canal (which he or she would know from your weekly check-ups), he or she may want to examine you. A rather rare but possible danger is that the umbilical cord can precede the baby's head in the birth canal (a condition called a *prolapsed cord*). This would threaten the baby's oxygen supply and warrants an emergency C-section. If the head has already dropped, however, you may be advised to stay at home until your labor picks up pace.

• **Possible other signs.** Less absolute, but pretty good tip-offs that labor is on its way include the following: In the days before labor begins, painless Braxton-Hicks contractions may become more noticeable and more frequent. Your abdominal area may feel sore, a bit like premenstrual achiness. A dull low backache is also common (though most women experience this throughout the third trimester). Some women notice sharp pains or soreness along their upper thighs for a day or two, caused when the pressure of the baby's head against the pelvis compresses nerves to the area. You may experience hot flashes—a warm flush that rises over your upper body and head, making you briefly uncomfortable, even sweaty.

Once labor is imminent, you'll probably feel the need to clear your bowels frequently or pass loose stool, possibly diarrhea. Despite these discomforts, a final burst of energy is characteristic a day or two before labor begins—an overwhelming, totally irrational urge to compulsively clean or make things ready for the baby, like organizing the linen closet or mopping the nursery floor one last time. (You can tell it's prelabor nesting if you're not much of a neat freak and suddenly can't help yourself.) *Don't* overdo it if this irresistible impulse strikes—you'll need all the energy you can muster for childbirth.

At the Hospital

Ideally, you've preregistered during your third trimester, allowing you to bypass time-consuming paperwork. On arrival, you'll be directed to the labor-and-delivery unit and given an identification band. Most women are given a hospital gown to wear, unless you've prearranged to wear your own nightshirt. (Remember, though, it may get stained beyond redemption.)

The first thing that happens is that a doctor or nurse does an internal exam to evaluate the progress of your labor, usually in a special exam room. If your cervix is not very dilated, you may be sent back home or instructed to walk around longer and return when contractions are more intense. If your water has broken, however, you're considered officially in labor and may be admitted without an exam.

A labor nurse will be assigned to you throughout her shift. Her job is to make sure you're comfortable, monitor vital signs, conduct periodic labor checks, keep your doctor apprised of the situation and execute his or her orders, and provide labor support. The nurse may be assigned to you exclusively or be monitoring as many as three other patients. Most obstetricians follow your progress through the nurse and check in with patients only briefly until the final stages of labor. If you have a midwife and/or a doula or coach, these individuals will be at your side throughout the delivery; with the exception of the midwife, though, they do no medical monitoring.

Depending on the facility, you may labor, deliver, and recover all in one room. Or you may labor in one place and be moved to a delivery room (which looks like an operating room) once the baby's head becomes visible (or *crowns*), then recover in a third location. All rooms designed for childbirth are equipped with special beds that have handles against which you can brace yourself, stirrups to elevate the legs during pushing, and adjustable positionings for the head and feet, since most women shift around periodically as they labor. The lower portion of such beds can break away to facilitate delivery. Some delivery rooms also offer high-tech birthing chairs or bars for squatting to aid an upright delivery. The best rooms will also have a rocking chair, a shower, and a Jacuzzi-style birthing tub to give you more options during labor. But don't feel confined to your assigned room. If you feel like walking around the floor during early labor, do so.

The preparations (or "preps") you receive on admittance to the hospital depend on the facility in which you're giving birth and its protocols, on your doctor or midwife, on your own preferences, and on the progress of your pregnancy. If you are expecting twins or have a high-risk condition such as gestational diabetes, for example, you may require more monitoring than someone in a routine delivery.

Some of the preps and procedures you may encounter include:

• *An intravenous line (IV)*. Once automatic, this is now optional at more and more hospitals. The purpose of an IV is to deliver fluid, nutrients, medication, or blood (in the event of an emergency) to the laboring woman. Having an IV in place can save valuable time, preventing injury to the baby in an emergency. A needle surrounded by plastic tubing is inserted into a vein in your arm or the back of your hand; the tubing connects to a bag of liquid (usually glucose, which is sugar and water) on a tall stand. If you've expressed a preference for an epidural, you will definitely be given an IV, whereas one may not be necessary if you're attempting a natural childbirth.

The problem with an IV is that it can restrict mobility or be cumbersome to move about with, unnecessary restrictions in a normal labor if the mother is receiving adequate liquid through ice chips or juice. Doctors sometimes insist on an IV "just in case." One compromise is a *heparin lock*, which is an IV needle and short tube inserted in your arm but not attached to tubing or a stand (the heparin is a local blood thinner that keeps the vein open).

• **Vaginal exams.** Your labor progress will be checked periodically by a nurse or doctor, beginning when you arrive at the hospital. To evaluate cervical thinning and dilatation, a medical staffer inserts two sterile gloved fingers into the vagina to determine, by finger measurement, how many centimeters wide the cervical opening is. It must expand to 10 centimeters, its maximum stretch, before you can safely begin pushing the baby out. (For example, you may hear the attendant say, "You're six," which is the shorthand for 6 centimeters dilated.) The doctor, nurse, or midwife also checks the baby's *station*. This is a measure of how far engaged the baby's head is into the birth canal, as compared to the pelvic ischial bones. A "minus station" means the baby is still high, above these distinctive bones. A "plus station" means the baby's head is below the bones. At plus-6, the head is crowning (or visible through the vaginal opening). Though they try to do the exam between contractions, lying still for it can be uncomfortable. Using your relaxation exercises can help. Be sure to ask for a progress report if the information is not volunteered.

• **Fetal heart-rate monitoring.** The medical team needs to track the baby's progress during the stress of childbirth. There are several ways to do this. (1) *Auscultation* is a simple, low-tech method in which the fetal heartbeat is intermittently listened to through the abdomen with a special stethoscope or handheld Doppler ultrasound device. You must remain still during the checkups only. (2) *External electronic monitoring* provides more detailed information on how the baby's heartbeat is responding to contractions. While you recline in bed, two cloth belts are placed around your abdomen. One belt records contractions and the other monitors the baby's heart rate. Measurements can be taken for 20 minutes of each hour or, in most cases, continuously. (3) *Internal electronic monitoring* is the most precise and can be done only after your water has broken. A small electrode at the end of a thin catheter is attached to the baby's scalp (through the cervix) to assess his or her heart rate. Sometimes another tube is inserted in the uterus to measure the strength of contractions. You have to stay in bed while being monitored internally. Exception: a *telemetry unit* allows you to move freely. A catheter is attached to the baby's scalp, but the portable telemetry unit, which sends radio waves containing the information to a video screen at the nurse's station, can be slung over your shoulder or carried by your partner. (The catheter is so thin it doesn't interfere with walking or urination.) The information gleaned from both external and internal electronic monitors is relayed to a machine that traces the intensity of contractions on a long, continuous sheet of paper and shows the heart rate on a video screen.

More than three-fourths of labors are electronically monitored today. It's done in part as a precaution to quickly detect fetal distress and partly as a way to ensure physicians better protection against malpractice. Women with epidurals or those who are attempting vaginal births after Cesareans are routinely monitored continuously. The risks to the baby are minimal, chiefly the possibility of infection from an internal monitor, although this is extremely rare and easily treated. On the other hand, several major studies indicate that electronically monitored labors are more likely to end in C-sections—and that the surgery is not always warranted, since the vast majority of the distress signals picked up are not life threatening. (For example, an abnormal heart pattern may not be caused by a lack of oxygen and therefore may not signal anything serious.) Electronically monitored labors, especially continuously monitored ones, tend to take longer because lying in bed often slows the progress of contractions. What's more, studies show that babies monitored by auscultation were found to be just as healthy as those monitored electronically. The bottom line: fetal monitoring is a low-risk way of catching some problems, but hasn't been shown to improve birth outcomes for women experiencing normal labors. If you're concerned about it interfering with your mobility when you're attempting a natural delivery and are low-risk, discuss your options (such as auscultation, intermittent monitoring, or telemetry) with your doctor or midwife before labor begins.

One plus to electronic monitoring is that you can use it to follow your contractions—when they're coming and when they've peaked—which can eliminate some of their fear-provoking mystery. Be aware that you don't have to lie perfectly still while being monitored. Changing positions in bed or lying on your side may cause brief blips in the read-out but are no cause for alarm.

• **Enema.** Thankfully this is no longer standard procedure, though some doctors recommend one to clear the bowels at the start of labor or if labor is prolonged. On the other hand, it's common for the bowels to empty naturally in early labor. Even if you defecate during labor, which is not uncommon at the pushing stage, no one will be offended and there's a minimal likelihood of infection, as the nurse will quickly whisk away fecal matter.

• **Pubic shave.** Also a bygone standard, once thought to reduce infection. Few women undergo this unnecessary procedure before a vaginal delivery anymore. In fact, razor nicks from shaving can introduce infection. Even before a C-section, it's not necessary to have a complete perineal shave; removing pubic hair along the abdomen from the navel to just above the pubic bone is sufficient.

• **Arm straps and leg stirrups.** Their very names conjure up images of confinement at odds with what's considered wise for a normal birth today. It's a rare hospital anymore that requires a woman's hands to be strapped to her bed to keep them clear of the sterile delivery site. If yours does, definitely refuse this unnecessary step. Stirrups, on the other hand, are a feature of every delivery bed. Using them is optional, though, and you may or may not use them during a vaginal exam or to help you push. But again, there's no need for feet or legs to actually be strapped in place in a vaginal delivery.

True Labor or False Labor?

Remember the motto "Longer, stronger, and more frequent." This will help you distinguish real contractions from the prelabor Braxton-Hicks practice variety. These simple tests can help you determine if your labor is the real thing:

TRUE LABOR	FALSE LABOR
How Regular Are Contractions?	
Occur at regular intervals that grow shorter over time (every 10 minutes, every 8 minutes, every 5 minutes).	Occur sporadically and without a predictable pattern.
Where Do You Feel the Contractions?	
Typically start high up in your abdomen, radiating throughout your stomach and lower back.	Typically centered in the abdomen or the groin.
Do Contractions Change When You Switch Position?	
They keep a steady pace whether you sit, stand, or move.	May stop or slow when you rest or shift positions.
How Long Does Each One Last?	
Contractions last about 15 to 30 seconds at the onset and get progressively longer.	Contractions vary in length and intensity.

Checklist: Alert Your Doctor If . . .

☐ You think you're in labor, even if you're not sure
☐ Your water breaks (even if you don't lose a lot of fluid or if you have no contractions)
☐ You're bleeding bright-red blood (not the blood-tinged discharge that marks a dislodged mucus plug in a woman at term)
☐ You experience severe, nonstop pain
☐ The baby has not moved for an unusually long time
☐ You experience any other symptoms the doctor has previously asked you to note (such as contractions a certain distance apart)

WHAT IF. . .

My water breaks and I'm out in public? It's a common fear, and it does happen, though pretty rarely. In just 10 percent of pregnancies do the membranes of the amniotic sac rupture before labor begins. Often, it happens in the evening or night hours when you're home, relaxed. But if you are out and about, onlookers will realize you're in labor, not incontinent. Stay calm and get help. Alert your doctor before making your way home.

I can't reach my partner? During your ninth month, your spouse as well as your labor partner, if they are not the same person, should make their whereabouts known to you, along with how to reach them at all times. Many couples rent a beeper or cellular phone to keep in touch. It's also wise to have a backup person ready to drive you to the hospital in case you need to get there quickly. If your coach doesn't show up while you're in active labor, the obstetric nurse can give you some support, but she may not be able to be at your side throughout labor. That's why, if there's a chance that your mate will be out of town when you deliver, you should investigate backup coaches.

I don't like the labor nurse assigned to me? Feeling compatible with, and supported by, your nurse is important because you'll come to depend mightily on this trained and experienced caregiver to guide you through labor, especially if you don't have a midwife or professional labor assistant. If you feel she isn't respecting your wishes or you clash somehow, ask to speak to the supervising nurse (or have your partner do so) and request a change. Be diplomatic but persistent. (Keeping your cool not only helps you achieve the change you need but spares you unnecessary, unproductive anxiety.) Unless the ward is full, you can usually be accommodated. You can also appeal to your doctor, who can help remedy the situation. Also realize that hospital nurses work in shifts that may not align neatly with your baby's schedule; you're apt to see two or more different nurses during the course of your labor.

Childbirth Basics

Every Labor's Different

Childbirth consists of three different stages. The first stage—dilatation—is by far the longest and the one on which most of your preparations have been centered. It can last anywhere from a couple of hours to a couple of days. Contractions must dilate the cervix to 10 centimeters, or about 4 inches, before the baby can be born vaginally. The second stage is when you push the baby out, usually lasting an hour or two, on average, for first-timers. The third stage is the delivery of the placenta, and takes less than half an hour.

The entire birth process lasts an average 14 hours for a first-time mother and 8 hours for a veteran mom. While every vaginal delivery will pass through these three stages, don't panic if they're not clearly identifiable to you and your labor partner. You may barely notice early labor, then progress swiftly to the pushing stage. Or your early labor may be very prolonged. Everyone's different.

Stage One: Dilatation

The first stage of labor typically lasts 12 hours for first-time mothers and about half that for subsequent vaginal deliveries. It's marked by three distinct divisions, each escalating in intensity:

1. Early (latent) phase. Initial uterine contractions cause your cervix to thin (efface) and open (dilate) to 2 to 3 centimeters in diameter. (Some of this is accomplished throughout the third trimester by Braxton-Hicks contractions.) This phase is when you're most apt to experience your water breaking, empty your bowels, or see a mucusy, blood-tinged discharge. Regular contractions begin mildly at 15- to 20-minute intervals and eventually come every 5 minutes or so. Each one lasts 30 to 60 seconds. At first, you may feel little more than your abdomen growing tighter and rock-hard, and you can talk easily. Gradually the intervals between contractions shorten and they become increasingly regular. As you realize this is the real thing—and there's no turning back—you'll feel both excited and apprehensive.

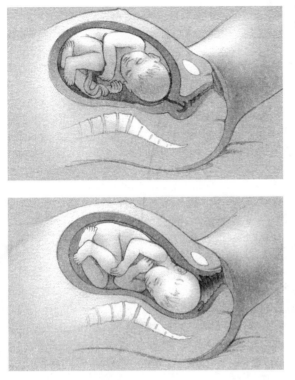

The cervix doesn't begin to dilate until the start of labor.

The first stage of labor is usually the longest, lasting 6 to 18 hours for first pregnancies and 3 to 10 hours for subsequent births. It begins when your cervix starts to open and ends when it's fully dilated.

What you should do:

- Monitor the frequency and duration of your contractions to help verify that you're in true labor. To determine how far apart contractions are, time them from the *beginning* of one to the *beginning* of the next.
- Alert your partner and/or labor support person.
- Don't go to the hospital too soon. If your early progress is slow, you may find it more peaceful to stay at home. Many hospitals won't even admit patients until they're in active labor.
- Sleep, if it's late and if you can, since you don't know how long you'll be laboring.
- Walk, if you feel rested, as this can help speed labor along.
- Relax. Breathe slowly and deeply during contractions. Try a warm shower or a bath if your membranes haven't ruptured. Play soothing music. Resist the temptation to call everyone you know.
- Eat a light, easy-to-digest meal—toast with jam, soup and crackers, yogurt and fruit—while contractions are still far apart. Afterward, hold off on solid foods (unless your doctor or midwife has previously okayed them) in favor of

broth, gelatin, and clear fruit juice (such as apple, not orange juice, which has pulp). Avoid dairy products (except yogurt), fats, and meat, since they're slow to digest. Freeze apple juice or lemonade in ice-cube trays for an energizing light snack.

- Drink water or juice every hour or so to prevent dehydration.
- Have your partner transfer your hospital gear to your car.
- Alert your doctor or midwife once your contractions meet agreed-upon criteria, or if your water breaks.

2. Active phase. As contractions become stronger and more frequent, your cervix dilates to 3 to 7 centimeters in diameter. Contractions are eventually 2 to 3 minutes apart and last 45 seconds, each one building to a peak of tightness and then easing off. The pain intensifies over time. It becomes harder, and soon impossible, to pay attention to other people during the duration of the contraction. The room seems to shrink, and you're aware only of your own body. Between contractions, though, you can still relax and converse. If this phase lasts a long time, or you haven't slept in a while, you may begin to tire. Periodic internal exams will be made to check the progress of your dilatation. This is the stage most women think of when they hear the word *labor*.

What you should do:

- Keep upright—walking, rocking, and so on—and change positions often, as the motion and positioning will speed your progress.
- Practice prepared-childbirth exercises for relaxation and breathing.
- Listen to your nurse, who may be able to advise you on breathing patterns or other tips you've forgotten.
- Ignore any questions or conversation until a contraction is over. Don't worry about being impolite—focus on yourself first.
- Suck ice chips, popsicles, or hard candies for refreshment and to moisten your mouth.
- Let your body relax between contractions. Some women like to keep their eyes closed.
- Urinate often—once an hour is a good rule of thumb—because keeping your bladder empty allows the baby's head to descend more easily. Some women prefer to spend part of active labor perched on the toilet, which is a comfortable height and requires a posture that is both comfortable and beneficial to labor.

GOOD POSITIONS FOR ACTIVE LABOR.

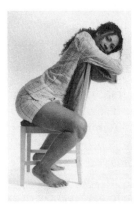
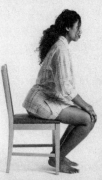

*Try sitting back-
ward in a
straight chair, or
sit upright in a
chair and rock.*

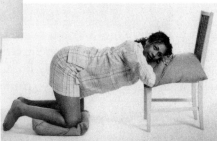

*Kneel and support yourself on a chair
or the wall.*

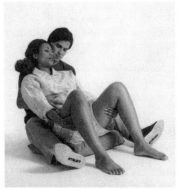

*Sit on the floor or bed, leaning back into
your labor partner's arms.*

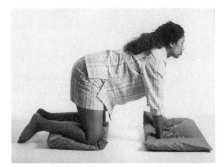

*Helpful for back labor: Kneel on all
fours, rocking through a contraction.
Don't arch your back.*

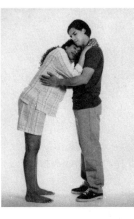

*Stand and lean
into your labor
partner, which
takes the weight
off your spine.
This position
eases back labor.*

- If you lie in bed, don't stay flat on your back, which restricts oxygen flow to the fetus. Try to recline on one side or with a pillow under one hip.
- If you're very uncomfortable, now is the time to request pain relief. This is the best time to get an epidural. Remember, however, that once you get an epidural you can no longer move around freely.

3. Transition phase (also called hard labor). During the transition from Stage One labor to Stage Two labor (pushing), the cervix dilates to its maximum width, from 7 to 10 centimeters. Contractions during this 30- to 90-minute phase last much longer, up to a minute or more, and come more rapidly, sometimes less than a minute apart. Each one may have several peaks before it subsides.

This is the most difficult part of labor, as you may be worn out just as your body demands more from you than ever. Your muscles seem to have a life of their own as they gear up to accomplish the enormous feat of birth. Nausea, chills, and sweats are common; steady breathing becomes more difficult and you may need to fight an urge to hold your breath. You won't want to be left alone. You may criticize or speak harshly to your labor partner. This is also when women get most irritable, panicked, or fearful that they "can't make it." But transition also tends to be the shortest phase. The pressure of the baby's head on your cervix may make you want to push. But if you haven't fully dilated to 10 centimeters, you'll be warned not to because the cervix could tear badly or swell.

Your unborn baby is working hard now, too. During a normal vaginal delivery, he or she enters the birth canal head-first and facing sideways, so that the widest part of the head (front to back) is lined up with the widest part of your pelvis (side to side). As the baby moves down, the face rotates toward your back, so the widest part of the head is aligned with the widest part of the birth canal (front to back). The baby's neck is also bent forward so that the chin rests on the chest, allowing the crown of the head (the *occiput*) to appear first.

What you should do:

- Continue relaxation and breathing techniques. You may need to switch to a different breathing pattern than you'd been using previously or need someone to pace you through the breathing verbally.
- Rely on your helpers to let you know when contractions are peaking, if you find that information helpful.
- Take contractions one at a time. Don't worry about what's coming next.
- Keep your mouth moist with ice and try to keep cool (with compresses, being fanned, or by changing or removing clothing).
- Resist the urge to push by using special techniques, such as blowing short bursts of air through your mouth.

- If the urge to push becomes uncontrollable and you make grunting sounds during contractions, continue to resist, but alert your coach or nurse so you can be checked.

Stage Two: Pushing and Birth

At last, you'll hear the much-hoped-for announcement that you're fully dilated—the baby has descended through the last part of the birth canal. The hair on your baby's head may be visible to your partner, or to you with a mirror. Now you can begin to push.

Though pushing is hard work, and can be difficult to get the knack of, many women get a second wind at this stage because they no longer have to fight the intensity of the contractions. Instead, to propel the baby out, you work *with* the force of the contractions, which usually slow slightly to every 2 to 5 minutes and last 60 to 90 seconds. You will also feel an overpowering urge to push, which is a very different sensation from that of ordinary contractions. For some women, especially those who have had long Stage One labors, pushing can be exhausting and frustrating—though tempered by the knowledge that childbirth is almost over. This stage lasts from 30 minutes to 3 hours for most first-time moms, and from 30 minutes to 1 hour for second-timers.

Compare which method of breathing works best for you while pushing: the traditional school (known as Valsalva pushing) says to inhale as the contraction begins, hold the breath and bear down hard as it peaks. Prolonged breath-holding can possibly promote perineal tears and exacerbate hemorrhoids, however, so it's increasingly considered better to exhale while you bear down. A newer method questions whether one giant push per contraction is necessary at all. It advocates slower, smoother pushes—as many as four per contraction—punctuated by a series of short breaths. Trust your body's instincts.

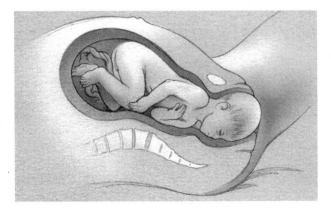

The second stage—which can last two hours or longer—commences when your cervix is fully dilated and continues until your baby is born. The last stage takes about 15 to 20 minutes and ends when the placenta is expelled.

EFFECTIVE PUSHING POSITIONS. Delivering your baby is easier if you're not fighting gravity. Compare these positions:

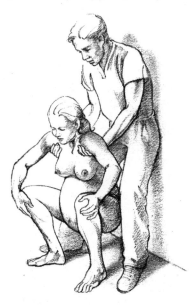

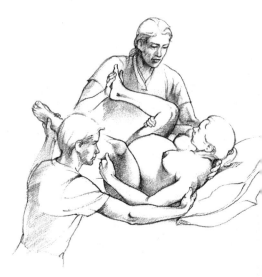

Squatting while supported is the most efficient position, since it uses gravity and the pelvic bones are most widely spaced. It helps to practice during pregnancy so your legs are strong enough to support you.

Semi-reclining (knees bent, feet supported or resting on someone's shoulders) is the most popular position and most convenient for birth attendants, because it give them unimpeded access to the vaginal area. But the baby is forced to descend the birth canal at an uptilt; what's more, the pelvic bones do not open as wide as possible when you're flat on your back.

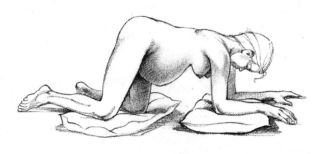

Kneeling is an effective alternative.

As relieved as you may be to get the green light to push, it may be difficult to shift your body into an effective position, especially if your contractions are still strong and fast. Let your attendants help you, and follow their suggestions as best you can; this is for your benefit as well as your baby's. The key to avoiding tearing is a slow, controlled delivery. A few extra minutes taken to ease out the baby's head give a woman's vaginal tissues time to stretch.

The hardest part—aside from getting the hang of how to move your muscles—is pushing out the baby's head, since that's the widest part of the body. You'll feel a powerful pressure on your rectum as the head presses against your dilated cervix on its way out. Some women feel sure they must be having a bowel movement, although the muscles involved are different. Others have a sensation of splitting apart. (Rest assured, though, that this is a biological impossibility.) As the head emerges, there is a sting and a burning sensation, sometimes referred to as a "ring of fire," naturally anesthetizing the tissues as it stretches them and blocks the nerve endings. Just try to relax when that happens—don't do anything. After the top of the head appears without slipping back (called *crowning*), you'll be asked *not* to push, so as not to tear the stretched perineum (the area between the vagina and anus) and to allow it to fully stretch naturally. Ideally, the doctor or midwife massages the area to help the tissues stretch (called *perineal massage*). Alternatively, this is when an episiotomy, an incision in the perineum to enlarge the vaginal opening, is performed.

With another contraction and either one big push or a series of shorter ones, the entire head is delivered. The baby faces the mother's back and immediately turns sideways, aligning the shoulders with the front-to-back width of the birth canal.

The doctor or midwife will suction any mucus from the infant's nose, mouth, and throat to help breathing. The baby's lungs, which have been getting oxygen from the mother's blood, must now draw their own supply from the air. If the umbilical cord is looped around the baby's neck, the doctor or midwife will gently uncoil it if possible. If not, you may be asked to stop pushing so it can be cut before the rest of the baby is delivered. During the next few contractions, first one shoulder and then the other shrugs its way out. The rest of the body slips out in a flash. Happy birthday!

You may be given the baby to hold even before the umbilical cord, which unites mother and baby, is cut. Some doctors will let the father "catch" the emerging baby or encourage him to snip the cord. The cord is usually cut within a minute of delivery, though this is not absolutely necessary. Some proponents of the LeBoyer birth method believe in waiting several minutes to cut the cord, until it has quit pulsating, so that it can supply the baby with additional oxygen.

The baby will be reddish and covered with blood, amniotic fluid, and possibly waxy white vernix (the substance that protected the skin in utero). Often the head appears misshapen (typically pointy), and the face may have reddish bruises, souvenirs of the narrow, bumpy ride past the pelvic bones. Usually the gender is obvious, but sometimes swelling can briefly obscure or confuse the answer to this burning question. (Some eager dads have been known to mistake the umbilical cord for a certain male part.) The doctor or midwife will set you straight.

Not all babies come out crying. When they don't, the doctor or midwife may massage the newborn's back or tickle the feet to stimulate the breathing reflex. (They don't dangle the baby by the ankles and swat the bottom to produce a cry anymore, though the purpose of that old-time practice was the same.) If your child was born in a delivery room, you'll be transferred to a recovery room for the next hour or two, or you may go directly to your room on the maternity floor.

What you should do now:

- Relax. The most painful part of labor has already passed.
- Ask for a mirror, if you want to watch the delivery. (Though you may get so involved in pushing that it's hard to see anything.) Ask for your glasses, if you wear them.
- Try to deliver in a relatively upright position, such as squatting or sitting while supported, which best widens the pelvic bones (see "Effective Pushing Positions," page 236).
- Take a cleansing breath before and after each push to signal its start and finish. Exhale slowly after a push to help the baby keep moving along.
- Think "Down and out" as you push, visualizing the baby's pathway.
- Don't push until you're asked to. Your doctor or midwife can tell at what point in the contraction it's best to try.
- Relax your pelvic floor as completely as possible. Resist the impulse to tighten your anus.
- To keep rested, go limp between contractions. The pause between contractions is now usually lengthier than it was during transition.
- Use your voice to help you move through a push, if it helps. No one will care if you grunt, groan, or scream.
- Don't feel rushed. Sometimes the pushing stage takes a while. As long as you are being well monitored and there are no signs of fetal distress, your baby can weather a long second stage of labor as well as a quick one. (The baby's heart rate slows naturally during contractions, but this is harmless even if pushing is prolonged.
- Ask to hold your baby right away after delivery. This can happen even before the cord is cut. Nonessential medical checks (such as weighing the baby) can be postponed until after this glorious moment of meeting face to face.
- Try to nurse. Newborns who are brought to the breast within the first hour of life have been found to suck better, making the initiation of breastfeeding

smoother for mother and baby. A newborn will instinctively root and latch on to the breast if held near it, and will be in an alert, receptive state to feed (if he or she hasn't been exposed to drugs during delivery).

- Thank the nurses who helped you. In the thrill of the moment, most new parents heap all the praise on their doctor or midwife. After all, you've known your caregiver for nearly 9 months. Just don't forget the hardworking (and typically underappreciated) labor nurses who may have made all the difference in your pregnancy's final hours.

Stage Three: After the Birth

Once the baby is born, the placenta, no longer needed, automatically separates from the uterine wall where it implanted 9 months earlier and is expelled. (The placenta and remaining tissue and fluid are referred to as the *afterbirth*.) Although the baby has been born, contractions continue, though less regularly and more mildly—in fact, in the thrill of meeting your baby face-to-face, you may barely notice them.

The doctor may lay a hand on your abdomen to make sure the placenta has separated and to cue you when to push, if necessary. Sometimes the placenta comes out through contractions alone. An attendant may massage or apply pressure to your abdomen to help. This can hurt. Through your IV or by injection, you may also be given oxytocin or another drug to help the uterus contract and to reduce bleeding. Delivering the placenta can take anywhere from 5 minutes to half an hour. The expulsion itself is painless, since it's all soft tissue and weighs about a pound. Ask to take a look at this remarkable organ, which nourished your baby for so long—it's a dark, matte red on the side that was attached to the wall of the uterus and a smooth, shiny gray on the side that cushioned the fetus. The doctor will examine the placenta to make sure all of it has been delivered. If any pieces remain inside you, they can cause bleeding and infection. At this time the doctor will also repair any episiotomy cut or any perineal tears.

Complications

The previous account describes a "textbook labor." Things don't always go according to plan, however. The following interventions are always possibilities. Knowing about them ahead of time can help make you and your spouse informed participants in the decision to use them.

- **Induction.** Efforts will be made to jump-start labor if a baby is overdue; if the mother has a medical condition such as diabetes or high blood pressure; or if

premature rupture of the amniotic sac has occurred but labor has not begun after a certain number of hours. The usual first course is for the doctor to use an
instrument to artificially rupture the membranes (*amniotomy*), if that hasn't happened yet. This is painless, and labor usually starts on its own within 12 hours.
Alternatively, or if the cervix hasn't begun to thin, a prostaglandin suppository
or gel may be applied. (Prostagel, a commonly used brand, is a synthetic form of
prostaglandin, a natural fatty acid that helps soften the cervix.) Several applica-
tions, a few hours apart, may be required. Prostaglandin can cause contractions
and may have side effects, including nausea, fever, or diarrhea. Once the cervix
is ready, labor can be induced.

To induce labor, small doses of the drug Pitocin, a synthetic version of the hormone oxytocin, are given intravenously. (This is informally known as a *pit drip*.)
Pitocin simulates the natural function of oxytocin to bring on contractions. The
normal stages of labor follow. For most women, contractions come more rapidly
and painfully in an induced labor, which can be more stressful for the baby. For
this reason, Pitocin-induced labors are continuously monitored electronically. Because Pitocin corrects insufficient uterine action, its use lowers the likelihood of a
C-section or infection. About 15 percent of pregnancies are induced.

• **Failure to progress.** Sometimes active labor stalls. The cervix dilates slowly
and weakly, or only to a certain point, where it plateaus for 2 or more hours
(even though contractions continue). Often the problem is exacerbated by modern medicine itself: a woman lying flat in bed, continuously monitored, is more
likely to have a slowed labor.

Several nonmedical measures may be tried to spur progress. The doctor may
break the water. Sometimes just moving around—walking, squatting, kneeling
on all fours—does the trick. (Though this may not be permitted if you've already
had an epidural or have been started on Pitocin and must be continuously monitored.) Nipple stimulation—by pulling them, using a breast pump, or rubbing
them with a warm, coarse towel—helps release natural oxytocin, which encour-
ages the uterus to contract.

If these measures fail to produce productive contractions, Pitocin is administered through an IV. As a last resort, a C-section will be recommended.

• **Fetal distress.** Signaled by alterations in the fetal heart rate (as revealed by fetal monitoring), this general term means the baby does not appear to be getting
enough oxygen. It can be caused by several things. The umbilical cord may be
wrapped around the baby's neck too tightly, or the cord may have a tight knot in
it. Other causes include anemia, blood pressure changes, severe infection, and a
deteriorating placenta. Some dips in the heart rate are normal and occur in most

babies. But if there is a continual pattern of drops or if the rate falls off suddenly, fetal distress is a possibility.

The doctor may draw a sample of blood from the fetus's scalp to determine if oxygen levels are low (called *fetal blood sampling*) and check the amniotic fluid for meconium. The amniotic sac must be ruptured and the cervix partly dilated to do this. Sometimes it's hard to be certain of a cause for fetal distress, and false alarms may occur. Even so, most doctors prefer to err on the side of caution and conduct an emergency C-section.

• *Episiotomy.* As the baby's head crowns, the doctor will determine whether the opening is large and flexible enough for the baby to pass through. An episiotomy is a cut that's made to enlarge the perineum (the area between the thighs, the vagina, and the rectum) that's made from the bottom of the vaginal opening down toward the rectum. Done in more than half of all first-time births, the incision is usually intended to facilitate delivery (considered a plus for the baby) and to prevent tearing (a plus for the mother). Local anesthesia is usually applied first (but not always, because the tissue is naturally numbed at crowning) and a local anesthetic is applied before the wound is stitched immediately following delivery. Absorbable sutures are used so stitches don't have to be removed later. There's no need to shave the area first, though public hair may be clipped to simplify stitching. The site may be sore for several days as it heals.

An episiotomy is not a routine procedure, however, nor should it be. Doctors perform episiotomies because a straight incision is better for the mother than a jagged tear, which can require more stitches. The surgery may also be performed if the baby's head is large or if a swift delivery is warranted in an emergency, such as fetal stress. But some studies indicate that episiotomies can extend into more severe tears than might have occurred otherwise. (Like fabric,

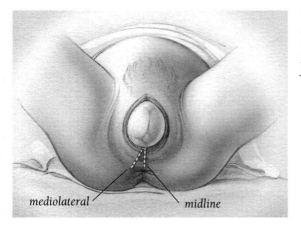

When your baby's head crowns, a small cut—either mediolateral or midline—may be made in the perineum to prevent the muscles from tearing.

mediolateral　　*midline*

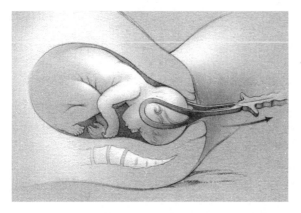

Forceps, which grip a baby's head, may be used to help pull him through the birth canal as you continue to push.

the skin tears more easily if you cut it first and then apply pressure.) What's more, newborns delivered without the surgery fare just as well as those born with it, and mothers without episiotomies tend to have stronger pelvic floor muscles and much less discomfort after delivery.

If you'd prefer to avoid an automatic episiotomy, let your doctor know well in advance of labor. The key to not tearing (and avoiding an episiotomy) is a slow, controlled delivery. It's important not to bear down or push once the head has crowned. This will allow the tissues to stretch naturally. Then push slowly and gently (with shallow panting, as opposed to one grand breath-holding push). Tears can also be minimized if the perineum is massaged prior to delivery. During the last trimester, perineal massage, along with Kegel exercises held for 20 to 30 seconds, can also improve the stretchiness and tone of these muscles. In labor, your doctor or nurse can further assist the tissue's natural stretching ability with massage.

• **Forceps delivery.** Forceps are a curved metal instrument that cradles the sides of the baby's head. They allow a doctor to carefully pull the baby out. It's used if the baby needs help descending, if the mother is too exhausted to push, or if she has received so much anesthesia that her abdominal and uterine muscles cannot push effectively. Sometimes the child's head may be bruised, and the cervix or vagina may tear during extraction. Increasingly, babies that are very high in the birth canal (and were once assisted out with forceps, known as a *high forceps delivery*) are delivered by C-section instead. Studies show that this use of forceps was associated with more complications for both mother and baby.

• **Vacuum extraction.** Used for the same reasons as forceps but beginning to replace it in popularity, a vacuum has a soft plastic or metal suction cup that's placed on the skull. The cup exerts a gentle pull to ease the baby out. There is a risk

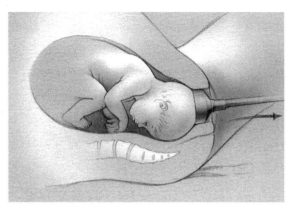

In a vacuum extraction, a plastic cup is attached to the baby's head and held in place by suction.

of tears or bruising during extraction. A vacuum or forceps is used in about 1 in 10 vaginal deliveries, particularly for women who have had epidurals. This is because the drugs can inhibit a woman's ability to actively or effectively push out her baby.

• *Prolapsed cord.* In the rare event that the umbilical cord descends out of the birth canal before the baby, the child's oxygen supply is endangered, as the cord can press against the bony ring of the pelvis. This may happen, for example, if the cord is long and a bit of it is pushed out with the sudden gush of fluid when the amniotic sac ruptures. Since a prolapsed cord can be life-threatening to the baby, this is considered an emergency situation. An immediate C-section is almost always required. If you are still at home, go to the hospital or call an ambulance immediately. If you are in the hospital already, alert a doctor or nurse.

• *Cord wrapped around neck.* It's common for a baby to be born either vaginally or surgically with the umbilical cord wrapped tightly around its neck. Usually this is no cause for alarm, but the newborn may need to be checked carefully by a pediatrician soon after delivery.

• *Stillbirth.* Nowadays an unexpected fetal death is extremely rare, because of advances in monitoring during pregnancy and labor. Any endangerment or cutoff of a fetus's oxygen supply is almost always detected and remedied by emergency C-section. If a fetus develops problems in the last trimester, it nearly always becomes less active or stops moving. This is why it's so important to keep track of the baby's movements. Lots of kicks and squirms are generally a sign that all is well. If your previously active fetus becomes calm and you don't count at least 10 movements in an hour, see your doctor. The baby may be fine, but your doctor will want to be sure.

Unexplained stillbirth is very rare in mid- to late-pregnancy. A vaginal delivery, while traumatic, is usually preferred because it is less risky physically to the mother. In such cases, labor is induced and the mother is carefully counseled before and after.

MOTHER TO MOTHER:
"My Speedy Labor"

Kimberley Kennedy, 36
St. Clair Shores, Michigan

At 36 weeks, and after several bouts with preterm labor, Kimberley's cervix had dilated to 2 centimeters, then stopped. Two weeks later, more intense contractions began. "I thought, 'Finally!' because we had run to the hospital at least five times before," she recalls.

Her doctor pronounced her in true labor and sent her to the hospital. At 4:30 P.M., with her cervix already 90 percent effaced, her water was broken. Kimberley and her husband Bill played cribbage, but, in less than an hour, she grew unable to concentrate. Contractions lasted 30 to 45 seconds each and came 2 minutes apart. "It was instinct taking over," she says. "I got up on the bed on all fours and rocked back and forth during contractions. I also tried squatting, sitting, rolling over, and walking."

After about 2½ hours of steady labor, the contractions came every 40 seconds, each one lasting nearly a minute. "They were right on top of one another. I'd hold my breath for a second, then remember I needed to breathe. When the pain was worst, my husband rubbed my back," Kimberley says. Although she had decided against an epidural because she dislikes needles and IVs, she changed her mind and asked for one at this point. The doctor told her she was already 8 centimeters dilated, too late for an epidural, so she soldiered on. At about 7:15, she was ready to push. Samantha was born at 7:56 P.M., less than 5 hours after her mother's first contractions.

Kimberley's tips for coping with labor:

• *Try to relax.* "If you get stressed about how long it will be, your labor probably will take longer."

• *Involve your husband as much as possible.* "Not only does it help him but it helps you know what's going on because he can talk to the nurses and doctor for you. And without my husband's encouragement, labor would have been much more traumatic."

• *Keep moving.* "I think my labor progressed quickly because I switched positions and walked a lot. Before I went to the hospital, I walked around the block to work through the pain of contractions."

• *Surrender to the moment as best you can.* "I just let my body tell me what it needed to do."

MOTHER TO MOTHER:
"My Labor Lasted Forever"

Belinda McCafferty, 23
Bloomington, Indiana

One Friday when Belinda was 10 days overdue, she began to feel crampy, like she was having a period. But the contractions came at irregular intervals and then stopped. The next morning, while out to breakfast with her parents, the pains started again. By the time she got home at 8 A.M., they were 10 minutes apart. Then her water broke, though the leakage was so slight that she wasn't sure at first what had happened.

"I called my doctor, who told me to come right in, and she confirmed that my water had broken," Belinda says. The obstetrician detected some meconium (fetal wastes) in the fluid, and sent her directly to the hospital. She was hooked up to a fetal monitor to check the baby, who seemed to be doing all right, and then got up to walk around a bit. "I looked at the other babies in the nursery and wondered how painful this was going to be and if I could do it," Belinda remembers.

By 4 P.M., she had only dilated 1 centimeter. "I thought I would have strong contractions and push and have a baby, but the process never went any further." An hour later, she was given Pitocin to prod her labor along. It worked. For the next couple of hours, sharp contractions came every 2 to 4 minutes. She used the breathing techniques from her childbirth class, focusing on pictures of her stepdaughter, husband, and cat. Around 8 P.M., 12 hours after her water had broken, she was given some Demerol to help her rest. The pains slowed again, as did her dilatation.

And so it continued through the night. "It was hard because I couldn't get up, and hadn't had anything to eat since the previous morning," she says. Finally, at 1 P.M. on Sunday, still only 1 centimeter dilated, her doctor told her they would need to do a C-section. At 2:50 P.M. the operation began. Daughter Tiffanie was born some 30 hours after her mom first thought "This is it!"

Belinda's tips for enduring a long labor:

• *Try to abandon your preconceived images about your delivery.* "People go in with certain ideas, but you don't always have the options you want. You should mentally prepare for all sorts of deliveries."

• *Plan some activities to pass the time.* "I brought a journal in which I wrote everything that was going on—it was nice to have it later to look back on. I also was able to read."

• *Use relaxation to keep up your energy.* "Having support was critical. I wish I had learned a little more meditation and that someone had given me a back massage."

• *Remember what you're there for.* "Long labors *will* end. Focusing on what was happening with my body and thinking about my baby helped me get through it."

MOTHER TO MOTHER:
"My Home Birth"

Geri Gossard, 31
Miamisburg, Ohio

Geri's first three children were born by Cesarean. For her fourth pregnancy, she was encouraged to consider natural childbirth at home by a midwife friend. "I wanted to be able to move around afterward, and to be in charge," Geri says. Her doctor advised against it (since three C-sections made her high-risk for a home birth), so she used the midwife for her prenatal care. Her husband was leery about possible complications, but she reassured him that they could go to a hospital quickly in an emergency.

At 1 A.M., Geri's contractions started. She began by sitting in the bathtub, with her midwife sitting on the rim of the tub and her sister nearby, talking to her and pouring water over her stomach. Her husband didn't fit in the small room, so he hovered outside. The midwife talked Geri through contractions. "I focused on her voice and that helped to relax me," says Geri, who was new to natural childbirth. "I thought about a grassy field and visualized the baby coming down the birth canal." Active labor lasted from 7 A.M. to noon. (Her husband got the older children off to school.)

"I tried to push in the bathroom, but I couldn't get situated," Geri says. "So I crawled into the living room." They spread a shower curtain and sheets on the floor. Geri's husband and sister held up her legs to help her push. "I never saw a baby immediately after birth, and it scared me a bit. He looked like a raisin," she recalls. "I just laid there and relaxed, then they cleaned him and I went to my bedroom. My husband got some blood on his shirt and said he was never going to wash it again."

At a hospital when you have drugs, Geri says, "It knocks the child out for hours and you can't nurse. Stephen was more alert and more mellow than my other kids were."

Geri's tips for a home birth:

• *Choose your midwife carefully.* "Pick a midwife who is confident and experienced, and with whom you have a good rapport. That's number one."

• *Weigh the positives and negatives.* "There may be complications, so you need to be sure a home birth is appropriate for you. At the hospital, I hadn't felt part of the birth—just the body the baby was coming out of."

• *Figure out what relaxes you.* "It was less stressful delivering at home. My family was there, and my sister sang to me."

FATHER TO FATHER:
"A Dad's View of Labor"

Joaquin Gonsalves, 33
San Diego, California

In childbirth classes, Joaquin learned breathing techniques, how to rub his wife Suzanne's back, and different positions for labor and delivery. "My role as a coach and supporter turned out to be what I expected," he says. "But I also felt helpless, because she was sick all night. I emptied bedpans and kept asking what else I could do. I learned that it wouldn't be a textbook birth."

He remained at Suzanne's side, talking and making jokes to relax her, and letting her squeeze his hand through contractions. "I felt nervous because at 12 hours it was such a long labor. I guess I thought we'd just go in, labor a while, and have the baby," he recalls. When she began to push, Joaquin was briefly bumped out of the way by the doctor, the anesthesiologist, and three nurses. "For about a second, I thought, 'Why can't I be there?' but I was mostly worried about the baby," he says. He repositioned himself in time to see son Stephen emerge: "He didn't come out screaming like in the movies. Once I got over the fear and knew that he and my wife would be okay, it was exciting."

Two years later, Joaquin had something even better than a front-row view of daughter Renee's delivery: the doctor let him "catch" her. "I was so excited. I didn't want to drop her. I cut the cord and she began breastfeeding right away. I told the doctor I'd send *him* a bill. What an incredible opportunity we dads have to be part of this experience."

Joaquin's tips for other dads at delivery:

• *Practice unselfishness.* "Think of her first—what she needs, what you can do for her. She's the one in pain."

• *Get involved as much as you can.* "Be a part of it. To see the baby's head coming out makes it 100 percent better."

• *Keep a clear mind.* "Just focus on what's going on at the moment, and don't worry about other problems in your life."

• *Don't stop being a coach once the baby gets home.* "You can't really prepare for the birth, besides taking classes and having some idea what to expect. But you can make the homecoming easier by cleaning up, having supplies ready, cooking food."

WHAT IF...

My husband faints or falls apart on me? Hard as it may be, don't worry about him. You'll have enough to think about as you work through contractions. The nurse will take care of a support person who gets ill, and can give him tips on avoiding hyperventilation, a common problem when partners breathe too rapidly while helping the laboring woman. If your labor is long, your partner should have a good meal by the time you're 5 centimeters dilated to avoid low blood sugar, the main reason partners faint. The labor nurse may also intervene with words of advice in the rare event that your coach is doing you more harm than good.

I feel sick? It's not unusual to vomit while in labor, especially during the transition phase or following certain medications. Just follow your body's cues.

I say or do something embarrassing? Don't give it a second thought. Childbirth taxes both body and mind. Laboring women have been known to cuss, shout, poop, leak urine, and blast their mates for "getting me into this fix." Rest assured that *nothing* you could do or say will surprise or offend your medical team, who've seen and heard it all.

That you're not supposed to eat during labor? This is controversial. Many obstetricians recommend only liquids (clear juice, soup, Popsicles) for laboring moms; some restrict patients to ice chips only. The reason is that your digestive system slows to a crawl during labor, and a heavy meal may make you nauseous or sick. Some doctors also believe that fasting in labor keeps your system clear in the event of an emergency C-section, since inhaling vomit during surgery can be fatal. (Glucose can be given via IV for sustenance.) On the other hand, these occurrences are rare and easily dealt with. And it can be hard to run a marathon of labor on an empty stomach. That's why some physicians and most midwives are more liberal about the matter. Your best bet is to eat small, frequent meals as your due date nears, and avoid going long spells without eating. Have a light, fortifying meal just as labor begins and follow your caregiver's advice thereafter.

That an episiotomy can interfere with sexual pleasure later? Sometimes. Generally, a stretched vagina, rather than a surgical cut or a tear, can alter the sensations of intercourse. But with a little time and a lot of Kegeling, even a slackened vagina should resume its original shape. Pain from stitches can persist for months, however.

That not all hospitals let you videotape the birth? Check policy ahead of time—many doctors will let you bend the rule if one exists, even for a C-section. The person filming must stay out of the birth attendants' way, of course. Note that Dad isn't the best candidate for extensive shooting anyway, since he ought to be coaching and comforting. Also, bright lights may distract the laboring mom-to-be. If she protests being photographed, *stop.*

All About Pain

What Does Labor Feel Like?

Now that you understand the mechanics of childbirth, you'll probably want to get down to the nitty-gritty: how much will it hurt and what can you do about it? Characterizing labor pain is tricky. One's individual tolerance for pain and the nature of one's labor vary greatly. What's more, stories you've heard, ethnic traditions, personal biases, and cultural trends all shape women's notions of what labor "should" feel like. In a study comparing women's expectations of labor pain in the United States and Holland, for example, American women were much more likely to anticipate a need for medication—and, indeed, ended up being much more likely to receive it.

Still, some generalizations are possible. Early labor often starts out like menstrual cramps that get more and more intense. The long muscles banded around your uterus are the most powerful ones in your body during labor. Imagine your body being tightened in a vise, then released, then gripped again, each time a bit more tightly. Typically, contractions begin high in your abdomen and radiate toward the back. Each contraction starts slowly as the uterine muscles begin to tighten (or contract). It builds to a peak and crests there as the muscles reach maximum pull. Then it fades away as the tension is released.

For most women, the duration and severity of each contraction increase gradually. Your tolerance builds with each one. Also, the intensity of contractions tends to ebb and flow throughout labor; each one isn't necessarily worse than the previous. Finally, you should know that all sensation of pain vanishes in between contractions. Labor pain is *not* continual. But make no mistake: By the time you reach active labor, you'll feel plenty.

It helps to understand where the pain is coming from. Uterine contractions are involuntary, like breathing or your heart beating. You cannot control the muscles' efforts. Each contraction is working not to push the baby out but to pull up the cervical muscles at the bottom of the uterus and thus widen the opening through which the baby can move out. Unlike the ordinary movements of your heart or lungs, as the uterine muscles tighten and pull, the pressure receptors in the neighboring nerves send messages to the brain. These may not start out as pain signals, but as the muscles tire and the contractions intensify, so does the perception of painfulness. External conditions can exaggerate the pain, including fear, tension, being alone, and a sense of helplessness. Childbirth counselors call this the *fear-tension-pain cycle*: the more afraid or nervous the laboring mother is, the more her muscles tense. The more tense her body is, the more the contractions hurt.

But pain isn't pointless or evil. It has a purpose. Just like the sear of touching a hot pan motivates you to cool the burning skin under running water, the pain of labor signals that birth is imminent and you should respond accordingly. You need to get to a safe place and be able to focus on the important work at hand. The escalating intensity of labor pain helps convey a sense of progress. And the pain can also communicate behavioral cues—if it gets very bad, it may be the body's way of telling you to change positions, relieve the bladder, walk or sit, or try to relax more.

No woman need labor in agony today. A wealth of knowledge exists about pain and how to ease it. Basically there are three points of intervention: (1) the site of the pain's origin (this is where massage helps); (2) the nerve endings that transmit pain signals to the brain (this is where medication helps); and (3) the brain itself (this is where distraction and breathing techniques help). Being informed and well supported *can* make a difference. Familiarize yourself with the full breadth of pain-easing options available, whether you'd prefer to labor naturally or be medicated. Many nonmedical pain-management techniques can benefit mothers who receive drugs. Whatever course your labor takes, never forget: giving birth is a tremendous accomplishment, no matter how you do it.

Nonmedical Pain Management

Pain-management techniques can help you stay on top of the intense feelings of a contraction. *They won't make the pain go away.* Although exceptions exist, for most women there is no such thing as a pain-free labor. But the relaxation and distraction offered by these tactics can provide your best weapon against the rigors of labor.

How does relaxation ease labor pain? The instinctive response to pain is tension. Unfortunately, tensing your muscles only makes the pain more acute. It slows the flow of oxygen in your system (including to the uterus), overstresses your body, wastes physical energy, and makes it difficult to think clearly or with focus. On the other hand, if your body can relax as it confronts pain, you experience less unnecessary discomfort and can work more constructively with a contraction to accomplish its goal. It will still hurt, but not as much as if you tighten up your muscles and panic. By relaxing in between contractions as well, you conserve strength. Your goal should be to relax your entire body, from your face to your toes, not just your midsection.

Unless there's a medical reason, most women are wise to begin labor without the assistance of drugs. In fact, doctors usually are reluctant to give painkillers until active labor is well under way. There are several reasons for this: (1) *Any* medication can potentially affect the fetus, so why take an unnecessary risk from the get-go? (2) You won't know how your body experiences labor until you've gone through it for a while, and you may be able to manage fine on your own. (3) Pain-relief medications can slow your progress, possibly making labor-promoting drugs or a C-section necessary, or prolonging pushing. (4) The introduction of pain relievers tends to snowball the use of further medical interventions, such as Pitocin and forceps.

The case for beginning childbirth naturally cannot be made without a few important caveats. It's equally important to enter labor open-minded about what eventualities might be in store. When your or your baby's safety is clearly at stake, it's no time to argue with the medical professionals attending you. A medical emergency may warrant a C-section, for example. A labor that goes on excessively long may exhaust you, making a shot of narcotic a welcome reprieve. You won't flunk childbirth if you take medication.

What works best for you may be a matter of trial and error. For example, you may find during labor that the idea of a shower suddenly strikes you as soothing—or revolting. Your best bet is to familiarize yourself with a variety of pain-management techniques, and then pick and choose among them when the time comes. Each tactic's usefulness may also vary during the course of labor, with some working best in early labor, and others having greater effect once you're further along.

The object of each method is the same: relaxation.

A good childbirth education class will drill you in the specifics of these tactics. Use the following as a supplementary guide:

• **Support.** Study after study confirms that continuous emotional support in labor soothes expectant mothers enormously. In fact, almost every culture worldwide traditionally provides laboring women with a constant companion, usually another mother. (In America dads have assumed that role, but midwives, other moms, and doulas can do the same.) All this familiar, reliable figure needs to do is be present, praise, project calm confidence, and respect the laboring woman. He or she should also help her breathe, keep her cool and comfortable, and do anything else that enables her to completely let go of the everyday world around her and surrender herself to the business within.

• **Breathing.** Every prepared childbirth course teaches one or more kinds of controlled breathing patterns, with the exact rhythm depending on the method being taught and the stage of labor. There's no single right way to breathe. So don't get jarred if you can't remember the exact mix of pants and blows—what's important is that you find a pace that calms you. The pattern may change at different stages of labor, as your mind and body are taxed in new ways.

Everyone relies on different strategies, but here are some suggestions:

During early labor. Breathe as normally as you can. If it helps, take slow, deep breaths from the abdomen, at about half your normal rate. Inhale through the nose, exhale through the mouth. You can even accompany the breath with thoughts or words: "Energy in, pain out." Relax your entire body as you exhale. Slow, deep breaths have the added benefit of ferrying lots of oxygen to your system.

During active labor. Switch from slow breathing only when it no longer lets you feel control over a contraction. Then try shallower breaths at a slightly escalated pace. Fixing your gaze on a focal point—a favorite photo, a spot on the wallpaper, your partner's eyes—can help rivet your concentration. Or close your eyes. Use a series of counted or rhythmic pants: "Hee, hee hee, long exhale. Hee, hee, hee, long exhale." Some women like to count or spell a long word as they breathe—their baby-to-be's name, for example—or chant an inspiring phrase such as "I-can-do-it" or "Health-y-ba-by." Take care not to breathe too rapidly or exhale too deeply, which can leave you hyperventilated. If you begin to feel lightheaded or your face tingles, revert to slow breathing to get back on track.

Alternatively, maintain deep, slow, relaxed breathing. Take a cleansing breath at the beginning and end of each contraction. Otherwise breathe naturally and slowly—the way you do when sleeping. As contractions get more intense, make the breaths a bit deeper, but always keep them slow. Keep your entire body limp; your partner should help you relax.

During transition. When resisting the urge to push, blow out short, gentle puffs of air—it's virtually impossible to bear down while doing so. This can be hard to sustain, though, so you could also try two or three short breaths (or pants) followed by a blow.

Take deep cleansing breaths at the start and finish of each contraction to signal their cycle to yourself and your partner. Inhale through the nose; exhale through the mouth. Don't hold your breath. It's rarely productive and restricts your intake of oxygen.

• **Movement.** Just about any activity is more comfortable than lying flat in bed—and movement has the added advantage of speeding labor. Try walking (at home or in the hospital), rocking, kneeling, or rocking your pelvis as you lean against your partner or the wall through a contraction. (See "Good Positions for Active Labor," page 233.)

• **Visualization.** Like daydreaming, this tactic involves transporting yourself to another place or circumstance through your imagination. You can train yourself to do it on demand. (You can practice this meditation throughout the last trimester.) Choose several soothing images, such as the lulling waves of a favorite beach or rocking your imaginary child in your ready-to-go nursery. Use all your senses to imagine the scene: What do you hear? What do you smell? In India, women picture the petals of a lotus flower slowly unfurling, an apt metaphor for the dilating cervix. You can combine visualization with patterned breathing, imagining the air entering and then exiting your body.

• **Massage.** Throughout pregnancy, you probably patted your belly in a light, circular pattern, an instinctive practice called *effleurage*. Touch during childbirth can be reassuring and relaxing as well. Between contractions, your partner can rub your temples, scalp, shoulders, soles, or other tension points. Counterpressure on the lower back, applied with the back of the hand, also feels great, whether or not you have a backache or back labor, and especially for the duration of a contraction. Use massage lotion or baby oil, but be aware that favorite scented lotions may not appeal to you in labor. Note: some women do not like to be touched at all during labor.

• *Music.* Soothing sounds help the body relax. Some researchers believe that they prompt the body to release pain-relieving endorphins. Bring your favorite tunes to the delivery room with you. They don't have to be ethereal and New Age-y, though they should be calming. If rock or Beethoven relax you, go for it. Record your favorite cuts, deleting parts of albums you dislike. Or try recordings of waterfalls, thunderstorms, and bird calls. Consider different music for the different stages of labor—perhaps something peppy for early labor and more gentle acoustic tunes later on. (Some women prefer the reverse: soothing strains early on and crescendos when they push.) A boom box or tape player is better than a Walkman, whose cords can become tangled. Earphones also prevent you from hearing your birth attendants.

• *Water.* A warm bath or shower massages and soothes tired muscles while refreshing the psyche. Immersing in a tub confers a welcome sense of weightlessness, too. You may literally feel tension float away. Late active labor and transition are good times to soak. In one study, women who spent part of their labor in a Jacuzzi-type tub had shorter labors, quicker cervical dilatation, less pain medication, fewer C-sections, and less reported pain than those who labored on dry land. Not all laboring women like to feel wet, however. Doctors disagree whether it's okay to bathe once your water has broken (for fear of infection), though birthing centers that routinely allow it see no increase in infections if care is taken. Don't overlook the refreshing sensation of having your face or limbs periodically wiped with a wet cloth.

• *Alternative methods.* Hypnosis, biofeedback, acupressure, acupuncture, and TENS (*transcutaneous electrical nerve stimulation*, also known as electrical stimulation) are other, less mainstream options for combating labor pain. All work in a similar way: they flood the brain with soothing signals that crowd out pain signals, similar to the way rubbing a banged elbow helps it feel better. If one of these methods intrigues you, it's best to investigate practitioners early in your pregnancy and to talk to other women who have used the method in childbirth. Clear the method with your doctor or midwife, too. If a professional practitioner is needed, be sure you have your doctor's and hospital's okay so you're not caught unawares on labor day. Find out how the technique can be combined with other pain-relief methods, from Lamaze to drugs. Note: many of these alternative methods are expensive (either to learn or to hire a professional's services) and aren't covered by insurance.

(For more details on relaxation methods, see "Relaxation," page 128.)

Medical Pain Management

For some women, particularly those who have a low tolerance for pain or who have very long labors, medical pain relief makes labor more bearable. Medication is also necessary for a Cesarean birth, of course. Sometimes epidurals (a procedure that provides numbing from the waist down) are recommended for multiple births in the event an emergency delivery is needed.

What if you're uncertain about medical pain relief? If your labor is not high-risk, try this: plan, with your birth partner, to wait 15 to 30 minutes after you feel the need before you make the request for medication. You may dilate a significant amount in that length of time and find that you can do without. Remember that once you have medication, you are generally confined to your bed, which you may find less pleasant than the pain.

If you choose medication, there are two basic categories of pain relief: *analgesics* (narcotics) provide some relief without a total loss of feeling or consciousness. *Anesthetics* numb part or all of the body completely.

• **Systemic narcotics.** Commonly used types include Demerol, Stadol, Fentanyl, Sublimaze, and Nubain. Since they affect the entire nervous system (rather than a specific body part), these analgesic drugs are usually given to take the edge off contractions and to help the mother relax. Each drug has slightly different effects from woman to woman, ranging from a pleasant buzz to drowsiness to dizziness and vomiting. If active labor is prolonged, narcotics can help you rest before the intense transition phase begins (alternately, you may be given a sedative such as Seconal or Nembutol for rest in early labor, which relaxes you but doesn't curb the pain as well as a narcotic). The drugs can be administered via injection or IV, with the latter providing more immediate relief. It's not always necessary to remain hooked to the IV once the narcotic has been given. Some hospitals allow women to self-administer premeasured doses of narcotics by pressing a pump attached to an IV line.

Ideally, narcotics shouldn't be given too early in labor (lest they slow its progress) or too late in labor (which might cause the baby to be born with some of the drug circulating in his or her body). The best time to administer narcotics is the middle of active labor when the mother is dilated 5 to 7 centimeters. That's because analgesics quickly enter the baby's circulatory system through the mother and can slow the child's breathing at birth. "Drugged" babies also tend

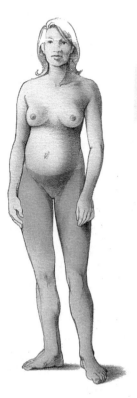

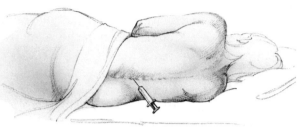

An epidural block, injected into the spinal column, relieves pain in the lower body. Shading (left) *indicates area of numbness.*

to be less alert and usually do not breastfeed as readily because their sucking reflex is depressed. It's easiest for the baby's system to break down the drug early in active labor, while the placenta can help flush it out.

• *Epidural block.* The drug of choice for modern American mothers-to-be is a regional anesthesia called an epidural, which is delivered just outside the spine. First the laboring woman lies curled on her side or sitting up in bed with her back rounded to make it easy to access the right spot on her back. An anesthesiologist numbs the area, then inserts a needle into her spinal column—specifically into the *epidural space,* a space around the dura, or spinal-cord cover between the vertebrae (hence the procedure's name). A plastic catheter is threaded through the needle and the needle is removed. For up to 24 hours after delivery, the catheter remains taped in place for later doses (you don't notice it). Then a cocktail of narcotics and anesthetic is injected through the catheter, blocking the signals that the nerves receive from the lower body, deadening pain. It's imperative to lie still, given the delicate placement of this needle, although this can be hard to do during a contraction. Sometimes bladder function is lost, so another catheter is inserted into the bladder to provide drainage. An IV is also required. There will also be continuous or intermittent blood pressure and electrocardiogram (EKG) checks. Finally, both mother and baby are electronically monitored continuously.

Relief is rapid. Within 5 to 20 minutes, sensation (including, of course, contraction pains) abates or vanishes from the chest to the toes, depending on the dosage. Every 2 hours or so, dosages are repeated or are infused continuously.

Another option allows the mother to control when she needs medication by pushing a button that releases a premeasured amount (called *patient-controlled epidural anesthesia*). Whereas epidurals once rendered the lower body leaden, the current trend is to use a smaller dose of anesthetic along with an analgesic, such as morphine, thus providing more control and enhancing the ability to push. Most women get great relief from an epidural. On the other hand, if the epidural is only partially applied, it's possible to retain areas of feeling.

An epidural is generally given during active labor once the woman has dilated 4 or 5 centimeters, so as not to forestall progress, but before she's in transition (7 to 10 centimeters), so as not to interfere with her ability to push. (See "Should You Have an Epidural?" page 259.)

• *Spinal block.* Like an epidural, a spinal block is a quick-acting form of anesthesia, though it's rarely used for vaginal deliveries these days because it only lasts for 1 to 2 hours and it prevents pushing by completely numbing the nerves that control the muscles required to push. A one-time injection, it's administered directly into the cerebrospinal fluid surrounding your spinal cord to reduce or eliminate pain. Unlike an epidural, all sensation in the lower body is fully numbed (though the woman remains fully conscious). It's done just once during labor, usually close to delivery, especially when forceps or vacuum extraction are needed, or before a C-section. A *saddle block* is a limited form of spinal block. Its name derives from the fact that it numbs only the parts of the body that would come in contact with a saddle.

• *Combined spinal-epidural block.* A newer form of epidural combines aspects of the epidural block and the spinal block. A narcotic is injected into the cerebrospinal fluid, and a catheter is put in place to provide further medication as needed. You can even walk around for the first few hours (hence the moniker the *walking epidural* or *walking spinal*). This is not always recommended, given your lack of complete control over your limbs. Like an epidural, it's offered after the woman has dilated 4 to 5 centimeters.

• *Pudendal block.* Medication is injected around the pudendal nerve, through the vaginal wall, to numb the vagina, perineum, and rectum. However, because it doesn't counter contraction pains well, a pudendal block is usually reserved for the second stage of labor or when forceps or vacuum extraction are required, or before an episiotomy. One of the safest forms of anesthesia, it has few side effects.

• *Paracervical block.* A local anesthetic is injected into the cervix, easing the pain of dilatation in the final stage before birth. It doesn't last long, however, and

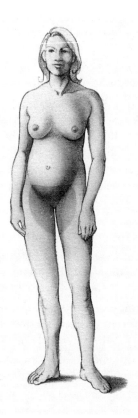

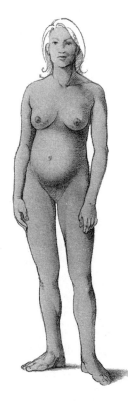

A pudendal block numbs the vagina, perineum, and rectum. But because it does little to temper labor pain, it's usually used only during forceps or vacuum extraction deliveries, or before an episiotomy.

Under general anesthesia you won't feel any pain, but you'll also sleep through the birth of your child; it's used only in special circumstances.

can depress the baby's heart rate. For these reasons, the paracervical block has fallen from obstetrical favor and is used less commonly than other anesthetics.

• *General anesthesia.* This option puts the woman to sleep for the duration of the birth. It's reserved only for C-sections in which the woman cannot have an epidural (in the event of a preexisting spinal injury, for example) or for rare emergencies when the baby must be delivered swiftly. The anesthetic may be delivered intravenously or by inhalation, or by a combination of both. Usually the baby is delivered before it is affected by the medication. Research shows that inhalant anesthetics can have longer-lasting effects on a baby's learning and motor skills than do other forms of narcotics.

Should You Have an Epidural?

Noting its reputation for almost pain-free labor, some women decide on epidural anesthesia long before their first contraction appears. Others prefer to avoid an epidural at all costs, either because they've heard stories of epidurals' side effects or because they prefer to labor with a minimum of medical interference.

Knowing the pros and cons of epidural anesthesia can help you make an informed decision.

Pros

- Once the medication kicks in, you feel little, if any, pain, although you may notice a tightening of your uterine muscle during contractions.
- The reassurance that pain will be minimal can help reduce fear.
- It offers a physical reprieve to a woman having a prolonged active labor.
- Today's dosages are adjusted in such a way that you can still maintain some muscle control for pushing and be able to walk soon after delivery.
- Less medication is thought to enter the baby's system than with other medical pain management options.

Cons

- By the time you feel you need one, you may already be in transition (dilated 7 to 10 centimeters), which is too late to offer real relief and could cause unnecessary delay in pushing and birth.
- In some cases, it hinders the progress of labor.
- Because it inhibits sensation in the hips and legs, effective pushing can be difficult. Forceps or vacuum extraction and an episiotomy may be required as a result.
- It requires an IV in your arm, a catheter in your bladder, and a needle in your spine—unpleasant if you're squeamish and also confining you to bed.
- It may not completely numb some parts of your abdomen or legs.
- Complications associated with the procedure (such as improper placement of the needle) can cause severe or long-lasting backache or headache.
- It requires increased monitoring of both mother and baby.
- It may affect the baby, slowing alertness and quickness to breastfeed.
- It's expensive (can add $500 to $2,000 to your hospital bill).

Checklist: Ways Coaches Can Help

In one study of twenty Lamaze-trained men assisting their wives' deliveries, only four actively fulfilled the role the way they were trained to do, four were helpful but needed to follow instructions, and the remaining twelve mostly just held the woman's hands and watched passively. Help your labor partner fall into the first category by having him or her read the section below.

Before Labor

☐ *Know what the laboring woman wants* before *labor begins.* Be sure you've gone over her preferences regarding use of an IV, fetal monitoring, positions for labor and delivery, and painkillers so you can back her up when dealing with medical personnel. Be familiar with her planned pain-relief methods.

☐ *Be prepared.* Have your own bag of necessities packed so you'll be able to fully concentrate on her when labor strikes—including snacks and refreshments, so you won't have to leave her side if labor is long.

In Early Labor

☐ *Remind her to rest.* In early labor, and between contractions throughout labor, encourage her to take it easy.

☐ *Remind her to empty her bladder.* Once an hour is best, throughout labor.

☐ *Be sensitive.* Don't eat a pastrami sandwich or gulp coffee in front of her if those sights or smells nauseate her. Many laboring women can't bear unpleasant odors, so bring along your toothbrush or breath-freshener.

In Active Labor

☐ *Anticipate her needs.* Don't wait for her to tell you what she needs. Once you've both figured out which actions best bring her relief—ice chips, a mop of the forehead with a cool washcloth, a neck rub—offer each one periodically. If she says her feet are cold, fetch another pair of socks. If the music stops, turn the tape over.

☐ *Time the contractions.* Check your watch or learn to read the fetal monitor printout to apprise her of each contraction's progress. It's easy—the labor nurse can show you how. Verbalize it for her: "You should be peaking now. Yes, it's easing up, going, going, gone! Great job!" At the same time, don't focus on the machine to the exclusion of the person. Stay in concert with her through the contractions—don't tune out.

☐ *Breathe with her.* Set the pace so that she doesn't breathe too fast. Counting aloud can help her concentrate, too. If she loses control of a hard contraction, encourage her to lock eyes with you, which can be a powerful psychological trick, and calmly continue the breathing pace.

☐ *Be upbeat.* She's nervous (or exhausted) enough. Don't complain or nag—accentuate the positive. Never criticize her actions or progress. Instead, phrase suggestions positively: for example, "Let's sit in the chair now" is better than "All this walking isn't helping, and you look tired."

☐ *Be flexible.* Her labor may not go according to plan and her preferred methods of breathing may not jibe exactly with the patterns you learned and practiced from childbirth class. Follow her cues.

☐ *Encourage movement.* Help her walk, if she can. Changing positions, even if lying in bed, can ease pain.

☐ *Keep her comfortable.* Add clothing or blankets if she's cold; remove layers or offer cool compresses if she's overheated.

☐ *Touch her.* Whether she prefers back massage or wants to grip your forearm, indulge this potent primal need.

☐ *Don't push medication.* It can be hard to see a loved one writhing in pain, but that doesn't mean she should be knocked out immediately. Let her ask for it first, and wait a few minutes to be sure she feels certain about her decision.

☐ *Try not to make her feel watched.* Be with her actively, not just as a passive observer. For some women, labor slows if they feel observed.

☐ *Don't disappear.* Make bathroom and snack breaks brief, and time them for between her contractions. Even if she says she doesn't want to be touched or talked to, your very presence provides powerful reassurance.

In Late Labor/Transition

☐ *Stay very close.* Most laboring women need extra strength and encouragement in the homestretch. Even though you may be tired, try not to show it. Offer praise for her hard work through each contraction. Don't leave the room or leave her side long to use the bathroom or to adjust a camera.

☐ *Discourage inhibition.* Never act embarrassed or censure a laboring woman for anything she says or does. On the contrary, encourage her to express how she feels. It's typical for her to lose all modesty in the later phases; support her nonjudgmentally.

☐ *Don't take it personally.* Laugh it off if your mate suddenly pushes you away or criticizes your efforts to help.

☐ *Recognize signs of panic.* During transition especially, a woman losing control over contractions may hold her breath, tense her face or upper body, and get a wild look in her eyes. If this happens, catch her gaze and hold it, praise her efforts, and help her refocus by calmly and commandingly telling her what to do (relax her shoulders, find her focal point, follow your breathing through the contraction, or so on).

☐ *Alert the medical staff when she expresses a need to push.* It may be time to check her cervix.

During Pushing

☐ *Follow the medical staff's cues.* Don't encourage her to push until she's told to.

☐ *Offer encouragement about the things you can see that she can't.* When you can see the baby's head, tell her. Reassure her that there's plenty of room for the baby to come out.

☐ *Resist the impulse to chant and cheer.* A woman in the second stage of labor doesn't need to hear "Come on! Push! Push!" as if she were a player in a ball game. Instead, offer quiet reassurances and provide concrete help. Remind her to take a cleansing breath at the end of a contraction and to relax between them.

• *Position yourself where she seems to want you.* Some women will want to hold their partner's hand during the hard work of pushing. Others will be so engrossed in the task that they don't mind if you're positioned down at their legs to witness the moment of birth—in fact, they may prefer that you see the baby being born.

For More Help: Pain-Management Resources

• National Association of Pregnancy Massage Therapy, 4200 Marathon Boulevard, Suite 330, Austin, TX 78756; 888-451-4945. Provides referrals to a therapist in your area.
• Biofeedback Certification Institute of America, 10200 West 44th Avenue, Suite 304, Wheat Ridge, CO 80033; 303-420-1706. Send a self-addressed stamped envelope for more information about easing labor pain.
• National Certification Commission for Acupuncture and Oriental Medicine, 1424 16th Street NW, Suite 501, Washington, DC 20036; 202-232-1404. Ask for its list of certified herbalists and acupuncturists.
• American Physical Therapy Association, 1111 N. Fairfax Street, Alexandria, VA 22314; 703-684-2782 or http://www.apta.org. Referrals to local physical therapists or a state chapter.
• (See also "Prepared Childbirth Resources," page 154.)

MOTHER TO MOTHER:
"My Drug-free Delivery"

Jennifer Herrin, 34
Tulsa, Oklahoma

Jennifer, a postpartum nurse, was motivated to attempt natural childbirth after seeing many patients who had had epidurals that resulted in long labors or C-sections. "I thought it was very do-able and that it would be better for me and my baby not to have any medication in our systems," she says. "I also didn't like the idea of an epidural because I wouldn't be able to move my legs. I hate it even when my foot falls asleep."

Four weeks before her due date, regular contractions began about 5 minutes apart. She arranged to see her doctor in 4 hours, at 3 P.M., to verify that she was in true labor, and walked around her house in the meantime. The doctor found her to be 5 centimeters dilated and sent her to the hospital. "It was the worst pain I'd ever felt, but I knew it wouldn't last forever and I thought I could put up with anything," she recalls. She and her husband practiced the slow abdominal breathing and relaxation exercises they'd learned in their Bradley-method childbirth class and in yoga. At 8 centimeters, her doctor broke her water and manually stretched her cervix the last bit. Daughter Phoebe was born a few pushes later, with Jennifer propped up in bed.

"Before my child was born, I was committed to natural childbirth and was looking forward to it," she says. "Afterward, I felt more strongly about it because labor wasn't so bad. I liked being able to get up right away and feel normal, and knew I could do it again. Going through this ordeal naturally is the most important thing I've ever done." Phoebe now has a sister Susanna, also born after an unmedicated vaginal delivery.

Jennifer's tips on natural childbirth:

• *Do yoga throughout your pregnancy.* "I did lots of squatting, which teaches you to concentrate on one part of your body and is good for pushing effectively. Yoga also helped my breathing."

• *Read about easing labor pain.* "For my second childbirth I didn't attend classes, but to refresh my memory I reread a lot of books that had been helpful the first time."

• *Bring reminder notes to labor.* "I made index cards with affirmations and tips that my husband could flip through. On each I wrote things that might be helpful, like "Open your mouth and relax everything else," "Go to the bathroom," and "Change position."

• **Don't equate pain relief exclusively with pharmaceuticals.** "I may not have taken any medication, but I did have powerful pain relief in the form of yoga breathing and concentration, hot showers, and unlimited mobility."

• **Have confidence in yourself.** "Women have given birth without medication for generations, but society doesn't push it."

MOTHER TO MOTHER:
"My Epidural"

Christine Lake, 28
Ramsey, Minnesota

Christine had no preconceived notions about epidurals, pro or con. She figured she'd see what happened as her labor progressed. At 9 days overdue, she went to bed to rest before her scheduled induction the next day. That's when contractions began, 6 minutes apart. She arrived at the hospital at 4:30 A.M., barely dilated 1 centimeter.

Over the next 12 hours, she only reached 3 centimeters. "We tried all the techniques for dealing with the pain—using a focal point, back rubs, walking, changing positions—but nothing worked. If I had been more determined to breathe, it would have helped me relax, but I couldn't focus," she says. "I just held my breath and lived through the pain, which you're not supposed to do."

Details of childbearing pain weren't discussed enough in her preparation classes, she thinks. "I wasn't dilating because I was tense with a sharp, back-to-front pain. I didn't know how to deal with it," she says. At 3:30 P.M., she readily accepted an epidural. "It was hard to lie perfectly still during the injection with all of the pain," she says. On the first try, only one side was numbed, so a half-hour later a second anesthesiologist finished the job.

"I had tubes sticking out everywhere, and couldn't get up and walk," Christine says. It was also hard to figure out when she was contracting, since she'd lost sensation. "But I felt better right away and was able to talk and smile again." She felt only a mild pressure in her rectum. Shortly after the epidural, she was also given intravenous Pitocin to speed her labor. From there she dilated quickly and 4 hours later, including 2 hours of pushing, son Zachery was born at 7:30 P.M.

Christine's tips about epidurals:

• **Trust your doctor's and anesthesiologist's skill.** "Even if you don't trust their judgment about whether you need an epidural, trust their ability once you decide to have one. They do them all the time—not just for births, but for regular surgery also."

• **Enlist help to push.** Listen to your birth attendant's advice on when to work with the contractions, and let others help you get in the proper position. "My legs were numb even though the epidural had been turned off so I could push. It helped to have my husband hold my legs."

• **Be as open-minded as you can.** "Originally, I didn't plan to have an epidural. But you don't know what will happen when the time comes. Don't have preconceived ideas; just do what you need to do to have a healthy baby."

MOTHER TO MOTHER:
"I Felt All My Labor in My Back"

Patricia Anderson, 34
Cincinnati, Ohio

Patricia took an all-day childbirth class to learn pain-management tactics and read a few books about labor. Still, she wasn't prepared when her pains all centered in her back.

Labor began at 9 P.M. on a Sunday night with mild contractions 10 minutes apart. The pace never changed, though, so she just tried to rest, leaning into each contraction to relieve the pressure on her back. Overnight, they advanced to 6 minutes apart, and she called her doctor. At 10:30 A.M., he found her to be 3 centimeters dilated and sent her to the hospital.

Once there, however, her progress slowed. "The pain is supposed to start forward and radiate to the back, but it never did that. It was all right in the middle of my back," she says. "My husband Larry rubbed my back very hard through every contraction. It's the only thing that got me through the whole day." She also found it helpful to stand up, lean over, and push into a wall while bracing herself with one knee. "Lying down on my side hurt. It also helped a little to sit up and hunch forward." By 4 P.M. she had dilated only to 4.5 centimeters, so her doctor broke her water in an effort to spur contractions. Getting tired and beginning to have trouble concentrating, she also received some Nubain by IV.

Finally, at 11 P.M., she dilated completely and began to push. "I don't remember as much back pain at that point," Patricia says. "But by then I was so tired, everything hurt." More than 2 hours later, at 1:38 A.M. Tuesday morning, a vacuum extractor helped son Joseph Arthur enter the world.

Patricia's tips on coping with back labor:

• *Prepare yourself for the possibility.* "Most books and classes don't gear the discussion to back pain. And you don't think it will happen to you."

• *Experiment.* "Of the ten different positions for normal contractions I had studied, only three or four worked for back pain. It was invaluable once we figured out that massage and leaning into the pain relieved the pressure."

• *Have someone with you who can provide constant counterpressure.* "I couldn't have done it without my husband."

• *Even though the pain is intense (and sometimes relentless), don't forget to relax.* "I used a lot of breathing techniques. If my body tensed up, my back hurt more."

• *Try refocusing the pain.* "I had to totally concentrate on something other than my back—for example, I'd imagine I'd smashed my finger, which allowed me to pull the pain to another place."

WHAT IF...

I change my mind about pain relief? Just say so. Nothing in the birth plans you've discussed previously with your doctor is set in stone. You can always change your mind about your preferences. The final decision may depend on your labor progress.

They say it's too late for the epidural I'd wanted? Usually this means that your labor is progressing so rapidly that you're near or at transition, and will soon be ready to push. Epidural relief might come too late to dull the pain as you dilate fully. It also may impede your ability to push well. Rather than despairing, congratulate yourself that you're having a swift labor and are almost through. This scenario points out why it's smart to learn nonmedical techniques for easing pain, even if you think you want to rely on drugs.

Special Situations

Cesarean Birth

One in 5 women delivers a baby surgically, through an incision in her abdomen and uterus. A Cesarean, or C-section, can be a planned event or an emergency decision. Nearly one-third of C-sections occur because of *dystocia*, an abnormal labor. This is a general term for a labor's failure to progress because of such factors as a cervix that won't dilate, arrested descent (the baby doesn't move through the birth canal), or *cephalopelvic disproportion* (the baby is too big to safely pass through the pelvis). Other common reasons include placenta previa (a placenta that blocks the baby's exit through the cervix), placenta abruptio (a sudden premature breakaway of the placenta from the uterine wall), a breech (upside-down) or transverse (side-lying) presentation of the baby in the womb, a prolapsed umbilical cord (which enters the birth canal before the baby) complications of diabetes or preeclampsia, or an active herpes infection.

A C-section is major surgery. In most hospitals you're transferred by gurney to an operating room. In preparation, an IV tube is inserted in your arm or hand (for the delivery of medications and possibly fluids directly into the bloodstream or in case a blood transfusion becomes necessary). Your upper pubic area is washed and may be shaved. To keep the operative field sterile, your arms may be strapped to the operating table and a drape raised, blocking your view. Your vital signs are monitored by the anesthesiologist, who is present throughout. In most hospitals, your coach is welcome and, indeed, you'll want his or her presence if you are conscious. (Both of you may be given scrubs and paper caps to wear.)

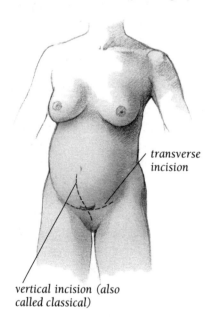

transverse incision

vertical incision (also called classical)

The incision made in the uterine wall for Cesarean birth may be either vertical or transverse. Transverse is preferred, however, because the resulting scar is less likely to tear during a subsequent delivery.

Two types of anesthesia can be used. Regional anesthetic, an epidural or a spinal, numbs you from the waist down; this is the most common practice. General anesthetic knocks you completely out; it's used almost exclusively in emergencies. A catheter is inserted in your urethra to continuously drain your bladder, which is located near the uterus and would be in the way if it were allowed to fill. You might feel a pinch during the insertion.

Once you can't feel anything, the obstetrician cuts through first the wall of the abdomen, then the wall of the uterus. The direction of the incisions depends on the position of the baby and the placenta. A low-transverse (horizontal) cut is used in the vast majority of Cesareans because it leaves a scar that's less likely to rupture during a subsequent labor than the old-fashioned vertical incision. The bladder is moved down so it's not damaged during delivery. The amniotic sac is punctured, and the baby is then lifted out through the incision. His or her nose and mouth are suctioned and the umbilical cord is cut and clamped. Then the placenta is removed.

Pitocin (synthetic oxytocin) is added to your IV to help the uterus contract postsurgery. If you are alert and feel up to it, you'll be allowed to hold your baby and breastfeed. The entire procedure generally takes 45 minutes to an hour, although the baby is actually born within the first 5 to 10 minutes. (The rest of the time is spent repairing the incisions.)

After surgery, you return to your room or to a recovery room, where your vital signs are monitored. If you feel well and the baby is healthy, there's no reason the two of you need to be separated after a C-section. To the contrary, seeing, touching, and breastfeeding your newborn right away can make a world of difference in your physical and mental recovery. (You may, however, be too exhausted if a long, hard labor preceded surgery, and that's fine, too. If you had emergency surgery, you will take longer to wake up from general anesthesia.) Your catheter is removed the day after delivery, but the IV usually remains in place for a day or two to prevent dehydration. Like any incision, the site will hurt for a few days and you may want painkillers. To minimize their exposure to your breastfed infant, take them after a nursing session. Hospital stays are usually longer than they are for vaginal births, about 2 to 4 days on average.

Get up and walk as soon as possible, even if it's only around your room. Abdominal surgery disrupts the digestive process and can result in horrible gas pains that may feel worse than contractions. These can be prevented if you walk even a little within a few hours of surgery. Always get help before first attempting to get up.

The chief objective of a C-section—which makes up for any discomfort—is a healthy baby. Sometimes, though, new moms are nagged by unexpected emotions ranging from dismay and disappointment to second-guessing whether there's anything they might have done to prevent surgery. These are common reactions, especially if your C-section was unexpected. They're born of a deep cultural prejudice in favor of vaginal deliveries and a tendency of childbirth preparation classes to accentuate empowerment and control, two things that

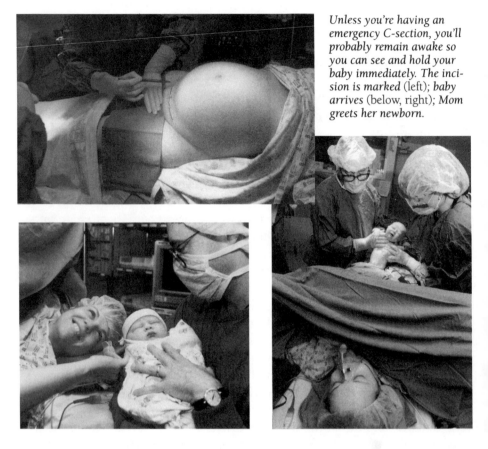

Unless you're having an emergency C-section, you'll probably remain awake so you can see and hold your baby immediately. The incision is marked (left); baby arrives (below, right); Mom greets her newborn.

sometimes get lost in the rush for emergency surgery. Feel good—not bad or guilty—if you need a Cesarean. It's hardly a cop-out, especially if it saves your life or your baby's! Tune out thoughtless observers who refer to your delivery as anything less than the real thing. You might find it helpful to review with your doctor the reasons the C-section was indicated and what this will mean for future deliveries, so you'll be prepared.

Some women question whether C-sections are always necessary. They take one look at the rapid rise in C-section rates in this country and wonder if American obstetricians aren't just a little bit knife happy. The American College of Gynecologists and Obstetricians credits C-section growth to technological advances in monitoring that permit earlier detection of problem deliveries, to a growing awareness that Cesarean births result in healthier babies than do prolonged or distressed vaginal deliveries, and to improvements in the surgery itself, making it a safer and more problem-free procedure than ever. After all, the ultimate goal of any delivery is a healthy mother and a healthy baby.

Although the C-section rate is much higher today, the number has dropped slightly from its peak in the late 1980s, as doctors have begun more carefully screening the circumstances under which they're performed. Forty percent of Cesareans are repeats, a proportion that has been falling as more women attempt subsequent vaginal births.

At the same time, critics argue that the total is still too high; that many are done unnecessarily for doctors' convenience, profit, and legal protection; or because physicians are trained to see birth as a series of potential disasters to be avoided, rather than as a natural event. Unnecessary surgery means exposing women to unnecessary risks. While the likelihood of maternal death is minuscule from Cesarean delivery, it's still four times greater than a vaginal birth. The causes include blood clots, infection, complications from anesthesia, and excessive blood loss. More likely, albeit also rare, are such complications as infection or damage to the bladder or bowels (because of their position relative to the uterus).

The healthiest mind-set to adopt about C-sections is to prepare yourself mentally and practically for the possibility *before labor starts*. That way, if one becomes necessary, you can rest assured in the knowledge that it was the right choice for this particular baby and this particular delivery. How can you get ready? Understand the possible reasons for Cesarean—don't tune out this important discussion in childbirth class or in the books you read.

Vaginal Birth After Cesarean (VBAC)

Forget the old saw, "Once a Cesarean, always a Cesarean." An increasing minority of women who have had a C-section attempt a vaginal delivery the second time around, known as a *vaginal birth after Cesarean*, or VBAC (pronounced "vee-back"). Several factors contribute to the growing popularity of VBACs. First, every labor is different. Just because baby number one was breech doesn't mean the same positioning is true of a second child. Or labor may progress more rapidly and steadily than it did the first time. Second, studies have proved that the likelihood of the old incision's scar tissue rupturing during the stress of labor (called *uterine rupture*), which once made doctors leery of attempting a trial of vaginal delivery, is always possible but relatively rare and with continuous monitoring can be diagnosed quickly. Third, the overwhelming popularity of the low-transverse incision, which has a rupture rate in VBACs of 1 percent, has further reduced that possibility. (A ruptured uterus is much more likely with a vertical incision.) Note: You can't tell whether you had the most advantageous incision by looking. It's possible to have a transverse incision on your skin (where the abdomen was cut), but a vertical incision in your uterus. The uterine incision is the one that matters most. That's why doctors need copies of your old C-section medical reports.

Why try a VBAC? If successful, you eliminate the risks associated with surgery, as well as the lengthy post-op recovery period. Although medications were once withheld from women attempting such vaginal deliveries (because of fear she would not feel the pain if her uterus ruptured while she was medicated), continuous monitoring has eliminated that problem. You can safely have an epidural during your VBAC attempt. It helps to have a supportive doctor, so be sure to ask his or her opinions about VBAC early in your pregnancy. Don't be shy about bringing up the possibility first. Even women with two previous C-sections can have safe vaginal deliveries. About 60 to 80 percent of women who attempt VBACs are successful.

Multiple Births

• **Twins.** The development of ultrasound has greatly simplified the delivery of twins because it's possible to monitor their position. Most twins are both head-down, allowing them to be born vaginally. Sometimes, though, one baby is born vaginally but the other requires a C-section, usually because it's breech. A breech twin can also be turned in utero, once the other has been delivered. Even for a vaginal birth, however, an epidural is advised in case something happens to warrant emergency surgery.

Mothers of twins tend to have slow labors, perhaps because the overstretched uterus doesn't contract as efficiently. On the other hand, the cervix has usually begun to dilate before a twin labor starts, which can make things seem to go faster. Twins also tend to be smaller than full-term singletons, making their delivery easier. The second twin, typically born 5 to 10 minutes after the first, is generally smaller.

• **Triplets.** More than two babies are almost always delivered by Cesarean.

For More Help: Special Delivery Resources

• C/SEC, 22 Forest Road, Framingham, MA 01701; 508-877-8266. Education and support.
• Informed Homebirth, P.O. Box 3675, Ann Arbor, MI 48106; 313-662-6857. Midwife referrals, support, and newsletter.

MOTHER TO MOTHER:
"My Two C-Sections"

Judy Gasarowski, 32
Freehold Township, New Jersey

Judy's daughter Jenna was born by scheduled Cesarean when it became clear that the baby's upside-down breech positioning wasn't going to budge. A year and a half later, Judy planned to deliver her next child vaginally, but after 24 hours of steady labor, the baby had not descended into the birth canal. So she headed for the operating room a second time.

As she was being wheeled from the birthing room to a surgery room four doors away, her epidural catheter fell out. "The anesthesiologist couldn't get it back in for 20 minutes," she says, which made for the most uncomfortable part of her marathon delivery, since she was already tired. Her husband Tim counted down the contractions for her so she could focus on his voice rather than the pain. Once the catheter was replaced, however, things proceeded quickly. Judy's husband sat near her head and told her stories as he watched the operation. Daughter Jillian was born 10 minutes later.

"The second delivery was worse because I was completely exhausted physically and mentally from the labor," she says. After the surgery, weak from fatigue and hunger, she began trembling (a common reaction), which made her panic a little. The staff gave her extra blankets and let her sleep for 4 hours. She still felt too weak to hold the baby and slept some more. She took no painkillers during the first 24 hours because she'd had an allergic reaction to a morphine-based drug after Jenna's birth. When Jillian was 11 hours old, Judy felt refreshed enough to excitedly cuddle and breastfeed her.

Judy's tips for moms having C-sections:

• **Be open-minded.** "Don't listen to anyone else's labor stories because no two are alike. Someone else's experience won't be yours."

• **Ask questions.** "If you're nervous about something, don't just go along. Be proactive."

• **Have a panic plan with your partner.** "Before labor, my husband and I decided he would be with me during my epidural and in the operating and recovery rooms. We also discussed things like, 'If I'm acting bitchy or grumpy, it's because I'm scared,' so he would know. Having a plan helped me feel a measure of control."

• **Rest.** It's not unusual if you don't feel like holding the baby right away. "I told my husband to look after the baby. I knew I needed rest."

• **Banish all thoughts of failure.** "I'd given it my best shot. The bottom line is that you're bringing a beautiful life into the world—that's something to be proud of."

MOTHER TO MOTHER:
"My VBAC"

Cathy Richard, 21
Westfield, Massachusetts

"After my daughter Danielle was born, everyone tried to tell me that it was too bad I would have to have C-sections with my future children," Cathy says. "Since I was fresh out of nursing school, though, I knew better."

Danielle had not been positioned properly for a vaginal birth. While pregnant less than a year later, Cathy read as much as she could about VBACs and discussed her goal with her doctor. "I also daydreamed about what I thought it would be like and reminded myself that others had done it, and so could I."

Overdue, she was scheduled to be induced when her labor began spontaneously. "During my C-section I didn't have to do much," she observes. "During my VBAC, I was much more in control and aware of what was going on. All through labor, the nurses kept asking me if the old incision from the C-section hurt, and it didn't," she says. The worst part was that it seemed to take so long. After 6 hours, she had an epidural, and a short while later began to push. "I thought the baby was stuck and would never come out of me," she confesses. But baby Amber did—and just fine. "I thought, 'I did it!'"

Cathy's tips to other moms considering VBACs:

• **Realize that pushing takes time.** "When I started to push I was so excited, but only for the first 10 minutes. Then I began to wonder if I could do it."

• **Have the right support.** "It was a better experience for me because both my doctor and my husband encouraged me the whole time."

• **Face your fear.** "It's common to be scared—of failing, of not knowing what to expect, of needing another C-section—but a vaginal birth is definitely worth it. While the pain is much more intense during a vaginal delivery, the recovery is much faster."

Right After Delivery

What Happens to Your Baby

Here's what you can expect regarding your newborn's care:

- **Immediate checks.** At birth, the baby's time of delivery will be recorded and the blood and whitish vernix will be cleaned off. To keep warm, the dried baby is wrapped in a clean towel or blanket and topped in a knit hat. Or the baby may be placed skin-to-skin on your chest with a blanket placed over top. One minute after birth, an Apgar evaluation is made to assess the child's overall condition. (See "Baby's First Test," page 281.) The baby receives an identity tag or bracelet and is weighed and measured. Finger- and footprints are also taken. (Ask to have an extra set of prints made right in your baby book; some hospitals provide a set made on paper with a peel-off backing that can be pasted into your baby's records.) Eye drops are administered to prevent infection.

The labor nurses usually conduct these initial procedures right in the delivery room. They can make you very impatient, though, as your partner gets a front-row view of the proceedings and you're left across the room, itching to get your hands on your new baby. But the procedures usually don't take long. Birth represents a stressful change of environment for your baby, and the medical personnel must make periodic checks over the first few hours of life to be sure the baby is making the adjustment well. The extremities, genitals, abdominal organs, breathing, temperature, and heart tones will all be assessed. If the baby gets too chilled—which, after leaving the cozy womb and getting wiped clean is common in a cool hospital—he or she may be placed under warming lights or given to you for skin-to-skin contact.

Except for the Apgar test, however, nothing needs to be done immediately. The aforementioned procedures can be postponed until after you get a chance to breastfeed, which has been shown to help the uterus contract. And if your newborn appears healthy, even the Apgar can be done while you hold the baby in your arms. Within a few hours of birth, a pediatrician will also evaluate the newborn's physical state, including the fontanel (soft spots in the skull where the bones have yet to fuse), the palate (for cleftness), backbone, fingers and toes, hip joints, spine, and reflexes. If the mother is Rh-negative, blood may also be taken from the umbilical cord to check whether Rh antibodies have formed (called a *Coombs test*) and to check the baby's blood type.

If there were problems at birth, such as the umbilical cord having been tight around the neck or if the baby inhaled meconium (fetal wastes), the newborn is

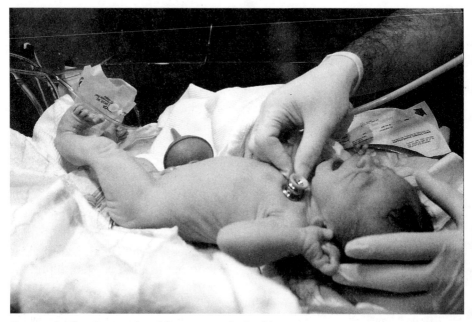

During the first hours after delivery, periodic health assessments are made to check your baby's well-being.

examined by pediatric specialists. If this must be done in a neonatal nursery, your partner can usually follow along and bring you an update. As soon as the baby is stable, you'll be able to hold him or her.

• **Meeting the world.** After birth, the newborn typically remains in a quiet, alert state for an hour or so, particularly if little or no medication crossed into his or her system. This makes for an ideal time to breastfeed. There's no reason not to let mother, father, and baby spend as much time together as they like.

If your child's head has a cone shape at birth, rest assured it will assume the typical round form within a few hours or days; the misshapen pointed look is just the result of the soft fetal skull having molded itself to the shape of the birth canal. Some parents also worry about puffy or squinty eyes at birth, or whites of the eyes that are flecked with red (from ruptured blood vessels). These effects, too, are the result of the narrow squeeze out the birth canal and will go away in the coming days. Newborn skin may be oily or appear to have acne, or it may be dry and peeling, especially on the hands and feet.

• **Tests before discharge.** A blood sample will be taken from the baby's heel. The blood is routinely tested for phenylketonuria (PKU, a rare, inherited inability to break down most proteins), hypothyroidism, galactosemia (an inherited inability to process galactose, a milk sugar), maple-syrup urine disease (or maple-sugar disease, an inherited disorder in which an enzyme needed to break down an amino acid is lacking), sickle-cell anemia if indicated, or other conditions as needed. Occasionally, a pediatrician may conduct a final physical assessment, including a battery of exams to test behavior and neurological state called the *Brazelton neonatal behavioral assessment scale* (after its developer, pediatrician T. Berry Brazelton) before the baby is released.

• **To room in or not to room in?** Rooming in—where your baby stays in your room in a portable bassinet—is a wonderful option, especially if you can't bear to be separated from your treasured newcomer. It's also been found to enhance the odds of successful breastfeeding. In fact, some hospitals no longer have general nurseries. But don't feel guilty about sending the baby to the nursery if one is available and you're worn out. That's what it's there for. Be sure to ask that your baby be brought to you for nursing every 2 to 3 hours and to specify that no bottles of water or formula be given to your baby, to prevent nipple confusion. (Breast- and bottle-feeding require different types of sucks.) You may also not wish your newborn to be given a pacifier for the same reason.

• **Postpartum paperwork.** Before checkout, you'll be given a form to fill out that will become the baby's official birth certificate. Depending on the state you live in, requested information includes parents' names, addresses, birthplaces, marital status, race, and education, and details about the birth itself. It's best to have the baby's name already selected, since it's more convenient and you may get charged a late fee by the state if you supply the name after the birth certificate has been filed. Check all spellings for accuracy, too—it can also be expensive to change a name (even if it was a mistake) once it's been filed. The hospital registers the birth certificate and, if you request it, the state sends you an official copy for a fee a few weeks later. The original is kept in state or county government offices. In most cases, the forms also allow you to indicate if you'd like to obtain a Social Security number for your child, sparing you the hassle of applying for one later. A Social Security card is sent directly to you within a few weeks. Your child must have a Social Security number so that you can claim him or her on your federal income taxes.

What Happens to You

What can you expect in the first days after giving birth?

• **Physical reactions—*vaginal delivery.*** How you feel right after childbirth
will depend on the nature of your labor and delivery. Most mothers who had
uncomplicated vaginal deliveries experience a surge of adrenaline and good
humor, no matter how long or hard they've just worked. You're also apt to feel
very hungry. Never again will hospital food and that first sip of juice (or especially cola, if you've just spent 9 months abstaining from it) taste so good. Because your body has just undergone a bit of a trauma, however, you may tingle,
shake uncontrollably, or feel very cold. The shakes are normal and will soon
pass. Ask for extra blankets if they're not offered right away.

For the first several days postpartum, you'll continue to feel contractions as
your uterus begins to shrink, a process called *involution.* More like bad menstrual cramps than the searing pain of labor contractions, they can nonetheless
be quite painful, especially within the first 24 hours of delivery. Involution
cramps intensify during breastfeeding because the oxytocin released in nursing
triggers the contractions. You may be offered medication (such as prescription-
strength ibuprofen) to ease discomfort.

You'll also bleed heavily after delivery, needing a change of sanitary pads
every hour or so for the first day or two. You may also pass clots, some the size
of small pancakes, in the first 24 hours. Called *lochia,* this discharge starts out
bright red and gradually subsides and fades in color over the next few weeks.

To get your circulation going, walk around as soon as you can. This speeds
healing, too. Be sure to have assistance the first time you try to get out of bed,
as you may be dizzy or unsteady on your feet. You may not be able to urinate
right away, since your bladder may be sore. You may not feel the need since
there is now more room for a full bladder to expand, but you will within a day.
Your bowels may also be sluggish, especially if it's been a long time since you
ate. If you had any stitching, the first bowel movement (within the first 1 to 3
days postpartum) can be as hard psychologically as physically because of soreness, but don't worry; you can't tear your sutures. A stool softener is usually
given. A cold pack helps relieve itching in the perineum for the first hours after
delivery; later, heat may feel better. Showers or warm sitz baths (in a special
shallow pan your nurse will provide) may help.

A mother with Rh-negative blood who has a baby with Rh-positive blood
will be given a shot of RhoGAM within 24 hours of delivery to prevent the formation of Rh antibodies that could be harmful to a future fetus.

• *Physical reactions—Cesarean delivery.* A range of physical responses is normal, though for all women the first day is the most difficult. You may feel considerable pain from your incisions and moving around in bed may be difficult. Nonetheless, get out of bed as soon after surgery as possible for a short walk to minimize severe gas pains caused by the buildup of gas in the bowels. You may not be steady on your feet, so don't attempt this alone. You'll need to master the art of getting out of bed and walking without using your abdominal muscles. The hospital staff will show you how. It also helps to shift positions as best you can in bed and to avoid carbonated beverages. Your bladder catheter usually will remain in place until the next day; when it's removed, you'll be encouraged to try to use the bathroom. Hunger is uncommon during the first day after delivery. You'll probably be kept on a liquid diet until your bowels recover and can function normally (in 2 to 3 days).

The uterus involutes just as it does following a vaginal delivery. Women who have had C-sections also experience postpartum bleeding (lochia), although the discharge may be lighter because the uterus was swabbed out during surgery.

• *Medical checks.* No matter what type of delivery you've had, like your baby you'll be closely watched by the hospital staff in the first hours after delivery. Your blood pressure, pulse, and temperature will be monitored repeatedly. Your uterus will be massaged to speed involution. You'll be checked for signs of excessive bleeding or infection.

Sometimes codeine or other medication is offered to relieve incision pain. Even an over-the-counter analgesic such as acetaminophen can help. Don't hesitate to take a painkiller if you need it; it can speed your recovery and will not interfere with your ability to nurse successfully.

• *Emotional reactions.* Most women (and men, too) experience one of life's peak highs right after childbirth. A wild mix of feelings courses through you: euphoria and incredulity that your baby is here at last, pride that your body accomplished such a feat, relief that the physical work is over, and an instant I'd-lay-down-my-life-for-you love more powerful than you may have ever imagined. Thoughts of your contraction pain vanish. Instead, you'll dwell on counting your baby's fingers and toes and trying to figure out who this new family member resembles.

You'll want to spread your news to family and friends. The conventional wisdom is to conserve your energy, and that's certainly wise. Some experts advise just telling a few close friends and relatives about the birth and letting them inform everyone else. On the other hand, you *will* feel keyed up in the first day and want to retell your birth story, so if you feel up to making a lot of phone calls and greeting visitors, indulge yourself. A day like this doesn't come around often in your life. *Important caveat*: Your partner must put some restraints on visitors. Your body will be tired, and a little bit of goodwill goes a long way in the postpartum period. Limit visits to no more than 15 minutes, and block off time for naps when no visitors are allowed. Some women prefer to just curl up with their newborn and their partner in a private bubble and not see anyone until after they're home. Also, your time in the hospital is so limited these days, you'll want to spend as much of it as possible learning about newborn care and breastfeeding, along with recuperating.

WHAT IF ...

I'm too tired to nurse right away? Though immediate nursing can speed the involution (shrinking) of your uterus, there's no rule of successful breastfeeding that says you must begin within minutes of delivery. Try as soon as you feel up to it, ideally within the first hour and definitely within the first 4 hours. On the first day of life, newborns can breastfeed up to twelve times and should nurse at least eight times, without restrictions. Ask a knowledgeable nurse or doctor to help you the first few times to be sure the infant is attached properly to the breast.

I don't fall in love with my baby right away? Sometimes overwhelming fatigue, residual medication, or pain leaves a worn-out new mom too preoccupied to feel much more for her newborn other than a relief that he or she has arrived at last. That's perfectly understandable. Other women harbor a lingering ambivalence about motherhood, or simply take longer to warm up to this new little being who is, in a sense, a perfect stranger. There's no right length of time involved in falling in love—sooner or later, you will.

My baby's born in the middle of the night—is it okay to call people up to tell them? It's your call, so to speak. While everyone is thrilled to hear about a birth, not everyone fully appreciates such news in the wee hours. Face it, few people beyond your parents and a select few others can possibly match your immediate postbirth high. You might make the essential calls right away, then force yourself to get some rest and tell others in the morning—when you've all had some sleep. (You'll probably get a more enthused reaction then, too.)

I want to stay in the hospital longer than my doctor recommends or the insurance company allows? Start by speaking up. Fatigue and nervousness don't count as legitimate medical excuses to stay, but if you're not feeling well, trust your intuition and tell your doctor. Be persistent. Likewise, tell your pediatrician if you're concerned about the baby, or if you want to stay in the hospital with the baby if you are being discharged before the child. Seek a second opinion. Often a doctor will appeal on your behalf to the insurance carrier. But if your doctor is still reluctant to extend a stay, you can always elect to pick up the tab yourself. Or go home but explore with the hospital discharge planner such resources as home health aides, visiting nurses, or temporary baby nurses.

Baby's First Test

When your baby is 1 minute old, he or she will be given an Apgar test. Named for pediatrician Virginia Apgar, this subjective measurement rates the newborn's response to birth in five areas: Appearance (color), Pulse (heart rate), Grimace (reflex), Activity (muscle tone) and Respiration (breathing). A perfect score is 10, though most healthy newborns score in the 7 to 9 range. Babies who score 4 to 6 usually require some assistance, such as suctioning the airways. A score below 4 indicates more serious problems that must be treated immediately. The test is repeated about 5 minutes later. The purpose of an Apgar is to give the pediatrician a quick snapshot of the baby's stress during delivery and progress outside the womb. Resist the temptation to read anything more into the scores than that: an Apgar doesn't predict IQ or future health.

Score	0	1	2
Color	Blue or pale	Extremeties blue/ body pink	Pink all over
Heart rate	Absent	Below 100 beats per minute	More than 100 beats per minute
Reflexes	No response	Grimaces	Coughs or sneezes
Muscle tone	Limp	Some movement	Active
Breathing	Absent	Weak	Good (crying)

IS IT TRUE...

That I should not miss the first minutes of bonding? If you and your baby are feeling well enough to cuddle or nurse immediately after birth, that's terrific.

Skin-to-skin contact in the first hours of life has been shown to give mothers and babies a head start on the delicious process of falling in love. But if you can't hold your baby right away, a perfectly healthy relationship is just as likely. Bonding is an often misused term that refers to parent-child intimacy and attachment, not to some sort of instantaneous postbirth mind meld. It's a long-term process that takes place over the first months, not minutes, of an infant's life. There's no evidence that mothers and babies who are separated in the hospital because of fatigue or medical emergency are any less close than those who immediately spend time together.

That boys weigh more than girls at birth? This is true, but only on average— exceptions abound. The typical full-term newborn weighs 7 pounds, 7 ounces and measures 20 inches from head to toe. The range of what's considered normal runs from 6 to 9 pounds in weight, and from 17 to 22 inches in length.

That the color of my baby's eyes at birth can change? Yes. Most babies of color are born with dark eyes that remain unchanged, but light-skinned newborns tend to come into the world with deep blue peepers. The color isn't fixed until after 1 year.

That my baby can't see well yet? Newborns used to be thought of as blind, senseless blank slates. Today researchers know that they can see fairly well up to about 12 to 18 inches (not coincidentally, the distance to a mother's face when cradled in her arms or when breastfeeding). In utero, a fetus can hear from about 22 weeks on. An hours-old newborn can even recognize Mom's unique smell.

That some babies are born with teeth? Supposedly Julius Caesar and Napoleon were among the 1 in 2,000 newborns who greet the world with one, and sometimes two, *natal teeth*. Usually a lower incisor, the tooth may be an actual primary (baby) tooth or a poorly rooted pretooth that will fall out and regrow at the usual time for teeth to appear, in the middle of the first year. Often natal teeth are pulled right away to prevent choking.

GOOD ADVICE: NEWBORN SECURITY

Everyone jokes about bringing home the wrong baby, but it can happen. Likewise, although babynapping is extremely rare, every year a half-dozen newborns are kidnapped from hospitals, usually by women desperate for a child themselves. That's why all hospitals give mothers and babies identification bracelets. Many hospitals band babies with tiny, lightweight security tags (at the ankle or umbilical stump) that can activate sensors at ward exits, the way department stores protect clothes. Though such nightmares are the last thing on your mind after having a baby, consider these precautions as your first foray into smart parenting:

- Consider rooming in throughout your hospital stay, which minimizes your infant's comings and goings.
- When your baby is in your room, keep the crib on the far side of your bed away from the door.
- Send the baby to the nursery or make sure someone else is in the room when you use the bathroom or shower.
- Always be sure hospital personnel show you identification before taking your baby (don't trust the look of the uniform alone). He or she should explain where they're going and why. If you're at all uncertain, ask for verification (such as by calling the nurses' station).
- Compare your baby's identification band number with your own when you're reunited—nurses should do this routinely.

Checklist: Are You Ready to Go Home?

Although federal law now mandates that new mothers be allowed a minimum 48-hour hospital stay, that's much shorter than in your mother's day. And for many new moms, the temptation is great to rush out of the maternity ward even sooner, perhaps home to an older child. There are, however, important reasons not to go home too quickly. Doctors want to monitor both you and the baby for unexpected complications. A longer stay also gives you more recuperation time as well as a crash course in breastfeeding, baby care, and how to identify potential conditions such as postpartum depression. Any mother who does leave a hospital or maternity center within a day of birth must have adequate follow-up care (for both herself and her baby) and help at home.

Mother

Before discharge, you should be comfortable knowing how to:

☐ Hold the baby
☐ Feed the baby

☐ Burp the baby
☐ Change a diaper
☐ Detect jaundice and dehydration
☐ Care for the umbilical stump and (if appropriate) circumcision site
☐ Get support or assistance at home; if you'll be alone, consider en-
listing in-home care by a visiting nurse or professional doula, and
have the number of a lactation consultant handy; find out about local mother support groups and breastfeeding groups, as well as
telephone help lines

If you've had a C-section, you should also be able to:

☐ Eat solid foods
☐ Urinate on your own
☐ Administer your pain medications
☐ Walk without too much pain
☐ Care for your stitches

Baby

Before discharge, a baby should:

☐ Be weighed and measured
☐ Be in stable condition
☐ Have urinated and passed one stool within 24 hours of birth
☐ Maintain a normal temperature
☐ Be able to suck and swallow
☐ Have received a heel stick for conditions such as PKU, hypothy-
roidism, and sickle-cell anemia

Checklist: Handy Items to Bring Home

Ask if these items can be taken home with you, if your hospital provides them to patients, or how to obtain them:

☐ Painkillers (or a prescription for them)
☐ Stool softeners
☐ A sitz bath

☐ A supply of peri pads (large sanitary pads) and light mesh underpants in which to wear them

☐ Tucks pads (gauze pads soaked in witch hazel to soothe the perineum)

☐ Anesthetic spray (for perineal care)

☐ A peri bottle (plastic squirt bottle for cleansing the perineum)

☐ Ready-to-use alcohol pads (for cleaning the baby's umbilical stump)

☐ Contact information for a follow-up home care nurse and a breast-feeding consultant

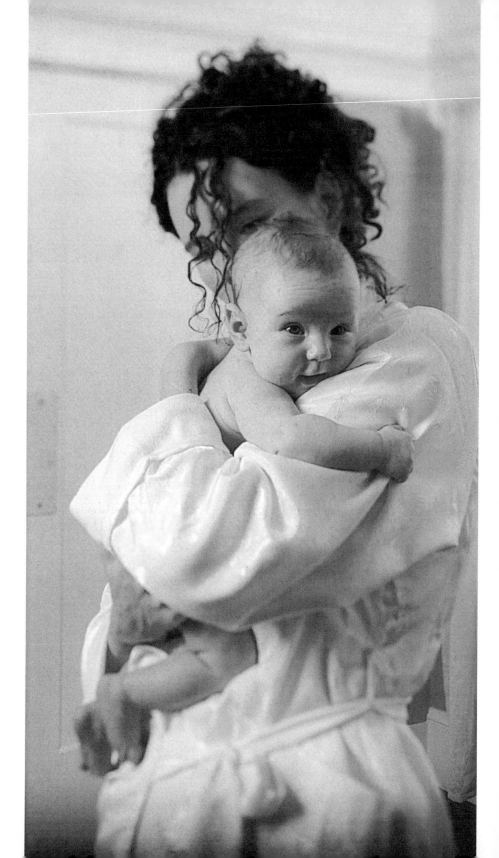

CHAPTER 5

YOUR "FOURTH TRIMESTER"

RECOVERY AND NEWBORN CARE

Unforgettable—that's the day you bring your newborn home from the hospital or birthing center. Even a familiar drive seems different, with your precious new cargo snuggled in an infant seat like some fragile, rare work of art. Maybe you'll photograph the grand entrance at the front door. Maybe you'll show your baby around the nursery. Almost certainly you'll spend a long time gazing into the bassinet, which so long had stood mysteriously empty, awaiting this very moment.

After that, though, the first weeks with a newborn tend to blur. Everything's new. Nobody except the baby sleeps (or at least not very much).

The pregnancy-related issues that had obsessed you for the greater part of the past year vanish. In their place spring forth new concerns—about taking care of your baby, taking care of yourself, and adjusting to your new life together.

What you need to remember now: Take it easy! Take it slowly!

Your body, after all, has just accomplished an enormous feat by growing and bringing forth a new life. Your physical recovery is the fountain from which all the other adjustments to motherhood flow. That's why doctors refer to the first 3 months after delivery as pregnancy's "fourth trimester."

What's Going on in Your Body

The Biology of Recovery

You don't go home from the hospital wearing your favorite old jeans. Nor will you bounce back to your former self right away. There are many reasons for this.

First, your body has just run a tremendous physical marathon. Over the past 9 months, your blood volume doubled, the capacity of your uterus expanded up to a thousandfold, and almost every major organ and blood vessel has been either squashed or working overtime to accommodate your baby's growth. Various muscles have lost tone, thanks to disuse (your arms and legs, if you've slacked off exercise), misuse (your back, from the havoc pregnancy often wreaks with posture), or overuse (your stretched-out abdomen and vagina). If you had stitches, either from an episiotomy, a perineal tear, or a C-section, you've got added healing to contend with. Yet even as your body craves time and rest in order to recuperate, it's taxed by the 'round-the-clock demands of a newborn who's making plenty of his or her own adjustments.

So how long does the physical recovery from childbirth take? That depends on your delivery, your level of fitness, the amount of help you receive in the immediate postpartum period, and whether or not complications develop. In general, most of the direct results of childbirth clear up in 6 weeks. Stitches heal, the uterus returns to its pre-pregnancy size, and bleeding stops. But side effects ranging from breast tenderness to perineal soreness can persist long afterward. Most startling may be the doughy condition of your midsection—for the first few weeks of motherhood, you'll still look 6 months (or more) pregnant. That's because your uterus is still enlarged and the abdominal muscles and surrounding skin are hanging slack after having been so stretched. You may bounce back in a few months. Or totally reclaiming your former figure may take up to 9 months or longer—as much time as it took to grow your baby.

Here are some of the most predictable after-effects of childbirth and what to do about them.

• **Vaginal discharge (lochia).** Bleeding after childbirth is normal as the uterus sheds its lining and the site where the placenta was implanted heals. The amount of odorless, bloody discharge gradually lessens and progressively lightens in color and consistency, from bright red and mucusy (for the first 3 or 4 days) to pink or brownish and watery, finally becoming yellow-to-clear within 2 to 8 weeks (about 30 days is average). Doctors aren't concerned about how long the discharge lasts, but whether or not it diminishes.

Use heavy-absorbency sanitary pads, not tampons, to absorb the flow. Change the pad every time you use the bathroom, or more often as needed. You should also avoid douching until the healing is complete.

• **Afterpains (uterine involution).** Beginning immediately after delivery, your uterus shrinks from the size of a watermelon to that of a small cantaloupe, a process called *involution*. The contractions that restore the uterus to its pre-pregnancy size help reduce postpartum bleeding as they clamp off blood vessels.

The contractions can feel mild or sharp, similar to menstrual cramps, and are most noticeable during the first postpartum week. Breastfeeding in the first weeks also stimulates uterine contractions, because the hormone oxytocin is released when the newborn suckles. That's why you may notice more intense contractions when you nurse. Breastfeeding speeds involution, causing nursing mothers to bleed less. In the hospital, medical staffers will press on your abdomen to be sure the uterus feels firm, rather than mushy, a sign that it's contracting properly. You can also massage the area to speed healing. A second-time mother, or one who had twins or more, tends to have severe afterpains because her uterus is more stretched, requiring more contracting.

You may be given pain relievers immediately after delivery (most are safe for nursing). Acetaminophen or ibuprofen are safe, common choices. Other ways to ease cramps are to empty your bladder frequently to give the uterus room or to lie on your stomach on a pillow or apply warm compresses. Also try whatever nonmedical tactics you've used successfully to relieve menstrual cramps, or use the relaxation and breathing exercises that helped you through labor contractions.

• *Perineal pain.* Recovery from an episiotomy or tear may be the most excruciating aspect of your physical recovery. Many mothers are surprised to discover that walking, and even sitting, is painful, especially if the stitches are extensive. That's because the skin in the perineum (the area between the vagina and rectum) tends to swell after trauma, tightening the stitches. Compounding the misery are common (albeit unwarranted) fears about straining the stitches during ordinary movement or elimination. Plus, it's hard to see the site and get a good mental picture of why you hurt so much. (The stitches dissolve on their own and do not have to be removed.)

To ease pain, keep the area clean. You'll probably be given a plastic squirt bottle (sometimes called a *peri bottle*) to fill with a special antiseptic or warm water for cleansing after you use the bathroom. Gently pat the area dry from front to back. You may also be given a topical analgesic spray or cold witch hazel compresses (such as Tucks pads). Acetaminophen or ibuprofen pills help too, and won't interfere with nursing.

Two other standard comfort measures for perineal pain are ice packs and sitz baths. To make a perineal ice pack, soak several large sanitary napkins in water and squeeze out the excess, then freeze. A sitz bath is a hot-water soak. In the hospital, you may be given a special shallow, plastic pan; it fits over the toilet and can be hooked up to a water dispenser to provide a constant flow of water. (Sitz baths are also available in pharmacies.) The pan and dispenser are filled with water as warm as you can tolerate, and you sit in the flow for up to 20 minutes. Some doctors recommend ice-cold sitz baths to numb pain. Repeated several times a day during the first week, a sitz bath soothes traumatized tissues. If toweling the area afterward (or after showering) hurts, try using a blow-dryer on a cool setting instead.

• **Hemorrhoids and constipation.** The same veins in the anal area that may have enlarged during pregnancy can worsen after the added strain of labor and delivery. While painful, they tend to disappear within a few weeks. Relief measures include over-the-counter topical ointments (such as Preparation H), witch hazel compresses, ice packs, and sitz baths. Although sluggish bowels are common for the first couple of days postpartum, constipation can result if pain causes you to hold in your bowel movements. You may be given a stool softener in the hospital to help minimize stress during a BM. Also, drink lots of fluids and eat foods that contain fiber (fresh or dried fruits, vegetables, bran cereal, 100 percent whole wheat bread) to keep your digestive system working smoothly. Drinking water, juice, and milk is especially important because your body is directing its fluid stores toward milk production.

• **Urinary problems.** A need to urinate frequently is normal. Fluids accumulated in your tissues during pregnancy must be shed. (Some women perspire profusely or have night sweats as well.) Don't assume that an increased need to use the bathroom is a sign to cut back on the amount of liquids you're drinking. To the contrary, continuing to drink eight or more glasses of water a day helps circulation, promotes milk production, and combats constipation and dehydration.

Some women also develop *stress incontinence*, a reduced ability to control urine flow, or a leakage of urine when they cough or sneeze. (If you had this problem during pregnancy, it may worsen postpartum.) To help regain control, empty your bladder frequently and practice Kegel exercises. Most postbirth incontinence clears up within a month; if not, be sure to inform your doctor at your postpartum checkup because it's easily remedied with Kegels, pelvic inserts to strengthen muscles, or medication. Surgery may be advised as a last resort.

• **Engorgement.** Expect your milk to come in about 2 to 4 days after you give birth. Before that, your breasts produce colostrum, a thin but rich liquid that is sufficient to nourish your baby even in small amounts. How will you know when the real thing kicks in? Your breasts will grow bigger, more tender, and hotter to the touch. Sometimes they overfill at first, a painful condition known as engorgement. When this happens, the breasts feel hard and tight. The best way to ease discomfort is to feed your baby on demand, at least ten to twelve times per 24 hours for the first few weeks. At first, it may be hard for the baby to latch on if the breasts are too full; if this is the case, try expressing a little milk manually or with a pump. (See "Expressing Breast Milk," page 310.) Ease the discomfort of engorgement with warm towel compresses or a warm shower. The problem clears up in a day or two as your baby begins regular feedings and the milk supply starts to regulate. The breasts then soften and feel more normal, although they will remain one or two cup sizes larger than they were during pregnancy.

You can prevent engorgement by not going longer than 3 hours between feedings, even at night, during the first week postpartum. Engorgement can recur anytime you go too long between feedings (or pumpings), but it's most common when milk first comes in and in the early weeks until a feeding pattern is established.

If you don't plan to nurse, your milk glands will cease production naturally. When no milk is used by an infant, the supply dries up. In the lag before this happens (usually several days), you'll experience some engorgement. The best way to avoid pain—which is also best for your baby—is to breastfeed at least for the first 2 weeks. Then taper off slowly, replacing breastfeedings with formula feedings (replace one feeding every 2 days or so). This not only prevents engorgement but also enables your baby to benefit from colostrum, the pre-milk substance that protects against disease. (The medication bromocryptine, trade name Parlodel, was once routinely given to nonnursing mothers to dry up the breasts and to treat engorgement. The U.S. Food and Drug Administration withdrew approval for this drug for these uses on the grounds that its risks, including stroke and death, outweighed its benefits.)

• *Sleep deprivation.* Not getting enough sleep because of 'round-the-clock feedings just as your recovering body needs it most can actually slow recuperation and cloud your emotions. Things that intensify fatigue include producing breast milk, postpartum anemia, poor nutrition (including a lack of potassium), and postpartum depression. (See "The Baby Blues," page 296.) You can minimize the ill feeling of sleep deprivation with catnaps, healthful eating, and fresh air. This is another reason postpartum helpers are so important.

Cesarean Recovery

All the rest-rest-rest advice chanted at new moms is doubly important if you had a Cesarean delivery, which is, after all, major abdominal surgery. Women who deliver surgically tend to lose twice as much blood as those who deliver vaginally. So in addition to allowing yourself a longer recuperative period, some special care considerations are in order. You'll need to:

• **Get help.** What's wonderful for any new mom—ready-made hot meals, help with the laundry—becomes essential after a C-section. Try to line up companions 24 hours a day for the first 3 weeks. Hire a nurse or postpartum doula if needed.

• **Take medication if you're in pain.** Don't tough it out. Use acetaminophen (without codeine if you're nursing) to relieve general soreness and pain. This can also make you feel less tense—which is a natural response to the tightness of your stitches.

• **Get moving.** You won't feel like it, but you need to get up and move around as soon as surgery is over, with a little help. Abdominal surgery causes the normal action of the intestines to stop, which can result in sharp gas pains. Short walks and frequent changes of position restore the normal movement of your intestines while promoting circulation, which speeds healing and helps prevent clots or swelling.

• **Rock steady.** Using a rocking chair for a half hour, several times a day, can relieve trapped gas, which can be excruciating if allowed to collect in your stomach. This is a pleasant way to spend time with your baby, too.

• **Simplify baby care.** Minimize the number of times you lift and set down your baby. Ideally, have someone bring the baby to you. You may find it easier to let the baby sleep by your side in bed at night. During feedings, place a pillow under the baby's body to cushion your abdomen when cradling him or her in your arms.

GOOD ADVICE: BEST REST IDEAS

How can you get the R&R you so richly deserve and need in the early weeks, when the baby's up all night, well-wishers are calling, and the dirty dishes are stacked higher than the laundry pile?

• Line up help—your partner, mother, sister, best friend—so that someone's with you all day and all night for at least the first 5 days. (It's no coincidence this is called the *lying-in period*.) Don't even think about going it alone.
• For the times when you can't enlist a volunteer, look into hiring a professional nurse or a postpartum doula. The latter option, growing rapidly in popularity, is a trained postpartum caregiver who takes care of the mother (cooking, cleaning, running errands, providing basic health assistance) so the mother can focus on the baby. Rates range from $20 to $30 an hour.
• Nap when the baby naps (it's the wisest maxim a new mom will ever hear).

- Wear your nightgown and robe all day long for the first week or two—nothing sends a more vivid signal to visitors that "I'm recuperating!" (Longer than 2 weeks, though, and you'll feel schlumpy, not pampered, by lingering in your sleepwear past noon.)
- Nap.
- Eat off paper plates.
- Nap.
- Do not play hostess to well-wishers. Don't clean up before they arrive, don't even offer them water. Nor should they expect you to serve them.
- Nap.
- When someone asks what they can do, follow up! Ask for a hot meal (home-made or take-out) or a hand with the laundry.
- Screen calls before automatically answering the phone.
- Nap.
- If you live in a house with more than one floor, set up a sleeping and diaper-changing station on each floor. A bassinet in the living room and a towel-covered ottoman next to a spare diaper pail will spare you unnecessary ups and downs. Keep extra diapers, wipes, baby clothes, blankets there, too.
- If you breastfeed, after your milk supply is established—within 3 to 6 weeks—express into a bottle before you turn in so your partner can take over at least one middle-of-the-night feeding.
- Keep the baby in a bassinet by your bedside initially, rather than making frequent treks to the nursery; or sleep in a spare bed in the nursery.
- Meet your baby's needs first, then your own. Let everything go after that—including use of the vacuum, oven, and dishwasher.
- Nap.

Checklist: When to Call the Doctor

Alert your obstetrician if you experience any of the following after delivery:

☐ Bright red bleeding with fever after your vaginal discharge has begun to pale (a sign the uterus isn't healing smoothly, perhaps because you've overexerted)

☐ Copious bleeding (soaking one or more sanitary pads an hour for 4 to 5 hours, which could indicate part of the placenta remains)

☐ Numerous large blood clots (another sign that the placenta didn't come out intact)

☐ Foul-smelling lochia (sign of infection)
☐ Painful urination (sign of infection)
☐ Fever higher than 100.4 degrees (sign of possible infection)
☐ Nausea and vomiting
☐ Feeling worse from week to week instead of better (you should be experiencing steady physical improvement)

What's Going on in Your Head

First Feelings

Gazing into your newborn's eyes and realizing that you're officially a mother can unleash a whirlwind of emotional reactions—some predictable and others that strike you like an unexpected thunderbolt. The range of normal responses is enormous. Little wonder. Having a baby is a major life transition, and one that impacts each individual differently. Your relationships and responsibilities are transformed overnight. And on top of all the other physical adjustments in your body, your hormones are packing an incredible wallop, even more dramatic than the hormonal surges you experienced back in your first trimester.

Reassure yourself that most feelings are common:

• *Pride and joy—or detachment.* Most mothers are thrilled to meet the baby they've fantasized about and obsessed over for 9 months. They find that they can't stop touching and looking at their newborn; even watching the child sleep seems fascinating. But not every woman experiences intense love at first sight. Especially if she's had a difficult pregnancy or delivery, or if the baby's condition or gender isn't what she'd envisioned, a woman may need longer to get to know and love her baby. Unconscious fears about babies or one's ability to care for a newborn can also cause some women to hold back. Don't feel guilty or remiss if ambivalence is your dominant emotion. It's no reflection on your suitability for motherhood. There's a lot going on right now. Give yourself time.

• *The need to relive the birth experience.* You'll find that you never tire of re-counting the centimeter-by-centimeter tale of how your baby came into the world. The most minute details about procedures, breathing exercises, and your labor support team are apt to stay with you for years. Whether it's a story laced with pride or disappointment, the compulsion to retell one's birth story is a universal phenomenon. In part, this is a crucial sorting-out process that helps resolve your feelings about the birth. Especially if the experience did not go exactly as imagined, reexamining all the details is cathartic, allowing a woman to grieve over what wasn't while coming to terms with what was. Likewise, reliving a positive experience can help cement a new self-image—as a strong capable person, as a mother.

• *Anxiety and inadequacy.* It's a big new job. Expect nagging self-doubts such as, "Am I doing this right? Will I be a good mother?" Your baby can further undermine your confidence, since newborns aren't terribly articulate about expressing their wants or giving positive feedback. Don't aspire to perfection, just try to get through each day as best you can. Your competence—and confidence—will grow right along with your baby.

• *Sensitivity (to criticism, to advice, to everyone).* If you thought you got a lot of tips during pregnancy, just wait. Opinions abound about baby care. The trouble is, your psyche is just a bit fragile now, making you ultrasensitive to the suggestions and actions of those around you. Self-consciousness about your new role, fatigue, and hormones can make your wick very short. Accept this (as those around you ought to be sensitive enough to do as well)—it, too, will pass.

• *Mood swings.* Don't be surprised if your elation over your baby is peppered with mild depression, weepiness, or plain ambivalence. It's hard for even the most contented mama to stay on a postbirth high through 2 A.M. feedings, sitz baths, and the 15th diaper change of the day. The mundane aspects of baby care can wear you down, especially in the anticlimatic weeks after the initial rush of calls and gifts subsides. A vague sense of letdown is also triggered by the jarring discord between your pregnant fantasies of motherhood (cooing babies, enthralled onlookers, trouble-free breastfeeding) and less rosy, more monotonous realities.

Anger is an extremely common, if seldom discussed, new-mother emotion. There may be plenty to be cross about, such as a disappointing birth experience, a colicky baby, lack of sleep, loss of freedom, isolation, episiotomy pain, or plain unrelieved boredom. The anger can be targeted at your doctor, your partner, your mother-in-law—even your baby, which in turn inspires guilt. The healthiest way to handle negative feelings is to confront them. By admitting what you're feeling, and understanding why, you can put such emotions in proper perspective, rather than allowing them to consume you. Only then can you reassure yourself—or get reassurance from your partner, friends, your childbirth educator, or others—that you're not crazy: You're a typical new mother.

• *Irrational fear.* Obsessive-compulsive thoughts about the baby's safety are pretty normal at first. Maybe you check on his or her breathing every hour, or you envision terrible car crashes or dropping the child. Such anxieties are a reflection of how seriously you're taking your new responsibilities and how appre-hensive you may feel about the enormity of parenthood. Such thoughts should fade in their extremeness as the weeks go on. If they don't, they may be a sign of deeper stresses about mothering or postpartum depression, and talking to others, such as in a new-mom support group, can be beneficial. Talk to your doctor.

• **Depressed body image.** Most new moms complain about neither looking nor feeling like "my old self." Especially if you're breastfeeding, you may not even feel like a separate person from your baby, so intertwined are the two of you by constant nursing. Some women rush into a diet, but this can have negative con-sequences, such as an insufficient breast-milk supply or postpartum depression. Exercising before your doctor gives the go-ahead can slow your recovery. Others simply are frustrated that, despite dissatisfaction with their appearance, they don't feel the least bit inclined to do anything about it, given their current pre-occupations. Grant yourself at least a month to wallow in new motherhood, be-fore gradually easing back into abdominal exercises and new hairdos. In the meanwhile, do simple things that make you feel fresh—a bath or shower, pulled-back hair, a new nursing top, a little cologne or makeup. Don't let your partner or anyone else pressure you to get back in shape before you're ready—physically and psychologically.

The Baby Blues

With birth, strangely enough, comes loss—the physical loss of the child from your womb, loss of sleep, loss of your old identity. You're also losing hormones: progesterone and estrogen levels plummet about 3 days after delivery, which can cause emotional changes. Add fatigue, pain, today's abbreviated hospital stays, and the stress of a crying baby to the mix, and it's little wonder that the upheavals of the first weeks of motherhood leave between 30 and 80 percent of new mothers experiencing the so-called baby blues.

The ways this type of depression makes itself known vary from woman to woman. For some, it may be a passing irritability that shows up around 3 to 5 days after giving birth. (Coincidentally, this is the same period during which your milk supply kicks in—hence the old term for postpartum blues, "milk fever.") Others experience moodiness, increased sensitivity, or crying jags over a period of 1 to 2 weeks.

For about 1 in 10 women, however, a more persistent form of postpartum depression (PPD) lingers. The first clue is its longevity. Most run-of-the-mill baby blues pass by the time the newborn is 2 weeks old. PPD can kick in at any time during the first 3 months and linger for a month to more than a year. Symptoms are usually more severe than those previously described and worsen with time, rather than improve. The woman may feel hopelessness, inertia, anxiety, obsessive worry, panic attacks, insomnia in spite of extreme fatigue, and a general lack of interest in daily life—including in her baby and her partner. A loss of appetite, energy, and memory are common, too. Often a woman first writes off these reactions as part of the normal craziness of new motherhood; as they persist, however, she may grow frightened by their intensity. She may feel guilty that she feels so down at what is supposed to be such an uplifting time of life. Any new mother can develop PPD, though risk factors include a blood relative who had it (ask your mother), colicky or hard-to-care-for babies, a prior bout with PPD or clinical depression, isolation, postpartum medical problems or a baby with problems, and a predisposition to self-criticism. (Breastfeeding has been found to reduce the risk of postpartum depression.)

Don't get hung up on trying to diagnose whether you're the 1 mom in 10 who experiences PPD. Symptoms, and their severity, vary widely. If your blues bug you enough, or if you have several of the symptoms, confide in someone, such as your partner, a friend, or your doctor. (Don't wait for your physician to ask about your emotional state at your postpartum checkup—not all do.) PPD is a recognized psychiatric disorder and not a figment of one's imagination, nor is it your "fault." Hormones plus stress are believed to be the major causes.

The earlier the symptoms are addressed, the less likely a woman—or her child—is to suffer from the effects of depression down the road. Sometimes just addressing the problem and taking steps to amend it, such as getting household help or joining a support group of other new moms, are enough to set women on a sunnier path. Or PPD can be treated with psychotherapy (seeing a psychologist or psychiatrist) and sometimes medication. These include antidepressants (such as Prozac and Paxil) and antianxiety drugs. Don't worry that you'll have to wean your baby; some antidepressants are safe for breastfeeding women.

Sanity Savers

The tumult of early motherhood is inescapable. To improve your odds of greater serenity, be sure to get:

• *Rest.* Fatigue exacerbates emotions. It also interferes with everything from breastfeeding to physical recovery, which in turn color your feelings. The new moms' rest credo is: instead of walking around, sit; instead of sitting, lounge on a sofa or recliner; instead of lounging, lie down.

• **Support.** This refers not just to day-to-day help with meals and diaper changing but also to the emotional support of your partner and others in whom you can confide your triumphs, fear, and irritations. Another new mom—especially one with a child just a few months older than yours—is the ideal person to compare notes with right now. Look into local mothers' groups, breastfeeding support groups, and postnatal exercise classes, or follow up with classmates from your childbirth preparation course.

• **Time for yourself.** Don't neglect your personal needs—physical and mental. Even though immersing yourself in your newborn can be galvanizing, it can breed resentment and fuel fatigue. Make an effort to recharge your batteries. At minimum, there's no excuse not to take a shower every day. (Five minutes crying in the safety of a crib won't hurt the baby. Or bring a bouncy seat into the bathroom so you can watch the baby while you bathe.) And while you don't want to overdo visitors in the early weeks, realize that isolation can be just as problematic as too much company. Aim for a healthy balance of companionship and time alone.

• **Outlets for venting.** Every new mom should have one or two "safe havens" where she can let out bottled-up emotions. Maybe this is a trusted friend, your mother, or your spouse. Maybe an electronic chat room, a support group, a parental stress line, prayer, or a journal works best for you. Whatever your outlet you should feel uncensored and unjudged—and unhurried, too. It doesn't help to confide in someone who tells you "Enough, already."

• **Knowledge.** Ignorance breeds fear, which is the last thing you need to deal with right now. Mothering is not all basic instinct—you have to learn how. In addition to reading books and magazines, seek out answers from your own mother, your ob-gyn and pediatrician, friends, and support networks in mothers' groups or on-line. Just bear in mind that there is no "right" way to parent. You'll make yourself crazy if you try to adhere to "the rules" about how to do things—not even the experts agree about every issue. Solicit lots of opinions and trust your instincts.

• **Relaxation.** This is not necessarily the kind delivered by visualization and breathing exercises. (Though those tactics may help you, too.) Rather, the kind of relaxation that new moms need most is the ability to go with the flow during these upside-down weeks. Lower your standards. Live in the moment and don't worry about should-do's. Pamper yourself with a rented video, a milkshake, or a bouquet from your garden. Listen to an inspirational or motivational tape. Above all, try not to obsess about your baby.

Checklist: Have You Been Good to Yourself Today?

Don't let yourself get lost amid the congratulations and emphasis on the baby. Ask yourself if you've managed these essential postpartum pampers:

- ☐ I napped when the baby napped.
- ☐ I showered.
- ☐ I took someone up on an offer to help. (Or, if no one offered—I called to ask someone.)
- ☐ I did something mindless (watched TV, read while nursing, stared out the window).
- ☐ I drank plenty of liquids.
- ☐ I treated myself to a favorite snack, then stuck to a pretty nutritious menu the rest of the day.
- ☐ I went outside, even if just for a few minutes.
- ☐ I made some notes in my baby's record book or took a picture of my baby.
- ☐ I ignored someone's advice in favor of my own instinct or my pediatrician's advice.
- ☐ I ignored all nonessential housework.
- ☐ I marveled at how wonderful my baby is.

For More Help: Postpartum Resources

- Depression After Delivery, P.O. Box 1282, Morrisville, PA 19067; 800-944-4773 or http://www.pleiades.net.com/org/DAD.1.html. Offers a packet of informative materials and contacts with women who have experienced baby blues and are available for telephone support.
- National Association of Postpartum Care Services, 11 Bronxville Rd., #1-C, Bronxville, NY 10708; 800-453-6852. Can refer you to a certified postpartum doula.
- Postpartum Assistance for Mothers, 510-727-4610. Support groups, phone counseling, referrals, and education.
- Postpartum Support International, 805-967-7636 or http://www.siup.edu/an/postpartum. Support, education, and referrals.

MOTHER TO MOTHER:
"I Had Postpartum Depression"

Staci Berner, 29
Rockville, Maryland

All her life, Staci had looked forward to motherhood. So she was shocked when a week and a half after her healthy son Adam Noah was born, she began to wish someone else would take over the job. "I didn't want to be alone with the baby. I wanted to give him back," she recalls. "I didn't feel bonded with him—I felt so distant."

That was also the point at which her mother-in-law, who had come to help out, returned home. Staci felt intimidated by the baby and lost both confidence and patience. Because she had always loved babies and had a lot of experience as a sitter, she felt even more scared. Her sadness grew worse when her husband left for work in the mornings because she couldn't bear to be alone. "At first, I wasn't about to tell anyone I was feeling this way. I didn't understand why this was happening," she recalls. At 3 weeks postpartum, she hired a baby-sitter to help her in the mornings—only to feel more depressed to discover that she didn't mind letting the sitter hold the baby rather than doing so herself.

Her husband thought she was tired and overworked. Her sister-in-law noticed something amiss, too. "She was doing my hair and I started to cry," Staci says. "She was considering getting pregnant and I advised her against it, which surprised her because I was the one who always wanted a baby."

Talking to her husband and her sister helped, but the real breakthrough came when she began comparing notes with other new moms. On-line, she conversed with a group of twelve women who'd had babies the same month. The chats helped her realize what was typical and what wasn't. They also gave her advice about developing routines for the baby. By 2 months, as her confidence grew and Adam began to sleep through the night, the worst of her anxiety passed.

"I never blamed it on my hormones because I didn't realize they were a factor," Staci says. "I see now that if I hadn't snapped out of it, I would have needed outside help. At the time, though, I knew something was wrong but I just figured it was normal."

Staci's tips to other new moms with the blues:

• *Confide in your partner.* "Talking about my depression brought us closer because we were both scared and needed each other."

- **Talk to other people, too.** "When you talk to other mothers, you realize what's normal and what's not."

- **Rest.** "Not getting enough sleep was a major factor in making me more depressed."

- **Initiate a routine to get control of your day.** "Once I put my son on a schedule, it gave me more confidence."

MOTHER TO MOTHER:
"Our Road to Sibling Revelry"

Cherie Spino, 32
Toledo, Ohio

Cherie's sons, Conor and Noah, were born 27 months apart. "We didn't say much to Conor about the baby until late in my pregnancy because I didn't think he would understand," she says. During her last trimester, she and her husband, Mike, moved their son to a new bedroom so the baby could use the nursery. "We were worried we hadn't left enough adjustment time, so we gussied it up by sponge-painting furniture with fun shapes and bright paint and putting Winnie the Pooh sheets on the bed," Cherie says. "We made a big deal about a big-boy bed, but we didn't connect it to the baby so he wouldn't resent him. He did beautifully."

At first, the big change was smooth sailing. Mike brought Conor to the hospital soon after his brother was born. "We had wrapped big-brother gifts—a toy cassette player and two books about new babies—for him to open at the hospital, and used them a lot when we got home," she recalls. "Conor was great. He wanted to take Noah everywhere with him and kept kissing him and patting his head."

By the time Noah was 3 months old, however, big brother Conor had had enough. "He became very clingy to me, and he liked to scream in the baby's face. When I breastfed Noah, Conor would jump on the couch for attention. And he no longer liked for the baby to come with us—'Leave Noah there,' he'd say."

Cherie and Mike let a lot of the older boy's behavior slide, but drew the line—with time-outs—when he'd try to harm the baby. As Noah got bigger and more sociable, things improved. "It helps now that Conor gets positive feedback from the baby. He can make the baby giggle when he dances, for instance,"

Cherie says. "It's so much fun to watch them together, and listening to him say 'my little brother' is heartwarming."

Cherie's tips for helping siblings adjust:

• **Line up special attention.** "We made sure Conor had plenty of visits with his aunts and cousins. I think at times he barely missed us."

• **Do double duty.** Take the older sibling for a walk while you wear the infant in a soft carrier, or try napping together. "While I was breastfeeding, I read to Conor at the same time."

• **Keep number-one involved.** "I let Conor open the baby's gifts and hold him while giving him a bottle."

• **Watch how you phrase things.** "Instead of bringing the baby into it all the time by saying, 'I can't—Noah needs me now,' I began to say, 'Let's do that together as soon as I'm done here.' "

Checkups and Tests

The Postpartum Exam

A new mother's first postpartum doctor visit is often called "the 6-week checkup" because that's when it's typically scheduled. Some doctors, however, prefer an initial exam 2 to 4 weeks postpartum, with a follow-up later. (A Cesarean incision, particularly, may be checked earlier than 6 weeks.) What's so special about the 6-week mark? By this time, the uterus has returned to its pre-pregnancy size, any episiotomy or C-section stitches are likely to have healed, and the vaginal discharge has usually changed from bright red to clear—all signs that your recovery is well on its way.

You'll have an internal exam to verify the uterus's size and position and to check the condition of your cervix and vagina. Your breasts may be checked and any stitches will be examined. By 6 weeks, you should also have lost 15 to 20 pounds or more (chiefly the weight of the baby, the placenta, and extra water and blood). Use this opportunity to discuss the resumption of intercourse, birth control, vitamins, and what kinds of exercise are acceptable. Mention how you're feeling, too. If you're having trouble with breastfeeding or postpartum depression, your doctor can refer you to sources of help.

One strange aspect of the postpartum exam is that, unless you're seeing a family or general practitioner, it represents an abrupt end to the close relationship many women develop with their practitioner during the prior 9 months of frequent visits. Your doctor or midwife was a central figure in the childbearing drama, and you may feel sadness that this person will no longer be a key player in your life. You won't need to see your ob-gyn for another year, until your next annual exam.

Some women also feel disappointment that the doctor isn't more congratulatory or curious about how the birth experience felt to them. While many women report that their doctor does make caring inquiries, the reality is that an obstetrician's training lies in helping women bear healthy babies. No matter how much he or she respects the miracle of birth, a patient's experience was not as personal to the doctor as it was to her. But if you feel a need to discuss the emotional details of your delivery with your caregiver, do bring the subject up. You'll probably engage your practitioner in a satisfying conversation that also provides some closure for you.

Feeding Your Baby

Breastfeeding Basics

One of your first official acts as a mother can be both nurturing and nourishing: breastfeeding your newborn within the first hour or two of life. Breastfeeding's benefits to baby and mother are impressive. (For details on why breast is best, see "Decisions, Decisions: Will you breast- or bottle-feed?" page 200.)

Although nursing a baby is the most natural thing in the world, that doesn't mean it comes naturally to every mother or every baby. Think of breastfeeding as a skill you both need to learn. As a result of today's relatively brief hospital stays, most new moms are back in their home rockers with a crying newborn on their lap before they've had adequate coaching on the fine points. And that's one of the main reasons that nearly 60 percent of mothers nurse in the hospital but just 21 percent are still breastfeeding at 6 months. What's more, not every baby gets the knack right away. So approach your first feedings with guarded optimism. Expect to muddle through a few frustrating sessions of trial and error. Just keep trying, and have handy the number of an experienced friend or a lactation counselor for free advice if you feel you need help. (Ask your childbirth educator, obstetrician, or pediatrician for a referral to a lactation consultant or check your phone book for the number of the local La Leche League.)

Breastfeeding your baby during the first weeks of life—and ideally, for 6 months or more—is the optimum. This speeds the healing of your uterus while passing on vital protection against infection to your newborn. It allows you both time to master the art of breastfeeding. Even if you ultimately decide not to con-

GOOD POSITIONS FOR BREASTFEEDING. These comfortable positions make it easy for your baby to reach the breast. Always make yourself as relaxed as possible. Support your back and use pillows to support your arms or the baby's body and to bring the head close to your breast. When seated, put up your feet on a low stool, which allows you to bring the baby closer. You shouldn't have to bend over to nurse—not only will hunching hurt, but the tension it causes can inhibit milk flow.

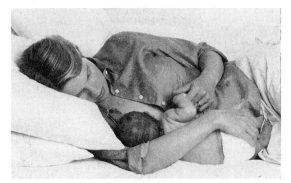

Lying down. *Lay the baby on the bed beside you, slightly turned to his side, as you turn sideways. Offer the breast closest to the mattress. This is an especially convenient position for middle-of-the-night feedings.*

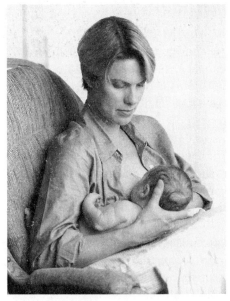

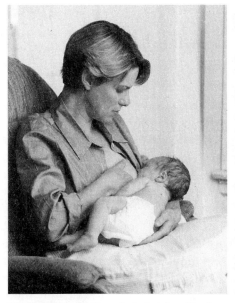

The football hold. *Support the baby's head with your hand and tuck your arm under his body so that his back is along your forearm and his bottom is at your elbow. This position makes latching on (to the breast on the same side as the arm you're holding him with) particularly easy for the baby and is great for mothers who have had C-sections, since it places no pressure on the stomach.*

The cradle hold. *Rest the baby's head in the crook of your elbow and guide your breast with the other hand. Hold the baby so his head is level with your breast and you can draw an imaginary straight line from his nose to his belly button.*

tinue nursing, doing so for the
first couple of weeks minimizes
the painful engorgement common to new moms who never
nurse, while providing special
immunities to your newborn.
With the right encouragement
and information, it's possible to
breastfeed whether you've had a
Cesarean, a preterm delivery,
twins, or even triplets. Some babies, particularly preemies, are
born with a poor sucking reflex
or health problems that preclude
immediate nursing. If the latter
case is true for you, it's still possible to breastfeed successfully by
pumping milk for feedings until
the infant can nurse on his own.
Working mothers can also continue to feed their babies breast
milk by expressing it into bottles.

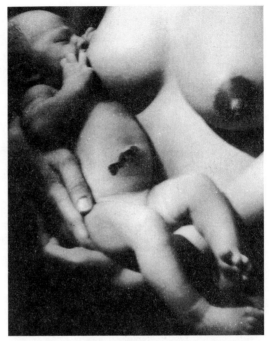

*A newborn has a tiny tummy. To keep him well
nourished, offer your breast at least 8 to 12 times in
a 24-hour period.*

Breastfeeding can be a won-
derful source of satisfaction and intimacy. Many women have little trouble getting started. For others, it requires a fair amount of commitment and
perseverance. If breastfeeding makes you tense or fraught with failure, even after you get support in the technical aspects, you shouldn't feel duty-bound to
continue. Feeding your baby is ultimately what's most important, not how you
feed him.

The first time you try, you may be surprised at how vigorously your newborn roots for your breast and begins to suck. Your job is to make sure the baby
does these things the right way so that the experience is comfortable for you and
nourishing for the baby. Start with how you hold the baby. Experiment with
what feels easiest at first. Then vary your positions from feeding to feeding to
avoid putting undue pressure on any one part of your breast.

Next you want to be sure the baby is positioned correctly on the breast,
called *latching on*. This is important so she gets enough to eat and so your nipples don't get sore. A baby who is latched on the right way takes as much of the
areola (the dark area around the nipple) as possible, as well as the nipple itself,
in her mouth. As she sucks, her tongue and gums squeeze the milk sinuses,

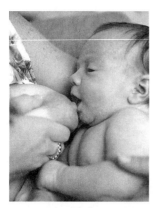 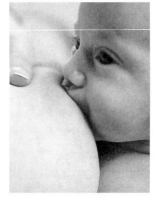 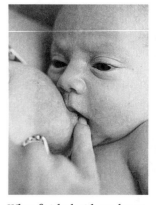

Hold your baby in a position that's comfortable for both of you. When you offer him your breast, cup it for support by placing your fingers underneath and your thumb on top. Then, to stimulate your infant's rooting reflex, try tickling his lower lip with your nipple until he turns toward it and opens his mouth.

Center your nipple in his mouth, making sure that his tongue is down. One way to tell whether your baby is properly latched on: His lower lip will curl outward.

When finished with one breast, place your little finger between your breast and your baby's gums. This will break the suction and avoid painful pulling on your nipple.

which lie behind the areola, and the milk comes out through multiple openings in the nipple. To get the baby to open her mouth wide, stroke her cheek or cup your breast between your thumb and forefinger or use the nipple to tickle the baby's mouth. Don't push her head forward toward your breast—that will only make her pull back and away. When her mouth opens, pull her stomach toward yours so that your breast is easily accessible. Slightly lift your breast and guide it into the baby's mouth. When latched on well, the baby's lower lip curls outward and the tongue lies curled below. The mouth should be centered around the areola and nipple. (If your breast is very full, you may need to gently press down on the top of it to make it easier for the baby to breathe.) If she has only the nipple in her mouth (you can see this, and it also feels uncomfortable), slide your pinkie finger into the corner of the baby's mouth to break the suction and start again. Always break suction first—pulling the nipple out will hurt.

The first food a baby gets in a feeding is called *foremilk,* a sweet, thirst-quenching liquid that pools in the sinuses just behind the nipple. Higher-fat, more nutritious *hindmilk* is released after about the first 5 minutes, when the baby's suckling stimulates nerve endings in the areola that signal the body to release prolactin. That hormone in turn triggers the production of milk in the *alveoli*, the glands within the breast that make milk. This is the *let-down reflex*, which many women experience as a pins-and-needles tingling. Others barely notice it. Upon let-down, the baby's sucking becomes slower and more rhythmic. The rush of milk may make the baby gag or sputter; if this happens, simply let your baby catch his breath and begin again. Wear a breast pad over the nipple you're not feeding from to absorb the slight flow of milk that will leak from that breast during let-down.

Once the first sleepy day or two has passed, your baby will seem to be hungry all the time. And he probably is, since his stomach is so small and breast milk is digested within 2 hours of consumption. Hunger signals include crying, rooting for the breast (or rooting around on anyone who happens to be holding him), smacking his lips, and sucking his fist or fingers. Feed your baby as often as he needs it. Schedules have no place in getting successful breastfeeding under way. This means, for the first 2 weeks or so, offering the breast about every 2 to 3 hours in the day and every 3 to 3½ hours at night, or more often as demanded.

The times your baby wants to eat may not space themselves out perfectly. Often babies *cluster-feed* in closely spaced intervals for part of the day, usually in the evening. Also, there may be one longer stretch in a 24-hour period—up to 4 or 5 hours—when your baby sleeps. During the first week, when the baby is regaining his birthweight (all babies lose a small percentage of their birthweight in the first day or two of life), wake him up for feedings at least every 3 hours; after that you can let him sleep. The baby may be very hungry and frantic upon awakening, though, making latching on and sucking difficult. So do pick up a sleeping newborn if he seems restless and is making sucking motions with his lips, or if he's had more than one long stretch of sleep in 24 hours. Dehydration is a risk in babies who don't nurse often enough. This, in turn, can cause them to sleep more, compounding the problem.

Each feeding should last as long as the infant wants to feed—at least 5 minutes per breast and usually 15 to 20 minutes per side. Burp your baby before switching breasts. In addition to making yourself comfortable during feedings by supporting your arms and back and elevating your legs, be sure to drink liquid while you nurse. Get in the habit of keeping an athletic squirt bottle of water or a glass of juice at the side of your favorite nursing chair.

Overcoming Common Setbacks

What are some of the typical problems—and their solutions—new nursing moms may face?

• **"It hurts."** Breastfeeding should be painless, although several situations—all correctable—can cause breast pain. In the first few days the tender nipples are unused to a baby's constant, vigorous sucking. You might feel discomfort while the baby is initially latching on, although this pain should dissipate after about 30 seconds. The nipples will toughen up by the end of the week. To help, after a feeding leave some breast milk on the surface of the nipple or apply a thin coat of pure lanolin (available at pharmacies). Let the breasts air-dry for 5 to 10 minutes; some women use a blow dryer on a cool setting. Also, let your breasts go uncovered when possible during the day to expose them to air. Keep breasts dry between feedings. Wear breast pads in your bra to absorb leakage and change them as soon as they feel wet. Avoid soap and alcohol (found in some perfumes and lotions), as well as witch hazel or other potential irritants that dry the skin.

If pain persists after the baby has latched on, he may not be doing so properly or may not be positioned correctly, causing the nipple to take the brunt of the sucking. Release the baby's suction and begin again, being sure his mouth is open wide and taking in the areola as well as the nipple. Never allow him to chew on the nipple. To further reduce nipple trauma, rotate among the different ways to hold your baby, and alternate which breast is offered first at each feeding. As a memory jog, some women put a safety pin on their bra on the side of the breast used last, or switch a ring from one hand to the other.

Yeast infections can also cause painful nipples. Signs include a mother's nipples that are red and shiny, a baby's bad diaper rash, or white patches on the infant's tongue or inner cheek. The white patches cannot be wiped off or will cause slight bleeding when you try to wipe them, unlike ordinary milk residue left in the mouth, which can be wiped away. These are signs of thrush, an oral yeast infection. See your pediatrician so both you and your baby can be treated. You can continue to breastfeed during treatment.

Sometimes a milk duct becomes plugged, which results in a very localized pain. Apply warm compresses to the area, massage the breast, and make sure it's emptied fully, either by the baby or by expressing manually or with a pump. A too-tight bra can also clog ducts. See your doctor if your breast is red, if you have a fever or flulike symptoms, or if the clogged duct doesn't disappear within 2 days. A clogged milk duct left untreated can cause a more serious problem, a breast infection called *mastitis*. The entire breast hurts, swells, and may be streaked red; the mother may also run a fever or think she's coming down with flu, thanks to chills, fatigue, nausea, and general body aches. Antibiotics and pain relievers safe for nursing are prescribed for mastitis—take the full course of antibiotics to prevent a recurrence, even though symptoms may disappear within 2 days. As is true of almost all breast pain, it's better to continue nursing than to stop, because the continued flow of milk can help clear up the problem and prevent an abscess, a buildup of infectious discharge. There's no chance of the nursing baby contracting an infection. Rest and drinking plenty of fluids are also imperative.

Always alert the doctor if your breasts are cracked and bleeding, if you have sore breasts accompanied by fever, or if breast pain persists.

• *"I have inverted nipples."* Even with inverted nipples, you can breastfeed successfully. Remember that what's important is that the baby latches on to the areola around the nipple. Some women can draw out their nipples on their own by simply pinching them between thumb and forefinger. Or you can consult a lactation adviser about special exercises to try. (Ideally you should do this prior to delivery, during the last trimester. If you do, get your obstetrician's okay first; women at risk for preterm labor, for example, should not do this as it can promote contractions.) The problem may also be easily remedied with one of the many available devices that draw out flat or inverted nipples. These include breast shells (plastic bra inserts worn between feedings to gently stretch the nipple), suction molds (a plastic device with a small cup on the end that uses suction to draw out the nipple), and breast pumps.

• *"My baby doesn't seem interested."* Try caressing a drowsy newborn's feet to interest him in a feeding, or removing his clothing so that you nestle skin-to-skin for a while. It's common for newborns to nurse slowly, with frequent pauses—that's because sucking is hard work. If your baby skips a feeding and doesn't seem enthused about making up for it at the next one, see your pediatrician. The doctor will want to be sure your baby is gaining weight adequately and is not sick.

• *"I don't produce enough milk."* Only about 5 in 100 women are truly unable to breastfeed. It can be difficult to tell how much milk you're supplying when it's not premeasured in a bottle. If you have any doubts, monitor your baby's elimination habits and weight gain. Keep a written tally so you're certain of the results. (See "CHECKLIST: Is Your Baby Eating Enough?" page 316.) Don't delay seeking your pediatrician's opinion.

Rest assured, though, that the vast majority of women are physically capable of breastfeeding. Breast size and nipple shape have nothing to do with it. Sometimes fatigue or anxiety can interfere with lactation, so be sure you're resting and relaxing. Breastfeeding within the first hours of life and not offering any supplementary water or formula will also establish a healthy milk supply. Breastfeeding on demand (when your baby is hungry, even if it seems like all the time, and including through the night at first) leads to more milk production, not less.

• **"I'm sick."** Babies rarely need to be weaned because of maternal illness. In fact, continuing to nurse can help protect your baby from the illness, since you'll be passing along the antibodies that your body is manufacturing. Even if you must take medication, many types are safe for nursing moms and their breastfed babies—including acetaminophen, ibuprofen, antibiotics, some anti-hypertensives, and thyroid-regulating drugs. Tell your doctor that you're breast-feeding, and double-check the drug's safety with your pediatrician.

• **"It's wearing me out."** Mothers who breastfeed report having less energy than those who exclusively formula-feed. That's not surprising, since a nursing mom is literally giving something of herself to her baby. Remember, though, that breastfeeding isn't the only cause of fatigue in the early months. Your body is still recovering from giving birth and your sleep-wake patterns have been dis-rupted. Rest and good nutrition are the best ways to restore yourself. Nursing moms need 300 to 500 calories a day more than before pregnancy, ideally from calcium and protein sources, such as milk, as well as plenty of replacement flu-ids. Within a matter of weeks as your newborn grows, 'round-the-clock feedings will end, too, boosting your energy.

Expressing Breast Milk

Most nursing moms invest in some kind of breast pump because sooner or later, they want to express milk. Reasons range from relieving engorged breasts to getting a few hours' sleep by letting someone else feed your baby from a bot-tle. As with breastfeeding itself, the skill takes practice. Always wash your hands before expressing or pumping. Get as relaxed and comfortable as you can. Most women have their best success early in the day and during or just af-ter a feeding.

Types of pumps include the following:

• **Manual pumps ($20 to $30).** These inexpensive, lightweight models are con-venient to have on hand for occasional pumping. But because they require squeezing a lever or pumping a piston repeatedly, they can be tiring to use. They empty one breast at a time and require two hands to operate.

• **Electric or battery pumps ($30 to $200).** The most affordable models express one breast at a time, while the high-end models can express both simulta-neously. These pumps offer varying degrees of portability, automatic pumping

Cost, efficiency, and portability are the main considerations when choosing a breast pump.

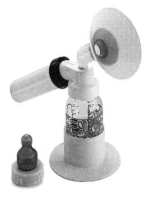

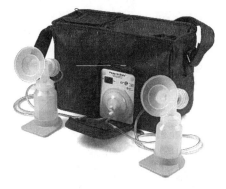

Manual
Brand: Natural Mother Breast Pump Kit,
from Evenflo
Cost: $19–$22
Contact: 800/356-2229

High-End Electric
Brand: Pump in Style, from Medela
Cost: $198
Contact: 800/835-5968

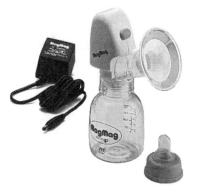

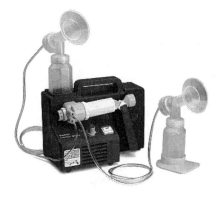

Electric/Battery
Brand: MagMag, from Omron Healthcare
Cost: $20–$30
Contact: 800/634-4350

Hospital Grade
Brand: Lactina Select, from Medela
Cost: $1–$2.60 per day rental
Contact: 800/835-5968

ability, and suction power. Manual and electric or battery pumps are sold at most baby-supply stores and drugstores, and some maternity clothing shops.

• *Hospital-grade pumps ($1 to $3 per day, rental fee).* Hospitals, hospital-supply stores, and lactation consultants rent heavy-duty double pumps, which are generally the most efficient and easy to operate. Most are not very portable, however—making them a good choice for the early weeks at home, after which a breastfeeding mother returning to work will want a portable version.

You can also express milk manually, though doing so may require a bit more practice. Before you start, lay a warm towel on your breast for a few minutes. To help get the milk flowing, relax and think about your baby. Remove the towel and place a wide-mouth bowl beneath your breast. Begin to massage your breast in a circular motion, especially around the areola. Then hold your breast the way you do when nursing, between your thumb and forefinger. Position your fingers at the edge of the areola and gently roll them back and forth to empty the milk glands. Rotate the position of your fingers so that you're emptying different ducts. Take care not to squeeze the breast—a gentle motion should be sufficient. Use a funnel to pour the expressed milk into a bottle without spillage.

After the effort you took to express it, breast milk can seem like save-at-all-costs white gold. But take care when handling breast milk. There are important safety considerations regarding how to save and reuse it. Always store expressed milk in the refrigerator or freezer (if you express away from home, carry the milk in an insulated cooler). Use it within 24 hours if refrigerated; otherwise freeze it. Frozen milk stays good up to 3 months. If you're not going to use it right away, label the bottle with the current date. Don't fill the bottle all the way to the top, since milk expands as it freezes. Refrigerated or frozen breast milk may look different in the bottle because the fat separates from the liquid. It's still good. Just warm the bottle under hot running water or place it in a bowl of hot water. Thaw frozen milk this way or in the refrigerator, not by leaving it out at room temperature. Don't heat it up in a microwave or on the stovetop, because the immune properties of breast milk are heat sensitive. The uneven heating of a microwave risks scalding the baby.

Always pump into a fresh bottle—not one that's been partially used. Left-over milk from a feeding can be saved in the refrigerator only until the next feeding (about 4 hours) and if not used then, it should be discarded. Never re-freeze partially used, thawed milk, or leave it out at room temperature for more than 1 hour.

Checklist: For Successful Breastfeeding

Reminders for improving your odds of sticking with it:

☐ Do you offer the breast at least eight to twelve times in 24 hours (about every 2 to 3 hours during the day, and every 3 to 3½ hours at night) for the first couple of weeks?

☐ Do you take care to ensure that your baby is latched on properly?

☐ Do you alternate which breast you start with first?

☐ Do you alternate among the various ways to hold your nursing baby?

☐ Do you put your feet up and support your back and arms with pillows?

☐ Do you keep a tall glass of water or juice at your side while nursing, and drink plenty of liquids throughout the day?

☐ Do you allow your nipples to air-dry after each feeding?

☐ Do you wear a pad to absorb breast-milk leakage (if this is a problem for you)?

☐ Do you know whom to call if problems develop?

Bottle-Feeding Basics

Enough can't be said about the health benefits, convenience, low cost, and intimacy of breastfeeding. Any new mother and baby who are both healthy enough ought to try nursing, at least for the first few weeks so the mother's natural immunities can be passed along. With persistence and experienced help, many women who are on the fence find that they're glad they've continued breastfeeding.

That said, bottle feeding is a valid, healthy choice for babies, too, either right from the start or after you've been breastfeeding for a while. If you're concerned about your choice, try to separate the medical facts from the political and cultural rhetoric. In the real world, there are plenty of reasons women choose formula, among them a baby with a poor sucking reflex (common in premature babies), prolonged mother-infant separation, the need to return to work (especially if pumping is inconvenient), extreme fatigue, or a desire to involve other family members in the feeding process. Whether you formula-feed exclusively or supplement nursing with formula, it's important to know that today's products are designed to nutritionally simulate breast milk as closely as possible. While they cannot pass along the resistance to infection that mother's milk does, formulas provide ample nourishment for a growing baby.

The type of nipple you finally settle on—orthodontic, traditional, or flat-tipped—will depend on your baby's preference.

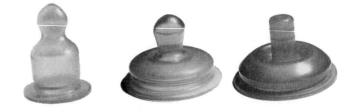

Solicit your pediatrician's advice in choosing a brand. Most formulas are based on cow's milk or soybeans. Most are fortified with iron, which is recommended to prevent anemia. (It does not cause constipation, as was once commonly believed.) You also have a choice of type: powdered (which you mix with a specific amount of water), concentrated liquid (which you dilute with water), and ready-to-feed liquid (which is the most convenient but also expensive). Premixed formulas are available in large cans, which you pour into bottles, or in ready-to-go 4- to 6-ounce baby bottles. Formulas must be used immediately or be refrigerated after mixing or opening, and used within 24 to 48 hours (check the labels).

Under no circumstances should you feed your infant cow's milk. Real milk is not recommended until the first birthday because it does not have the proper nutritional components needed by a growing infant and can trigger digestive trouble.

Bottles and nipples come in an even more dizzying array of options than types of formulas. Nipples, for example, can be bought in orthodontic, traditional, and flat-tipped shapes. They also come in different sizes (according to age) and flow rates. Bottles are made in several sizes and shapes; some feature disposable liners. They all work well, so don't get hung up on finding the perfect system. You may want to buy just a few of a given product type until you decide what's most convenient for you and most acceptable to your baby. In general, the smaller (4-ounce) bottles work best for the first few months, as a newborn won't take more than that per feeding.

Sterilize bottles, nipples, and rings (the plastic apparatus that attaches the nipple to the bottle) before first using them. To do this, boil them in a pot of water for 5 minutes (or however long it says in the directions that come with the bottle), then remove them and allow them to dry on a clean paper towel. After that, a good cleansing in hot soapy water or the dishwasher is sufficient. Handy gear includes a special dishwasher basket that holds nipples, rings, and caps, and racks that hold inverted bottles for drying on the counter. Most baby-supply stores carry these items. Caveat: If your home tap water supply is supplied by a well, repeated sterilization may be best.

You don't need to sterilize the water used to mix formulas unless your pediatrician recommends it in the rare event that a contaminant is present in the local supply. (If you have well water, you may also be told to sterilize or use bottled water.) To save time, prepare an entire day's worth of water in the morning. When you're ready to feed your baby, add formula to the bottle. Warm it in a pan of hot water or by running it under the tap; you can also buy a bottle warmer device designed for this purpose. Never use a microwave or boil the bottle, which can cause a breakdown of the nutrients. The formula should drip steadily out of the nipple—if it pours out in a stream, the hole is too big and the nipple should be discarded. If liquid barely comes out, the nipple ring may be attached too tightly. Check nipples periodically for signs of wear, such as discoloration or thinning, and replace worn ones, which could break and become a choking hazard.

As with breastfeeding, most experts agree that rigid schedules are futile in the early weeks, though you may be able to work out an approximate pattern for feeding within a month or two. Offer the bottle every 2 to 3 hours at first, or as the baby seems hungry. Until the baby reaches about 10 pounds, she'll probably take 1 to 3 ounces per feeding. Don't force more than she seems ready to eat. Your pediatrician should advise you about suitable amounts for your baby as she grows.

BURPING BASICS: When babies suck breast milk or formula, they also swallow air. This can cause uncomfortable gas, which makes a baby fuss and, in turn, gulp more air. That's why it's essential to burp your baby during and after feedings—either after each breast or after every few ounces from a bottle. Sometimes it's enough just to walk around holding the baby upright with her head at your shoulder. Keep a burp cloth (a cloth diaper or a towel does the trick) handy to catch spit-up. Other positions to try:

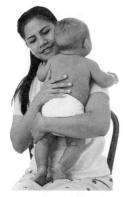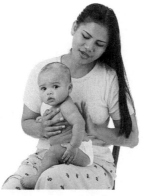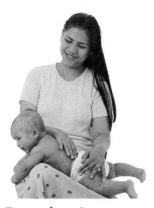

Over the shoulder: *Hold your baby upright and gently rub or pat the back.*

Sitting: *Prop your baby into a sitting position on your lap, with his chin resting in your hand, and gently rub or pat the back.*

Tummy-down: *Lay your baby across your lap and gently rub or pat the back.*

If you hear a lot of noisy sucking sounds while she drinks, she may be taking in too much air. To help your baby swallow less air, hold her at a 45-degree angle. Also, take care to tilt the bottle so that the nipple and neck are always filled with formula. Never prop a bottle. This can cause a baby to choke.

If you plan to supplement breast milk with formula, or to express milk, an ideal time to introduce the bottle is at 3 to 4 weeks. By then, nursing will be well established but the baby is not so old as to be resistant to the new kind of nipple. (Breast and bottle require different types of sucking.) Someone other than the mother should give the first bottles, since the baby will be able to smell her milk and may refuse anything but her nipple. When formula is used just for occasional feedings by a nursing mother, use no more than one bottle per day to avoid inhibiting milk production.

Checklist: Is Your Baby Eating Enough?

Dehydration in newborns is rare, but it's important to know the signs of a healthy eater so you can consult your pediatrician if anything seems amiss. Your baby is getting enough breast milk or formula if he or she:

☐ Eats at least every 2 or 3 hours (eight to twelve times per 24 hours) for the first 2 to 3 weeks. (The interval between feedings is measured from the start of one session to the start of the next.)

☐ Spends 10 to 20 minutes per breast (or takes 2 to 4 ounces of formula) and swallowing can be heard.

☐ Wets six or more diapers a day (once your milk has come in). You can usually tell if disposables are wet by the way they feel, but if you're unsure, try putting a small piece of paper towel in the diaper each time you change the baby.

☐ Has at least four bowel movements a day (tarry, green-black meconium the first few days, then loose, yellowish stool after your milk comes in if you're nursing, or darker stool if formula-feeding).

☐ Regains birthweight in 10 to 14 days. A newborn loses up to 10 percent of his birthweight in the first few days after birth, and breastfed babies tend to lose more than those on formula. After 3 or 4 days, a newborn begins to gain at a pace of 4 to 7 ounces (or more) per week, or about 1 pound a month.

☐ Has good color and firm skin (if you pinch a dehydrated baby's skin, it will stay pinched).

WHAT IF...

My breasts leak all the time? Leaking is most common before a regular feeding time or when you're thinking about your baby; also during a feeding, milk in the unsuckled breast will let-down. Manual stimulation—from the accidental rub of a shirt or towel or from sexual foreplay—can produce breast milk, too. To absorb leaks, lay in a good supply of breast pads and change them often to keep the areola and nipple as dry as possible between feedings. Sometimes you can stop leakage by applying gentle pressure to your breast with your hand when you feel the pins-and-needles sensation of milk flow. Excessive leakage usually stops within a few months, once feeding patterns are more predictable.

My baby falls asleep after nursing on the first breast? It's best to empty both breasts at a feeding in the beginning. But if your baby snoozes right through burping and a diaper change, it's okay to occasionally let her sleep mid-feeding. Just start the next session on the other breast. After a few weeks it's common for a baby to feed on just one breast at each feeding.

Breastfeeding arouses me? As unexpected and guilt provoking as this experience can be, it's not unusual. Arousal is a natural response caused by the way women are wired—the stimulation of sucking connects to the clitoris via nerves. Some women even experience orgasm. (Similarly, during sex it's common to leak milk upon orgasm.) It's nothing to be ashamed of.

I have breast implants—can I nurse? Depending on where the surgical incision was made, women who have had surgery to enlarge their breasts should be able to breastfeed. Some women with implants have difficulty producing ample milk, however. If you want to try, inform your pediatrician about your implants so that he or she can closely monitor the baby's weight gain. Also be aware that it remains unclear whether silicone and other by-products that may be released by ruptured implants can contaminate breast milk. But many experts believe that the amount of silicone leakage is so slight that the benefits of mother's milk outweigh any risk.

I've had breast-reduction surgery—can I nurse? The answer depends on the technique used in your surgery. Your plastic surgeon can tell you if the milk ducts were left intact and functioning.

IS IT TRUE...

That nursing will make my breasts sag? Actually it's pregnancy, more than lactation, that tends to alter the firmness and shape of a woman's breasts. Heredity, age, and weight gain play a role, too.

That some babies need solid food earlier than others? Your mother or grandmother may urge giving a large or fussy baby "pablum" to help him sleep through the night, but solids aren't necessary until around 4 to 6 months of age. Nowadays few pediatricians recommend anything but breast milk or formula before then. (The too-early introduction of solids may not harm a baby, but can cause him to become overly fat. It's simply not useful or necessary and has not been proven to improve how long a baby sleeps.) Babies typically go through growth spurts at 3 weeks, 6 weeks, and 3 months of age. For a period of one to several days, it may seem like your baby is hungrier than usual and wants to nurse more frequently. Indulge him or her with breast milk, not with solids.

That drinking a beer stimulates the let-down reflex? Studies have disproved this belief, along with another old saw that says beer enriches mother's milk. Whether nursing mothers should drink at all is still debated in medical circles, though, and therefore an individual choice. According to the American Academy of Pediatrics, an occasional glass of beer or wine, ideally consumed right after a feeding, isn't going to harm your baby, since the alcohol exits the body in 3 to 4 hours. (And while it won't cause let-down, the alcohol might help a tense or frazzled mom relax.) You could also pump before drinking. Keep up your fluid intake, though, since alcohol is dehydrating. More than one drink at a time is unwise, since the alcohol could enter the baby's system and may inhibit milk production.

That I should wear a bra while nursing? Even if you're normally small-chested, a nursing bra (with handy access openings) provides comfortable support for milk-heavy breasts. A bra also lets you wear pads easily (to absorb leakage) and helps prevent shirt stains. Be aware that, although you may feel that you need the support of an underwire—and many nursing bras have them—this style can compress the breast, leading to clogged milk ducts. A wireless model is best. If you're very large, look for one with wide support bands at the shoulders and beneath the cups. Avoid too-tight bras as well.

That nursing can cause jaundice? Breast milk isn't the cause of jaundice, an extremely common newborn condition characterized by a yellow cast to the skin. Not getting enough milk can exacerbate the problem, however, leading to something known as *breast-milk jaundice*. What happens is that a baby who doesn't get enough milk takes in fewer calories and therefore has fewer bowel movements, making it harder for her system to rid itself of the jaundice. The stool normally carries out bilirubin, a natural chemical formed during the body's normal processing of red blood cells. But if there are infrequent bowel movements, the bilirubin gets reabsorbed and worsens the jaundice.

Giving a baby supplementary bottles of water or sugar-water can exacerbate the problem because she gets filled up on water (which does *not* make the infant have BMs) and wants less milk. Breast-milk jaundice is now thought to affect 10 to 30 percent of newborns during the second to sixth week of life. Minimizing breast-milk jaundice is easy: experts advise nursing ten to twelve times per 24 hours during the first few days, beginning right in the delivery room, and avoiding sugar-water supplements. (See "Jaundice," page 352.)

That giving a breastfed baby a bottle or a pacifier while nursing will confuse him? Experts are divided on this question, and the answer is that it probably depends on the baby. The concern is that a plastic nipple or pacifier (even if orthodontically shaped) is so different in shape and texture from a mother's nipple that the baby will forget how to suck from a breast, which requires different motions by the tongue and mouth. Some lactation advisers suggest waiting until breastfeeding is well established, usually 3 to 4 weeks, before introducing a pacifier or a bottle. On the other hand, if you wait too long, the baby may refuse a bottle altogether. Many babies have been fed interchangeably with both breast and bottle from birth, or given a pacifier from birth, with no apparent confusion.

That I should also give my baby water, especially in summer? There's no need to give a newborn water regularly. Breast milk is nearly 90 percent water, and frequent nursing will prevent dehydration. Besides, the baby risks filling up on the water, which contains no nutrients, and thus becoming less interested in feedings. This could hamper your milk supply. Formula-fed babies can be offered a little water between feedings in warm weather, since formula is saltier than human milk, though it should never be forced; always check with your baby's doctor first.

That I should warm up milk or formula before giving it to my baby? It's true that breast milk is naturally warm, so a breastfed baby may prefer temperate formula or expressed breast milk. But there's no health reason to feed a baby warmed milk. Indeed, if you can get the baby accustomed to drinking it at room temperature or slightly cold, you save yourself the time and hassle of preheating bottles, especially when she's crying to be fed—right now!

That I should quit breastfeeding once my periods return? Menstruation doesn't alter the taste of your breast milk, as was once believed. Nor does the monthly blood flow make a woman too weak to nourish a baby.

MOTHER TO MOTHER:
"I Had Trouble Nursing at First"

Margret Bower, 32
Silver Spring, Maryland

Margret always planned to breastfeed. But a C-section and the pain medications she took afterward meant that she didn't get a chance to try until 36 hours after son Noah's birth. "He latched on well in the hospital, but when I'd ask for more help from the nurses, they'd stay for 30 seconds and then leave," she says. One nurse even told her (incorrectly) that her son was too big to nurse. "I know they were busy, but they could have been more supportive."

Her frustrations increased at home, when she began to have mysterious breast pain every time she nursed. "I thought it would be a simple, pain-free process," she says. "Breastfeeding is such an emotional thing. I felt pretty bad at first—I was obviously doing something wrong and couldn't figure out what it was." When her obstetrician couldn't diagnose a problem and she couldn't match up her symptom to any common complaint described in books, Margret gritted her teeth through feedings and expressed milk with an electric pump when the suckling was too painful.

When Noah was 1 month old, his pediatrician put her in touch with a lactation counselor. The woman suggested that Margret not hunch forward and look down so much when she nursed, and she also advised using a heating pad on her breasts before and after a session to make them feel better. Margret found that a warm shower helped, too. She also found a local hotline for nursing moms that she could call for encouragement.

"I'm glad I stuck with it," she says. "At 5 months, Noah is gaining weight and has not gotten sick. When it's going well, it's such a nice time with him."

Margret's tips for other nursing moms having trouble:

• ***Visit a doctor sooner, rather than later.*** He or she can check for medical problems and provide needed emotional support. "I was depressed at first and felt too tired and stressed to talk about my breastfeeding problems. But my doctor is the one who put me in touch with the lactation counselor who helped me."

• ***Be persistent about getting support.*** Ask friends to help, and tune out naysayers (such as relatives who don't believe in nursing). Recognize, too, that some hospitals are more pro-breastfeeding than others. A good sign: A staff lactation adviser on the new-mom floor. "If one doctor or nurse doesn't help, find another."

• **Know where to find ongoing help.** Many towns have support groups for breastfeeding mothers. There are also many professionals or experienced moms who will advise novices. "I found a hotline for nursing moms I could call for encouragement or if I had questions."

• **Get a good pump.** "Mine was a lifesaver. Sometimes at first I found it less painful to pump than to breastfeed."

• **Don't get down on yourself.** "When I was in pain, I'd just pump. Nor is it the end of the world if you sometimes give the baby formula. Don't feel guilty. You need to balance your needs with your baby's."

GOOD ADVICE: PUBLIC NURSING

It's sad but true that such an everyday, natural act as breastfeeding still garners cold stares and even occasional requests to button up and move somewhere else. It's also ironic, especially in a culture where bouncing breasts are readily seen on sitcoms and in advertisements. A number of states now have laws on the books protecting the rights of mothers to breastfeed in public. (But the practice is perfectly legal everywhere.) Here are more confidence builders:

• **Be upbeat.** Your attitude can make a huge difference. If you're convinced that you're doing what's best for your baby, convey that with a smile and self-assured body language.
• **Be confident.** Some women are more self-conscious than others. Practice opening your shirt and offering the breast to your baby in front of a mirror.

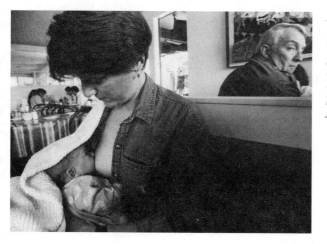

At first you may be self-conscious breastfeeding outside the home. With practice, however, it's possible to do it discreetly. Some states now have laws that protect your right to breastfeed in public.

- **Be comfortable.** You don't have to perch on the edge of a potty in the nearest ladies' room. (In fact, that's the least hygienic place to go.) Find a place to sit where your back gets good support—even sitting on the floor against a wall works.
- **Be discreet.** Toss a receiving blanket over your shoulder as you nurse or breastfeed while wearing a baby sling. Most onlookers probably think the baby's sleeping.
- **Be conveniently dressed.** Any front-opening blouse or easy-to-lift T-shirt will do. But stylish, confidence-boosting nursing clothes also abound; a variety of ingenious, easy-access openings makes discreet nursing easy. Check your local maternity store or look for mail-order advertisements in the backs of baby-care magazines. The Motherwear catalog is a wonderful source.
- **Be sensible.** Make nursing in public as easy on yourself as possible. Schedule outings right after feedings when possible. If you're shopping, try nursing in the car (where you're guaranteed a comfortable seat) before you enter the store. Know where the lounges are. In restaurants, consider booths for greater privacy.
- **Be calm, but firm.** If someone does complain about your nursing, maintain your composure. Pleasantly apologize for disturbing them but don't let yourself be intimidated by other people's hangups. You're not being impolite. Calmly explain that you have the right to feed your baby wherever you choose.

For More Help: Lactation Resources

- La Leche League International. See page 213.
- International Lactation Consultant Association, 4101 Lake Boone Trail, Suite 201, Raleigh, NC 27607; 919-787-5181. For referrals in your area or general information on breastfeeding.

What Should I Eat?

Losing Weight

After 9 months spent carefully nourishing a fetus, many new moms trade in their former preoccupation with eating right for a new goal of simply losing weight. That's certainly understandable. Unfortunately, it's not wise—not yet. Good nutrition is essential during the postpartum phase to fuel a healthy physical recovery and to put yourself in the best possible mind-set for mothering. Don't even think the word *diet* for the first 6 weeks. You'll be too busy adjusting to the demands of a new baby and learning to function on little sleep to burden yourself with self-recriminations about your looks.

How quickly you revert to your pre-motherhood shape (or close to it) depends on many factors, including your pregnancy weight gain, your diet, your activity level, your build, your metabolism, whether or not you're breastfeeding, and heredity. Realistically, it takes 3 to 12 months, with the average being 9. No matter how impatient you are to shed pounds, go slowly. Losing more than 1 pound a week isn't recommended. (Ignore fantastic tales of friends who wore their pre-baby blue jeans to their postpartum checkup or actresses who showed up at awards ceremonies in slinky gowns while still suckling twins. Rest assured they're in the minority.)

At delivery, most women immediately drop about 10 to 12 pounds—the combined weight of the baby, the placenta, and amniotic fluid. Another 5 to 10 pounds are shed over the next few weeks as your body loses the water and blood stores it accumulated during pregnancy. That usually leaves you with about 7 to 12 extra pounds, if you gained the recommended 25 to 35 pounds (more if you gained more). If you're nursing, your enlarged breasts will account for some of that weight. But your muscle tone is apt to be more slack, particularly around your middle, making you feel bigger than the scale indicates (which is a good reason not to get on a scale during the first few days after delivery). Also adding as many as 8 pounds to your weight are things like epidurals and IVs, which can cause fluid retention. This excess water will disappear through urination in a few days.

Nutrition Now

As a basic template for postpartum nutrition, stick to the rules you followed during pregnancy, with these modifications:

• **If you're breastfeeding,** you should consume slightly more calories per day than during pregnancy to fuel your recovery and the manufacture of milk. Your daily total should be about 2,500 a day, with the exact amount depending on your build. To speed weight loss, you can trim this amount a little after the first 6 weeks (once you're fully recovered and your milk supply is established), but only if you're consuming a balanced diet with enough of the nutrients needed to fuel milk production and recovery. Aim for three servings of protein and four to five of calcium each day—one to two servings more of dairy products than during pregnancy—as well as two servings of vitamin-C–rich foods (such as orange juice or melon). As important as how much you eat is how much you drink. Nursing mothers produce 20 to 30 ounces of breast milk daily, which means they lose more body fluid than normal. Drink whenever you feel thirsty, especially water; if your urine isn't running pale to clear, you may not be getting enough. Milk, juice, and water are better choices than cola, tea, or coffee, although small amounts of these beverages won't hurt.

• *If you're formula-feeding,* you'll need about 2,000 calories per day. Balance your diet among the food groups to keep up your energy, including two servings of protein, three servings of calcium, and one serving of vitamin C.

• *Downsize your portion size.* Many pregnant women eat more because they're hungrier. After the baby's born, however, their serving sizes remain big and their snacking stays constant, even though their appetites aren't as large. If you ate with abandon during pregnancy, take care to scale back your eating habits now.

• *Don't substitute lack of time for lack of nutrition.* Nobody feels like cooking during the early weeks, and you probably won't be out sampling gourmet restaurant fare. Take care not to overdo fatty fast food and order-in pizza. Stock up on healthful, quick-fix foods, such as fruits and vegetables, yogurt, eggs, bread, soups, lean meats, and easy casserole ingredients.

• *Keep easy, nutritious snacks handy.* Cut up fruit slices or vegetable crudités in the morning so you can grab them quickly throughout the day. Many groceries sell precut produce. Other good choices for quick snacks are juice, low-fat cheeses (such as string cheese), cold cereal, peanut butter and graham crackers, bagels, pretzels, and yogurt.

• *Beware "low-fat" and "fat-free" foods.* Chips, crackers, muffins, cookies, ice cream, mayo, and other foods labeled as such still have plenty of calories.

• *Sample some banished favorites, if you like.* If your taste for coffee and chocolate has come back, go ahead and incorporate them—in moderation—into your diet. The amount of caffeine in one or two 5-ounce cups of coffee a day or fewer will not cause a problem for most breastfeeding mothers or babies. (Sticking to decaf is wiser still.) Just be sure to consider all your sources of caffeine in your daily total. A baby who's getting too much tends to be wide-eyed and fussy, and doesn't sleep long; if this is the case, try cutting out caffeine for 2 weeks or so. An occasional alcoholic drink is also safe for nursing mothers. (See "IS IT TRUE . . . ," page 317.)

TRY THESE RECIPES!

Spinach and Ricotta Lasagna

Preparation time: about 50 minutes
Cooking time: 30–40 minutes

This hearty, calcium-rich recipe prepares enough for three meals—useful during the first months with a newborn. It can be made up to 48 hours ahead of time, covered, and refrigerated until ready to use, or frozen for a month before cooking.

2 pounds fresh spinach, stems removed
3 teaspoons olive oil
1/2 cup chopped onion or shallot
Salt and freshly ground black pepper
1/4 teaspoon ground nutmeg
9 strips uncooked lasagna noodles
2 eggs
2 cups ricotta cheese, whole milk or low-fat
Salt and freshly ground black pepper
3 cups tomato sauce, homemade or bottled
2 cups grated mozzarella cheese
1 1/2 cups grated Parmesan cheese

Wash the spinach well and place in a large pot with the water still clinging to the leaves. Steam over high heat until tender, stirring frequently, about 6 minutes. Drain in cold water to stop the cooking process and keep the spinach green. Drain well and finely chop.

In a medium skillet, heat 2 teaspoons of the oil over moderate heat. Add the onion and sauté 3 minutes. Add the chopped spinach and sauté with the salt, pepper, and nutmeg for about 5 minutes. Meanwhile, bring a large pot of salted water to a rapid boil. Add the lasagna noodles and boil for 8 minutes. Drain and place the noodles in a bowl of cold water to keep them from sticking to each other. Set aside.

In a medium bowl, whisk the eggs. Whisk in the ricotta, salt and pepper, and 1/2 cup of the tomato sauce.

Add 1 teaspoon oil and 1/2 cup of the tomato sauce to the bottom of a 13 × 9–inch pan. Place 3 lasagna strips (dry them off first on a tea towel) on the bottom of the pan, lengthwise. Add half the ricotta mixture and a third of the mozzarella and Parmesan. Add 3 more strips of lasagna (dried off) lengthwise and top that layer with the sautéed spinach. Top with the remaining ricotta mixture and another third of the cheeses. Add the remaining 3 strips of lasagna and top that with the remaining tomato sauce. Sprinkle the top of the lasagna with the remaining cheese, drizzle on the remaining teaspoon of olive oil and add a grinding of fresh pepper. (The recipe can be made ahead up to this point.)

Preheat the oven to 400 degrees. Place the lasagna pan on a cookie sheet (to catch drips) and bake for about 30–40 minutes, or until hot and bubbling. Yield: 6 to 8 servings.

Quesadillas

Preparation time: 5 minutes
Cooking time: about 3 to 4 minutes

A quesadilla is a corn or flour tortilla with melted cheese and a variety of other toppings. This is a master recipe—you can add any number of toppings listed below. Great for a quick dinner, snack, or lunch, depending on how simple or fancy you make them.

2 corn or wheat tortillas
About 1/3 cup grated cheese (a sharp Cheddar, Monterey Jack, or any hard cheese)
Toppings of choice: sour cream, chopped pitted black olives, finely chopped cilantro, chopped tomatoes, chopped cucumbers, finely chopped scallions, finely chopped ripe avocado, cooked black beans, caramelized onions, sautéed mushrooms or olives, grilled shrimp, cooked sausage slices, or salsa

Place a large skillet over moderate heat. Add the tortillas and heat about 10 seconds. Flip the tortillas over and sprinkle each with half the grated cheese. Let the cheese melt, spinning the tortilla around every few seconds to prevent it from burning or sticking, until the cheese is completely melted, about 3 minutes. Add the topping of your choice. You can either fold the tortillas in half or place one tortilla on top of the other and cut into quarters. Yield: 1 to 2 servings.

Oriental-Style Brown Rice Salad

Preparation time: about 15 minutes

Make this salad with leftover cooked rice and add any combination of vegetables you have around.

The Vinaigrette
1 tablespoon tahini (sesame seed paste) or smooth peanut butter
1 teaspoon minced fresh ginger, or 1/2 teaspoon ground
4 tablespoons peanut, vegetable, or olive oil
2 tablespoons rice wine vinegar, balsamic vinegar, or wine vinegar
1 teaspoon roasted sesame oil
1 teaspoon soy sauce

The Salad
2 1/2 cups cooked brown rice
1 scallion, thinly sliced
1 carrot, finely chopped
1 celery stalk, finely chopped
6 fresh mushrooms, thinly sliced
1/4 cup coarsely chopped peanuts, walnuts, or pine nuts (optional)

In a small bowl, mix the tahini and ginger. Add the remaining vinaigrette ingredients and stir until smooth. Taste for seasoning.

In a large bowl, break up any clumps of rice. Mix in the scallion, carrot, and celery. Gently pour in the vinaigrette and toss. Mound the salad in the center of the bowl and scatter the mushroom slices around the sides. Sprinkle the nuts on top, if desired. Yield: 4 servings.

Note: Tahini is available in most groceries and specialty food shops.

Orange and Ginger Rice Pudding

Preparation time: 25 minutes
Cooking time: 15 minutes

Rice pudding is one of the ultimate comfort foods. This version is a bit more sophisticated than most and full of good, fresh flavors.

1/2 cup raisins
1/4 cup orange juice
2 large eggs
1 cup milk
1/3 cup maple syrup or honey
1 teaspoon vanilla extract
1 teaspoon ground ginger
1 teaspoon grated orange zest

1/2 teaspoon ground cinnamon
1/8 teaspoon ground nutmeg
2 cups cooked white rice, warm or cold
2 tablespoons brown sugar mixed with 1 teaspoon cinnamon
1 cup heavy cream (optional)

Preheat the oven to 350 degrees. Generously butter an 8-inch square baking pan. In a small bowl, soak the raisins in the orange juice for 20 minutes.

In a large bowl, vigorously whisk together the eggs with the milk, maple syrup or honey, and vanilla. Drain the raisins and add them to the mixture along with the ginger, orange zest, cinnamon, and nutmeg. Mix in the rice, stirring well to break up any clumps. Pour into the prepared pan and bake for 15 minutes.

Sprinkle the brown sugar and cinnamon on the pudding and bake another 10 minutes, or until set. Serve hot, warm, or cold. If desired, pour cream on top. Yield: 4 to 6 servings.

Is It True...

That breastfeeding is a good way to lose weight? Nursing does burn calories, which helps some women shed pregnancy pounds. (One theory holds that the reason nature has made extra pounds cling to a new mom's frame is to fuel breastfeeding.) On the other hand, you need to consume some 300 to 500 extra calories per day to properly produce milk. For some women, nursing does speed weight loss, while others find that pounds melt off more quickly after their babies are weaned.

That if I drink milk my baby will be colicky? A few babies are, in fact, allergic to dairy products and can fuss and cry when they are exposed to them through their mothers' breast milk. The fussiness would occur only after a feeding. If this is the case, as a test you could try to eliminate all dairy products from your diet for a week. If the fussiness subsides, talk to your pediatrician about the possibility of the baby having a dairy allergy. But more commonly, newborns have colic for unknown reasons and will cry regardless of what you eat or drink. Your dairy intake can't *cause* such an allergy. To the contrary, nursing moms need to drink milk (and consume other dairy products) to bolster their calcium levels.

That I shouldn't eat spicy foods if I'm nursing? It depends. If you've always eaten a spicy diet, your baby will probably feel no ill effects. Think about breast-fed babies in different cultures around the world, whose moms eat hot or spicy foods routinely. Strong tastes such as garlic and cabbage can alter your milk's taste. But basically, you don't need to eliminate any food from your diet unless the baby seems to get sick or fussy or develop a rash, in which case you should consult your pediatrician.

I still need a prenatal vitamin? Since your prenatal vitamin supplies the iron your body needs in the stressful first weeks with a baby, it's a good idea to keep taking it until your postpartum checkup, unless advised otherwise. Then your doctor can recommend what's best for you. Many women are encouraged to continue taking the supplements as long as they breastfeed. Vegetarians who consume no animal products should continue a B_{12} supplement and possibly take added zinc, calcium, and vitamin D.

Fit for Motherhood

First Exercises

Most physicians feel it's unwise to begin a vigorous exercise program before 6 weeks postpartum, unless you were active throughout your pregnancy and had no complications. Even then, you should get a doctor's green light that you've healed properly. Anyway, you'll probably find yourself too worn out during the first weeks to bother with leotards and sneakers.

There are some simple exercises you can do as early as the day after giving birth, however, to begin restoring muscle tone. (If you've had a C-section, ask your doctor first.) They include:

• *Kegels.* By increasing blood flow to the perineum, these pelvic-floor strengtheners promote healing. They also help to regain vaginal tone and prevent incontinence. (See page 132.) Start Kegel exercises immediately.

• *Deep abdominal breathing.* Take a deep breath, then exhale slowly as you pull in your stomach muscles. Repeat throughout the day. You can do this while lying in bed, sitting, or walking to help restore abdominal tone.

• *Basic stretching.* While lying in bed or standing, stretch your arms over your head and extend your legs out as far as possible. When you feel up to it, you can also resume the pregnancy stretches on pages 129–132.

• *Pelvic tilts.* This exercise improves abdominal tone and posture. (See page 132.)

• *Walking.* Start in the hospital by simply ambling down the hall to the nursery. Slowly increase the distances you cover, as well as your pace.

Working up to Workouts

Once you and your doctor feel you're ready for more vigorous exercise, you can begin figuring out what kind of routine best suits your lifestyle now. Studies show that active new moms report feeling more like their old selves much more quickly than sedentary mothers. You'll feel more energetic, too.

Still, a few considerations are in order. If your lochia (postpartum vaginal discharge) turns bright red, you're probably overexerting. Wear a supportive bra if you're nursing. Always stretch beforehand—in fact, this may be all you manage for the first few weeks, and that's fine.

Finally, be realistic about what kind of progress to expect. Most new moms continue to wear their maternity clothes, or clothes in an in-between size, for the first few months postpartum. Not only your weight but also your physical proportions are apt to be rearranged—notably, larger breasts, wider hips, a bulging stomach, and possibly larger feet. You may not feel completely ready to resume a workout routine for many weeks, and once you do, your pace may seem so slow as to be useless. Rest assured, though, that any exercise is better than none and will help speed your path to your pre-baby figure.

Some good postpartum exercise options include:

• **Walking.** It's the best first exercise a new mom can try. Walking requires no special equipment, and your baby can come along (in a carriage or strapped into a chest carrier). In inclement weather, you can walk in a shopping mall. Aim for a brisk 20-minute outing, three times a week.

• **Postpartum exercise classes.** The type of exercise varies; postpartum yoga or baby-and-mom yoga are especially rewarding ways to get back in touch with your body. If it's an aerobics class, choose low-impact over high-impact classes until your recovery is complete. Check your local YMCA or YWCA, community rec center, or health club for classes, or ask your childbirth educator or doctor. Some postnatal classes incorporate babies into the routines (as weights to lift, for example); other programs provide childcare or simply expect and encourage infants' presence. Bonus: Postpartum classes are a great way to connect with other new mothers and swap tips and experiences.

• **Exercise videos.** The advantage here, of course, is convenience. Look for tapes prepared especially for new moms.

A POSTPARTUM AB-DOMINAL WORKOUT. The following simple, ballet-inspired moves can help firm a postpartum stomach. Each movement targets the four major abdominal muscles (abs) that are stretched and weakened by pregnancy and childbirth. Get your obstetrician's okay before beginning such a program.

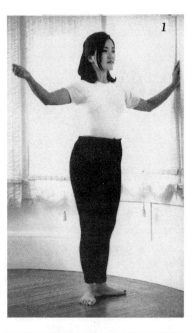

1. First Position. This exercise helps you understand your body's alignment and find your center of gravity. Stand up straight, shoulders back, tailbone tucked under, abdominals contracted, and rib cage lifted. Your heels should be together and toes pointed out so that your feet form a "V." Using your left arm to balance against a wall, hold your right arm extended out to the side, elbow slightly bent. Pretend that there is a balloon on a string attached to the top of your head, pulling you up so your spine is straight. Take deep breaths and concentrate on the inner abdominal muscles. Hold the position about one minute.

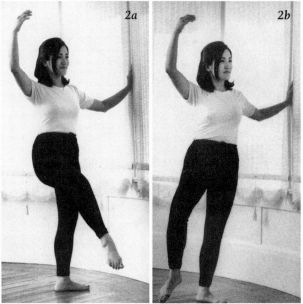

2. Attitudes. Stand in first position (described above) with your right arm over your head. With your right knee slightly bent and toe turned outward, slowly lift your right leg halfway to hip level (photo 2a). Tighten your abdominals as you slowly return to first position. Do 8 slow repetitions, then 8 fast. Repeat the motion with your right leg turned to the side (photo 2b). Concentrate on contracting your abs during the lowering phase. Repeat 8 times slowly, then 8 times fast. Switch sides and repeat with your left leg.

3. Battements. Stand in first position with your right arm over your head. With your toes pointed and your leg straight, extend your right leg in front, as high as the thigh muscle will allow without compromising your posture (photo 3a). Hold for two counts. Contract your abs as you slowly lower your leg to starting position. Do 8 slow repetitions. Then repeat, this time lifting your right leg out to the side, keeping it straight and your toes pointed (photo 3b). Do 8 slow repetitions. Switch sides and repeat both movements with your left leg.

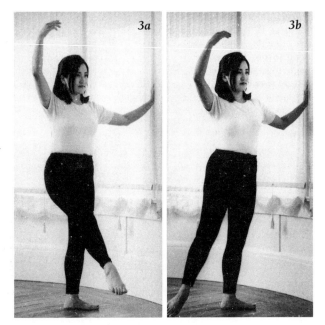

4. Seated Attitude. Sitting in a chair, lift your upper body through the torso; your shoulders should be down and relaxed, your spine straight, your abdominals contracted, and your feet flat on the floor (or on books if you need to raise them). Arms should be overhead. Lift your right leg out in front, with your knee slightly bent and your toes pointed. Lower your leg, contracting your abdominals. Repeat 8 times slowly, then 8 times fast. Repeat using your left leg.

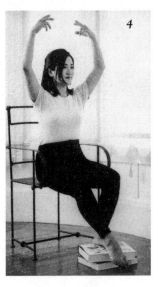

CRUNCH TIME: *Before progressing to the basic crunch, do the following check to make sure the gap in your stomach muscles has closed: Lie flat on your back with your knees bent and your feet flat on the floor. Place the fingers of your left hand, palm facing you, just above your belly button. Inhale, and as you exhale lift your head and shoulders off the floor, and slide your right hand down your thigh toward your knee. This will make your abdominal muscles tighten and you should be able to feel a gap between the two edges of the muscles. If the gap is three or more finger widths, you're not ready for crunches. Once the gap narrows to one or two finger widths, it's safe to proceed.*

5. The Basic Crunch. *For the basic crunch, lie on your back as described above. Place your hands behind your head, elbows out to the sides. Keeping your lower back pressed against the floor and your neck relaxed, contract the abdominal muscles so that your head and shoulders lift naturally an inch or two off the floor to the point of resistance without pulling your neck—not very high. Keep the movement very small and exhale as you lift. Hold for two counts. Inhale as you slowly lower to the starting position. Repeat 20 times.*

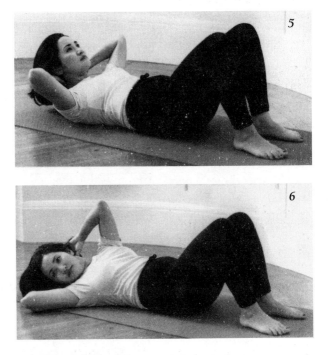

6. Crunch with a Twist. *With both shoulders on the floor, arms behind the head, exhale and slowly raise your left shoulder, twisting your torso toward your right knee. (You should feel the twist in your midsection, not in your lower back or elbows.) Inhale as you return to starting position. Do 10 twists on each side, alternating left and right.*

WHAT IF...

I had a C-section—when can I start to exercise? A Cesarean delivery is major surgery. Wait at least 2 weeks before attempting even simple stretching exercises, and get your doctor's advice about when you can begin abdominal work (usually 4 to 8 weeks postpartum). Begin slowly, with deep breathing or isometric exercises. If your incision hurts or pulls at any time during exercise, you're probably doing too much, too soon.

IS IT TRUE...

That exercise can inhibit breast milk production? On the contrary, women who exercise postpartum may have higher milk volume than their sedentary counterparts. Just be sure to drink plenty of water before and after exercising.

That I should avoid walking up and down stairs? It's hard to believe that a generation or two ago, new moms were sometimes delivered home by ambulance, carried to their bedrooms, and admonished to stay put for weeks. Today, many hospitals send mothers off without so much as a wheelchair ride to the door. Unless you've had a C-section, taking the stairs is perfectly fine. If you've had a severe episiotomy or tear, though, minimizing all movement for the first week is smart.

MOTHER TO MOTHER:
"How I Got Back in Shape"

Valerie Becker, 34
Mill Valley, California

Before becoming pregnant, 5-foot 4-inch Valerie weighed 110 pounds. She played a lot of tennis and took long hikes to stay fit. By the time she delivered her son, Daniel, she had gained 35 pounds. "When I was pregnant, I worried that I'd never fit back into my pre-pregnancy clothes and that my stomach would be flabby," she recalls. "I didn't want to go out in public much because I felt misshapen."

Though Valerie was determined to get back to her old shape, she waited 6 weeks to recover fully before starting, so as not to jeopardize her health. Because she was breastfeeding, she didn't want to crash diet. Instead, she tried to eat sensibly and focus on exercise. Three days a week, she attended a postnatal class for 1-hour sessions that featured a lot of sit-ups and weight training to tone her abdomen and arms. "I'd bring Daniel with me, and exercise while holding him."

When her baby was 6 months old, she reached her pre-pregnancy weight, although it took a little longer to fit back into her old clothes. Then a cold and a vacation led her to quit the exercise class. Instead, Valerie began pushing Daniel in his stroller for at least an hour every other day, in a park, on a trail, or in a shopping mall.

Valerie's tips for getting back in shape:

• *Keep up the emphasis on nutrition that you had in pregnancy.* "Have a balanced diet with lots of fruits and vegetables so you won't succumb to fatty temptations."

• *Rest as much as you can.* "If you are well rested, you will have more energy for exercise. Just getting out of bed is a chore when you're tired."

• *Have an incentive.* "I was determined to get back into my old clothes because my maternity ones were so ugly. A friend of mine motivated herself by taping pictures of women whose figures she admired on the refrigerator."

• *Exercise regularly.* "Be consistent. Just go out and do *something* every other day for 20 minutes."

• *Be patient.* "How you lose weight is very individualized—it depends on your body and how conscientious you are. Don't be discouraged if it goes slowly—it's just a matter of time."

What About Sex?

When to Resume?

Most doctors recommend that women not resume intercourse until after their initial postpartum checkup, which is usually 4 to 6 weeks after delivery. That's so the doctor can rule out any medical problems that might interfere. But if you have had no perineal tearing or only minor perineal stitching, and no complications, intercourse is physically safe as early as 2 to 3 weeks postpartum. Intercourse is not advised before that time because of the risk of uterine infection or damage to stitches (though orgasm is okay at any point after delivery).

But Do I Have To?

In fact, most women don't feel ready for sex within the first 2 months after giving birth. Or if they do engage in sexual intercourse, it's less often than before. To start with, as soon as the placenta is delivered, the hormones that had been nourishing it rapidly vanish. Libido plummets, and the vaginal lining thins to a menopause-like state, making it drier and more susceptible to irritation or infection. Lactation can exacerbate this condition because the hormone prolactin (which stimulates milk production) inhibits estrogen (which normally provides lubrication), so sex sometimes hurts. And this can last as long as you nurse. Breasts may leak or no longer feel like an erogenous zone. Also, although episiotomy stitches or tears heal within 3 or 4 weeks, soreness in the area can persist for months. On top of physical recovery, there's sheer exhaustion. Sleep deprivation. Needy older siblings. Returning to work. The result is major stress, which can further delay healing and sabotage desire.

On a psychological level, much of a new mother's sexual energy gets funneled into nurturing, which can be hard for a man to understand. When they're not feeding or handling the baby, most new moms just want to sleep. Many women also report feeling "touched out" at the end of the day—they want their bodies to themselves. Others, drowning in a constant flow of breast milk, spit-up, baby wastes, and lochia, get turned off by the very idea of any more bodily fluid. There's also the strange sensation of suddenly seeing yourself as your own mother—and who tends to think of their mother in a sexual context? Changes in your physical self, from a squishy belly to milk-swollen breasts, can take some getting used to for either partner. (Though many couples find post-pregnancy voluptuousness a turn-on.)

Given all these changes, it's little wonder that couples can take 6 months or longer to fully regroup sexually. One major study of nearly 600 couples found that just 17 percent had resumed intercourse at 1 month postpartum; 89 percent by 4 months (though frequency tended to remain lower than before pregnancy). Women who were nursing resumed sex later and reported less sexual satisfaction than those who did not breastfeed. If lack of desire persists longer than 6 to 12 months, it may reflect underlying marital problems not wholly related to childbearing, and a couple may benefit from counseling.

Making Sex Better

The first time out, you may be apprehensive about whether it will hurt. Some new mothers experience an involuntary clenching of their vaginal muscles (a reflex called *vaginismus*) that's triggered by anticipation of pain. It can help to visually inspect the area with a hand mirror for signs of swelling or irritation, or to insert a clean finger to test for soreness. It's also a good idea for the man to see and touch the scar, if the woman had an episiotomy or tearing, to better empathize with his partner. He should also avoid deep thrusting at first. In fact, you may feel better limiting your initial sexual encounters to nonpenetrative play, such as gentle oral or manual sex.

Vaginal dryness can cause painful intercourse *(dyspareunia)*. To relieve dryness, use extra lubrication. A water-soluble lubricant (such as K-Y jelly or one of the made-for-sex alternatives such as Astroglide or Aqua-Lube, which tend to last longer) is less irritating. Avoid nonsoluble types, such as petroleum jelly (Vaseline). If you use condoms, buy the lubricated type. Equally important is prolonged and gentle foreplay. If you're breastfeeding over several months, a temporary vaginal thinning can occur that causes itching, burning, or dyspareunia. This is easily treated with a vaginal estrogen cream, prescribed by your doctor that is safe for nursing.

The missionary position can be painful, especially after an episiotomy, though a pillow under the woman's buttocks can relieve pressure. Also try variations, such as side by side or the woman on top. And if inexplicable pain persists, always discuss it with your doctor.

Finally, remember that intimacy is about more than sex, even about more than touching. It's being able to talk frankly about your strange new feelings. It's about taking turns walking a colicky baby. It's about realizing that you're parents together. It can be hard for men, especially, to understand the many disruptions that having a baby brings to a woman's sexuality, especially if he's already waited out 9 months of vanished wifely *amour*. But don't feel guilty or pressured. Sexual interest, like a growing fetus, can't be rushed. In time, you'll feel ready. And in the meantime, your new baby represents a good reason to feel close to your spouse.

Birth Control After Baby

Since ovulation typically occurs 2 weeks before you menstruate, don't wait until your period resumes to discuss family planning with your doctor. Here's how contraceptive options stack up for postpartum use:

WHAT IT IS	FOR NURSING MOTHERS?	EFFECTIVENESS	CONSIDERATIONS
The Combination Pill			
Oral contraceptive combining estrogen and progestin that suppresses ovulation.	No.	97%.	Should not be started until 2 to 6 weeks postpartum. Best for nonsmokers. Reduces breast milk production.

continued

What it is	*For nursing mothers?*	*Effectiveness*	*Considerations*
The Mini Pill			
Oral contraceptive containing progestin only.	Yes.	96–98% (for nursing mothers; 80% if not nursing).	Should not be started before 4 to 6 weeks postpartum. Has no effect on breast milk production. Can cause vaginal spotting and irregular cycles. Effectiveness declines when breastfeeding is supplemented.
Norplant			
Six match-size plastic progestin capsules inserted by a doctor under the skin of the upper arm; the capsules suppress ovulation for up to 5 years but can be removed at any time and fertility is restored within days.	Yes.	99%.	Best not started before 6 weeks postpartum when breastfeeding is established. Expensive if used for fewer than 3 years. Possible irregular periods for the first year.
Depo-Provera			
Injections of synthetic progestin, given every 3 months to suppress ovulation.	Yes.	99.6%.	Best not started before 6 weeks postpartum until breastfeeding is established. Can take 10 months or longer for fertility to return after usage is stopped. May cause weight gain that's difficult to lose, irregular periods, or breakthrough bleeding.

What it is	For nursing mothers?	Effectiveness	Considerations
Condom			
Male condoms fit over the penis to capture sperm; they are made of latex or polyurethane. The female condom (brand name Reality) is a sheath with a closed inner ring that fits over the cervix like a diaphragm and an open outer ring that rests outside the lips of the vagina.	Yes.	84% (male); 79% (female).	Best used with spermicidal jelly or foam (they appear to have no effect on breastfeeding).
Diaphragm			
A round rubber dome that fits inside a woman's vagina and covers her cervix.	Yes.	82%.	Proper fit is essential. After childbirth, a woman who previously used a diaphragm should be refitted, but not until 6 weeks postpartum.
IUD			
A small plastic device placed in the uterus to prevent fertilization or the attachment of a fertilized egg to the uterine wall; most last one year.	Yes.	98–99%.	Unlike the old Dalkon Shield model associated with infection and infertility, today's IUDs (ParaGard and Progestasert) are considered very safe and a good choice for women who have children but don't want permanent sterilization. Wait until 6 weeks postpartum before insertion.

continued

What it is	For nursing mothers?	Effectiveness	Considerations
Natural Family Planning			
Method of avoiding intercourse during peak fertility by monitoring body changes (also called *periodic abstinence* or the *rhythm method*).	No.	80%.	Unpredictable. Relies on ovulatory changes that may be difficult to detect postpartum. After menstruation is clearly reestablished, it's best for women with very regular cycles.
Sterilization			
In a woman, a tubal ligation involves blocking or severing her fallopian tubes so that sperm cannot reach eggs. In a man, a vasectomy cuts and seals his sperm ducts.	Yes.	99.2–99.6%.	If you want your tubes tied in the delivery room, you should discuss this with your doctor well in advance of your due date, as consent needs to be signed early.

WHAT IF ...

My husband doesn't seem interested in sex? Often a woman blames her partner's hesitancy on her changed appearance, but this is rarely the real cause, psychologists say. He may be struggling with the conflicting images of his partner as both a sexual object and a maternal one, or may feel uncertain how to relate to her sexually after the tumult of pregnancy and childbirth. The problem can be compounded if either partner feels ambivalent about parenthood. Frank talk about the problem is essential—and usually leads to a closer relationship. But sometimes such feelings are so deeply rooted that counseling is the answer.

I feel stretched out? The vagina is an elastic organ and shrinks remarkably quickly after delivery. Breastfeeding hastens this process, too. But the best way to rebuild pelvic muscle tone is to work at it. Even if you sluffed off your Kegel exercises during pregnancy, it's not too late to start them now.

I'm too tired? Sex requires both physical and psychic energy, resources sorely lacking when you're tending a newborn. Obviously, your need to rest and replenish is a priority. But take care not to squander your energy, either. In the big scheme of things, marital intimacy is more important than a clean floor. You'll probably be too tired to think about sex once a week, let alone actually engage in it. So you may need to make a concerted effort to stay close to your partner. Consider initiating some ritual into your sex life, such as planning ahead and making sex dates. But don't feel pressured to perform like the last of the red hot mamas—focus on loving, not lovemaking.

IS IT TRUE...

That I can't get pregnant if I'm still nursing? Don't rely on breastfeeding for birth control. There's no way to know when ovulation will resume. It's true that ovulation tends to restart later in nursing mothers (on average, at 17 weeks, compared with at 10 weeks for nonlactating mothers). But there's no way to determine *exactly* how long breastfeeding will suppress ovulation and the chance of getting pregnant again. Some women who nurse exclusively get their periods within 2 months of delivery, while others remain period free even long after their babies have begun solids.

Exception: There is a form of contraception known as the *lactation amenorrhea method (LAM)*. This method is considered 98 percent effective during the first 6 months. According to LAM, you can have unprotected intercourse without conceiving if you meet three conditions: (1) if the infant is exclusively breastfeeding; (2) no more than 5 hours elapse between feedings; and (3) your period has not yet resumed. LAM is not very forgiving of deviations from this formula, however. One drawback is that some babies start to sleep through the night (as long as 6 to 8 hours) around 6 weeks. Another is that supplemention is out, and many babies begin solids at 4 months. And all women using LAM need a backup plan for when their baby reaches 6 months or when they get their first period (which can happen within a month or two of delivery even if you're breastfeeding).

That I should wait until my bleeding stops? It's generally safe to resume intercourse around 3 weeks after a complication-free delivery. But waiting until lochia discharge completely stops (generally between 3 and 6 weeks) is a prudent way to assure yourself that the uterus is sufficiently healed. The risk of having intercourse too soon is that, if the site where the placenta attached to the uterus hasn't had a chance to heal, bacteria may be introduced that can cause a uterine infection.

"Give It Time"

Yasmen Mehta, 36
San Francisco, California

Like most women, Yasmen's interest in sex declined during her pregnancy. "I was sick a lot during the beginning. Sometimes I would be in bed by 6 P.M. I felt too lazy and too big," she recalls. "But my husband and I didn't consider it a big deal, so it didn't put a strain on us."

Six weeks after daughter Roxana was born, Yasmen got her doctor's okay to resume intercourse. But it was nearly 3 months before her desire bounced back. "Not only was my body not ready, but I was also adjusting emotionally to having a little one around me," she says. "All of your energy goes into caring for your baby, especially if it's your first child. Everything else gets put on a back burner." There was also the practical roadblock of finding time when Yasmen and her husband were both awake and the baby was asleep.

The couple expressed their love in many nonsexual ways, such as taking walks and sharing baby care. The long disruption in their sex life has been frustrating sometimes, but it has a silver lining, she says. "In a way, sex is even better now, because we've gone through so much together."

Yasmen's advice on postpartum intimacy:

• *Take it slowly.* "Cuddle first. You can be in bed and do fun things besides intercourse."

• *Say "I love you."* "It's reassuring and it doesn't take any special energy."

• *Let your partner know that your disinterest isn't a sign you're rejecting him.* "It's important to make a conscious effort to show your husband you still care for him."

• *Encourage your husband to be involved with the baby.* "It's endearing and appealing to see my husband play with our daughter. He'd also put her to sleep when my arms were aching. Things like that are signs of great intimacy and love."

Newborn-Care Basics

Sleeping

Most newborns seem to do nothing but eat and sleep. In fact, they average 16 to 17 hours of slumber a day, though only for 3 to 5 hours (or less) at a stretch.

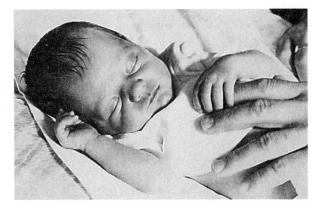

To reduce the risk of sudden infant death syndrome (SIDS), make sure to always put your baby to sleep on her back.

Starting at about 6 weeks, most babies begin to sleep for one longer period (4 to 6 hours or longer) at night. By 3 months, a baby drifts toward 15 total hours of sleep and a more predictable schedule, including three or four naps.

All you can do during the early weeks is go with the flow. Let your baby sleep when she seems to need it. She may doze off right after a feeding or while you're rocking her, and that's fine. It's too soon to think about establishing a schedule for her. That's because a newborn's circadian rhythm—the 24-hour internal clock of wakefulness and sleepiness that all humans follow—isn't fully developed yet.

By about 6 weeks, you can gradually begin to help your baby fall asleep on her own. Try putting her down when she seems tired, usually after she's been awake for about 2 hours. Some babies start to sleep through the night (for 6 to 8 hours) on their own around 6 weeks—sometimes just for an isolated night or two and, gradually, on a consistent basis. You can start to reinforce the idea that night is for sleep by keeping night feedings quick and quiet. To avoid further unnecessary stimulation, you can even begin to skip middle-of-the-night diaper changes unless the baby is uncomfortable or you smell a BM. One good habit to develop right from the start is to maintain a normal household noise level while your baby naps (don't turn off the TV and radio or avoid running the dishwasher, for example). That way she'll learn to sleep through routine activities. A minority of babies are particularly sensitive to environmental noise, but they are the exception rather than the rule.

Always put your baby to sleep on her back. Numerous studies have confirmed that this reduces an infant's risk of sudden infant death syndrome (SIDS), a medical enigma that's the leading killer of children between 1 week and 1 year of age. No one knows what causes SIDS, and there is no surefire way to prevent it. Thankfully, the incidence of this unspeakable tragedy has dropped dramatically in recent years as more risk factors are identified and avoided.

Don't worry that sleeping on her back will cause a baby to choke should she spit up; that's unlikely in a healthy child. (The only thing that sleeping position is likely to cause is a flat or bald spot on the back of the baby's head, and that will disappear over time.) Your child should also sleep on a firm surface—not on a comforter, sheepskin pad, beanbag, waterbed, or other soft bedding—without any pillows or stuffed animals in the crib. If you bring the baby in bed with you, keep her head away from your pillows and comforters and make sure that your mattress is firm, too. Note: Smoking increases the risk of SIDS. Expose your child to as little smoke as possible, including secondhand smoke from visitors or in public places. Breastfeeding reduces the risk of SIDS.

Crying and Colic

Crying is your baby's chief way of communicating with you. A cry can mean, "I'm hungry," "I'm wet," "I'm tired," "I'm hot," or "I'm cold." Cries can also signal boredom or overstimulation. At first, you may fear you'll never decipher this complicated Morse code. As you and your baby settle into some semblance of a schedule, however, you'll be better able to gauge probable times for hunger or fatigue. Trial and error will help you solve other cries, such as a quick diaper check to verify that discomfort. Eventually, you may even be able to distinguish the tenor of the cry—a hunger cry, for example, starts slowly and builds to a rhythmic, piercing wail designed to wake you from the deepest slumber. A cry of pain, in contrast, is more shrill and punctuated by long pauses while the baby catches his breath to scream again. Personality is also encoded in your baby's cries. Some babies sound off frequently and loudly, while others mostly whimper. Infants have distinct temperaments, too, so what upsets one child may not bother another.

The general rule is to respond quickly to a baby's cries. Forget the old saw about spoiling your child this way; it's virtually impossible for a newborn to be held too much. You're also building the baby's trust in you. In fact, one study found that babies who are carried for at least 3 hours a day (in someone's arms or a baby sling) cry less than babies who aren't held as much. Research has also shown that parents who respond swiftly to a baby's cries in the early weeks tend to have children who cry less at 6 months.

Often babies who cry a lot are said to be colicky. It's certainly true that many infants have fussy spells, especially in the evening, even when all their basic needs are met—it's thought that they simply need to discharge tension by crying it out. Bona-fide colic, however, follows a fairly common pattern. If your baby has this mysterious syndrome, you'll know. Characterized by long bouts of inconsolable crying, usually beginning in the late afternoon or evening, colic strikes around 2 to 3 weeks of age and lasts until about 3 months. The baby may draw up his legs as if experiencing gastric trouble or extend his body rigidly. Each session lasts at least 3 hours, though the next day, the baby is usually sunny and agreeable again. There is a broad range of variations on that general theme, however, depending on the baby's personality. Some babies fuss and cry day and night. About 10 to 20 percent of infants show colicky behavior.

Colic is exasperating because there's no surefire fix except waiting for him to outgrow it. It's also frustrating because experts don't agree on the cause. Theories range from an easily agitated temperament to a sleep-wake cycle that's out of sync with other body rhythms, to an immature nervous or digestive system. Gas is most commonly blamed, but studies show that colicky babies are no gassier than noncolicky ones; if anything, the crying may cause the gas, rather than the other way around. Nor is breast milk the cause of colic, so weaning is pointless. Cow-based formula is not a cause, either. (A dairy allergy can make a baby cry, but this would occur after any feeding, not just in the evening.) One thankfully disproven theory is that a mother's anxiety somehow is to blame.

Enduring a baby with colic or a colicky disposition is enough to make a parent cry. Try the techniques recommended in "Good Advice: Soothing Baby's Cries," page 358. Keep trying to read your baby's cries when she's not colicky and adapt soothing routines during those noncolicky times that she can get used to. Often, however, nothing will work. The baby just needs to cry it out. Since you're already tired from recovery, nursing, and a lack of rest, it's easy to blame yourself or to succumb to the criticisms of those who insist there must be something wrong. Tune out this unhelpful chorus. (What they'll say: "You're holding him too much." "What are you eating that's giving him gas?" "He needs cereal." "Your milk must be bad.") Tell your pediatrician that you suspect colic so you can have the peace of mind that the child is otherwise healthy. And in the meantime, be good to yourself. Get friends or your partner to share the baby-walking burden with you during colicky spells. Go for a walk. Put the baby down for a few minutes—he's already crying; it won't hurt him. Know that colic's relentlessness can make new moms feel angry at their babies or overwhelmed. That's only natural. Admitting your frustrations to a friend can help. Finally, reassure yourself that colic is just a fact of life for some babies. Though 90 days of it may seem like an eternity, it *will* be outgrown.

Swaddling

Many newborns prefer the security of being enveloped in a blanket the first few weeks. If you didn't watch closely enough when the nurses swaddled your baby in the hospital, here's how to master this comforting, snug wrap:

HOW TO SWADDLE

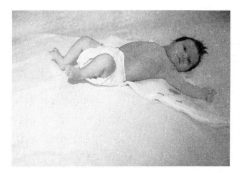

Fold down one corner of a receiving blanket. Then place your baby diagonally on the blanket. Her head should be perched just above the fold line.

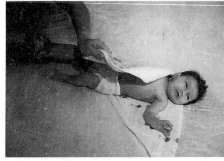

Place your baby's right arm next to her body and pull that side of the blanket snugly across her chest.

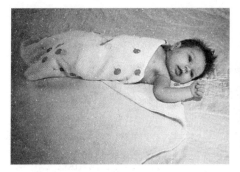

Tuck the folded side of the blanket under your baby's mid-section. Her arm should be nestled inside.

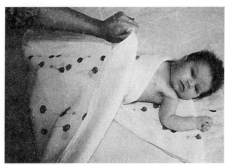

Then fold the bottom of the blanket up, making sure the excess fabric doesn't cover her face.

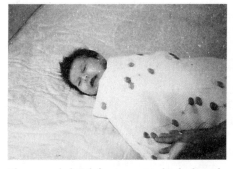

Place your baby's left arm next to his body and pull the other side of the blanket snugly across his chest.

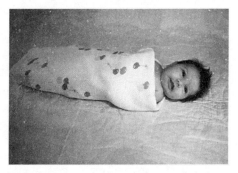

Tuck the remaining fabric under your baby's back to create a tiny bundle.

Dressing

If, like most new parents, you're showered with welcome-baby presents, your little one already has a bigger wardrobe than you do. These guidelines make dressing a snap:

• *Start with easy-access clothes.* For the first weeks, when your baby's body is smallest and floppiest—and when you're changing diapers nonstop—skip the cute outfits with a million snaps at the crotch. The easiest layette items to maneuver are sleep sacs (with gathered or drawstring bottoms), kimono-style shirts that snap in the front, snap-front one-piece suits, and pants that pull on and off.

• *Cover her head.* Top your baby's topper with a cotton knit cap for the first several months when you go outdoors, even in summer, and longer than that in cooler months or if your baby has little hair. A brimmed hat shields her eyes and face, though such hats tend to work best after the baby gains head control. Starting out early with hats also helps your baby get used to them—helpful later for protecting a tot from sun or cold.

• *Add one layer more than you dress yourself in.* If you're fine in shirtsleeves, for example, add a sweater for your baby. Premature babies and those under 10 pounds, especially, may need the added insulation of an extra layer. To retain body heat, the best item of clothing next to the skin is an undershirt or a one-piece suit that snaps at the crotch. Layers atop this, including a blanket, can be easily removed (or added) as the temperature changes.

• *Choose cotton.* It's more comfortable next to the skin and it breathes, minimizing heat rash. One hundred percent cotton clothing is even safe as sleepwear if it is close fitting (such as a one-piece jammie); it's also less scratchy than the old flame-retardant polyesters and more practical.

• *Know the tricks.* Stretch neck and sleeve openings with your hands before putting them on. To get your baby's arm in the sleeve, first slip your hand into the opening from the outside and connect with your baby's arm. Then, with your other hand, wriggle the sleeve up the baby's arm until his hand comes out the opening.

Diapering

One's first fumbling attempts can make it seem hard to believe, but in a matter of days you'll have so mastered the art of changing a diaper that you can do it in your sleep. And given that the average newborn runs through ten to twelve diapers in 24 hours, you probably *will* be half-asleep through many changes. It's important to change a newborn's diaper promptly to minimize rashes caused by the urine and feces against the tender bottom skin.

Set up several diaper-changing stations around the house in the rooms where you'll be with your baby most. This spares you treks up and down stairs or from room to room. Any flat surface will do; cover it with a waterproof mat and a clean towel. Store all your supplies within arm's reach. *Keep one hand on the baby at all times and never turn away,* even if you use the buckled strap on a changing table. After removing a wet or soiled diaper, wipe the baby from front to back. It isn't necessary to apply diaper-rash ointment after every change unless you see telltale signs of a coming rash (redness or slight pimpling).

For the first few days, a newborn's stool looks like greenish black tar. This thick, sticky substance is called *meconium*, an accumulation of fetal wastes gathered in the womb. After the mother's milk comes in, a breastfed baby's stools are mustard colored and odorless, with a consistency that can range from loose and watery to slightly thick and mushy or flecked with seedy particles. Formula-fed babies' stools are firmer, smell like adult BM, and vary in color from pale gold to brownish. Iron-fortified formulas or vitamin drops will add a green to dark brown cast. Stool color and consistency can vary from day to day.

Cord and Circumcision Care

The dark, clamped stump of the umbilical cord that's left on the baby's abdomen usually falls off in 1 to 3 weeks (occasionally longer) and the spot beneath becomes the navel. Clean all around the base of this stump, which is the area most prone to infection, after each diaper change by gently applying rubbing alcohol. Use a cotton swab (Q-tip), rolling it as you clean.

Keep the area dry. Fold down the diaper so that the stump isn't covered. (Some brands of newborn-size disposables feature a cut-out area for this.) Don't immerse the baby in water until the stump falls off.

Never remove the stump, even if it's barely hanging on. Signs of infection—redness on or around the navel, pus, or swelling—should be evaluated by your pediatrician. You may see a small amount of blood; if it can be easily stopped with mild pressure, it's probably just a sign that the stump should be handled more gently. The area may also bleed slightly after the stump falls off or remain raw for a few days. Keep the raw spot clean and dry, with the diaper folded down to prevent infection. If the stump doesn't show signs of healing within 3 weeks, your pediatrician can painlessly cauterize (seal) the tissue with silver nitrate.

If your baby was circumcised, the site just needs to be cleaned and watched for signs of infection until it heals (in about 1 week). Check the penis at every diaper change. For the first few days, apply petroleum jelly directly to the incision area to keep the penis from sticking to the diaper. If a plastic ring was used for the circumcision, be sure it has not slipped onto the shaft of the penis. Some yellow or whitish coating on the head of the penis is normal; don't remove it. But if you see any bleeding, redness, or swelling anywhere on the penis, alert your baby's doctor.

Note: An uncircumcised penis requires no special care. Don't attempt to retract the foreskin. That will occur on its own over the next 3 or 4 years or often longer.

Bathing

Until the umbilical cord and circumcision are fully healed, babies should be given only sponge baths. Afterward, they can graduate to a bit more water in a portable infant tub or the kitchen sink. (Both options are easier on you at first than bending down to a big tub.) Some moms find this a pleasurable time with their babies, but it's not necessary to bathe a newborn daily—after all, they don't get very dirty. As long as you keep the baby's bottom clean and occasionally wipe the face and hands—the "topping and tailing" method—you can limit baths to once or twice a week.

How to give a sponge bath: Wrap the baby in a towel and lay him on a flat, waterproof surface or in a plastic infant tub lined with a towel but no water. Have on hand 2 containers of lukewarm water—one for washing and the other for rinsing your washcloth—along with several cotton balls, a washcloth, soap, shampoo, and another towel for drying off. (Lotion and powder smell good but aren't necessary. Also, powder can be inhaled and harm a baby's lungs.) First, use the moistened cotton balls to wipe the baby's eyes, mouth, ears, and chin. Next put a drop of shampoo on a wet washcloth and rub it on his scalp. Rinse the washcloth and rewet it to remove all the shampoo. You can also hold your baby in a football hold, with his head over the tub, and wash and rinse the scalp with your free hand. A weekly shampoo is sufficient; just rinse the hair on other days. If your baby has cradle cap, wash his scalp more often and use a soft baby brush. Dry his head immediately and cover it with a hooded infant towel. Finally, soap and wash your baby's body, being sure to get inside all the folds of skin. Uncover half the baby at a time, so he'll stay warm and comfortable. Dry him off carefully so that the crevices between skin folds and between fingers and toes are all dry.

HOW TO BATHE A NEWBORN

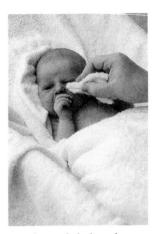 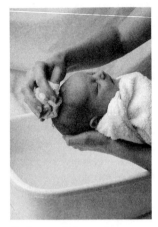 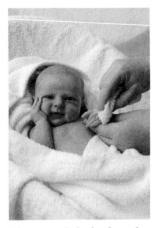

Dip the washcloth in the warm water and gently wipe the eyes to remove any discharge, starting from the inside corner and wiping outward. Then use the washcloth to clean the rest of his face. Pat dry.

Tuck your baby under one arm, using that hand to support his back, neck, and head. Hold him over the basin and use your free hand to wet, shampoo, and rinse his hair. Gently dry his head with the towel.

Place your baby back on the padded surface. Wash his neck, chest, arms, and legs, moving the towel to expose only one area at a time. Rinse with a wet washcloth and pat dry.

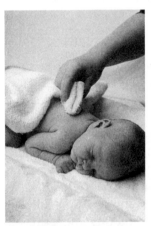 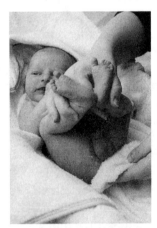 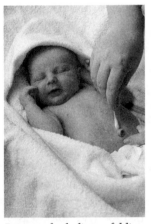

Carefully lay your baby on his stomach. Wash the back of his neck and his back. Rinse with a wet washcloth and pat dry. Turn him over.

Remove your baby's diaper and gently wash the genital area. (Keep soap off the circumcised penis for the first few days.) Wash your baby's bottom last. Rinse with a wet washcloth, wiping from front to back, and pat dry.

Put on a fresh diaper, folding it down in front to expose the umbilical stump. Dip a cotton swab in rubbing alcohol and wipe around the base of the cord as well as the stump itself.

To bathe a baby in a tub, follow the same routine, except that the baby is fully naked and sitting in 2 or 3 inches of water, with you propping her up. Most babies find this very relaxing, making just before naps a good time for a bath. Some, however, dislike the water and will howl straight through. Remember that babies are SLIPPERY WHEN WET. Always support your baby's back and neck in the tub—if the shape of the tub alone isn't sufficient, line it with a towel and place one hand behind her neck. You might find it helpful to wear a terry-cloth bath mitten or cotton gloves (available at pharmacies). Some parents like to bathe with their baby.

Outings and Visitors

When can you take your baby out in public? Sooner than you may think. After all, you safely navigated the trip home from the hospital, didn't you? It's impractical (not to mention mentally unhealthy) to cloister yourselves away from the world. As soon as you feel able—even in the first week or two postpartum—you can take your baby with you to a restaurant or store or for a short walk. You can even go out in extreme cold or heat, provided the baby is adequately dressed.

During the first month, take extra steps to prevent exposing your baby to germs. Although a breastfed newborn receives many protective antibodies against certain diseases like strep throat, the baby is still very susceptible to viruses such as colds. Avoid crowds in close quarters such as malls. Encourage strangers to look but not touch, especially during cold and flu season. It's perfectly fine for healthy people, including children, to hold your baby, though they should wash their hands first. Designate a special spot on the baby, such as a foot or knee, where a child can kiss her.

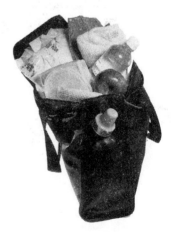

When leaving home, you'll need a well-stocked diaper bag, which contains four to six diapers, wipes, a prepared bottle (if you're formula feeding), breast pads (if you're nursing), a plastic bag (for dirty diapers), a change of clothing, a baby sweater for layering, changing pad (or waterproof lap pad), burp cloth (to protect your shoulder), receiving blanket (to warm your baby or help you breastfeed discreetly) and snacks and bottled water for you.

With a baby in tow, leaving the house empty-handed is out of the question. A well-stocked diaper bag is a new mom's best friend.

Jaundice

Virtually all newborns arrive in the world with some degree of jaundice (*neonatal hyperbilirubinimia*). In about half of the cases, the skin (and sometimes eyes) becomes yellow-tinged by the second to fifth day of life. Jaundice is caused by too much bilirubin, a substance formed during the normal breakdown of blood hemoglobin by the liver; it builds up when the newborn's immature liver can't yet process the bilirubin efficiently, and the circulatory system deposits it in the skin and mucous membranes, giving them a yellow cast. Premature babies are especially vulnerable.

Jaundice is usually detected in the hospital but can develop at home, especially in the event of discharge within a day or two of delivery. This is why many pediatricians like to re-check newborns around the fourth day of life. Always get a doctor's input when you suspect jaundice. How can you tell? For Caucasian babies, gently rub the baby's skin between the knee and ankle. The skin will have a yellowish cast if jaundice is present; if the baby isn't jaundiced, the skin should resemble the tone on the back of your hand. For babies of color, check the whites of the eyes; if they're yellowish, the baby may have jaundice. Be sure to check the baby in the clear light of a window, away from yellow walls or curtains. Blood tests (usually a prick in the baby's heel) can confirm a suspected case and are also used to monitor bilirubin levels.

The most common type, physiologic jaundice, usually clears up on its own as the liver matures and the condition corrects itself within 10 days. If a more serious case is left untreated, though, a baby can be at risk for brain damage. When treatment is warranted, however, it's easy and almost always successful. The most common cure is *phototherapy*. This consists of exposure to special ultraviolet bili-lights or a fiber-optic pad that transmits light, in order to chemically alter the bilirubin and speed its excretion. This is typically done in the hospital before discharge. Home phototherapy equipment may also be provided, though the practice is declining. The levels of bilirubin considered acceptable have changed recently, and some cases that were once treated with bili-lights no longer are. Instead, parents are often advised to let their baby lie naked in a warm, sunny spot near a window and to feed her frequently.

Checkups

Your pediatrician will advise you of his or her preferred schedule of well-baby checkups for the first year. Many doctors like to see babies at 4 days, 4 weeks, and then monthly thereafter until 6 months, then at 9 months and 12 months. The baby's growth and general health are assessed at each visit, and this is also when immunizations are given. An innoculation against hepatitis B is given at birth.

Not Quite Picture-Perfect?

Even after a newborn has been cleaned up in the delivery room and brought home, many new parents feel shock or worry upon detecting some common, but unexpected aspect of their baby's appearance. To ease your concerns, check this guide:

CONDITION	DESCRIPTION	CAUSE	CARE ADVISE	CAUTIONS
Blocked tear duct	One or both eyes tear repeatedly.	The tears normally produced to keep the eye moist usually drain from the eyes through ducts in the nose; in some newborns, this drainage path isn't fully developed, so they drain continually down the cheeks instead.	Your baby's doctor may show you how to massage the duct area to unblock it. This may not have any effect, however, and the duct may simply need to mature on its own (in as much as a year or two).	Eye infection can result—watch for yellow discharge, redness, or swelling. Antibiotic drops may be prescribed. In the case of repeat infections, surgery may be recommended to open the duct.
Soft spots on head (*fontanels*)	A newborn's skull has two soft places—one in the front and one near the back.	The bones haven't yet fused in these places (which helped the head pass through the birth canal more easily and allows allows brain growth after birth).	They require no special care—don't be afraid to touch, brush, or wash these areas.	A sunken fontanel is a sign of dehydration, while one that bulges can indicate serious illness. Tell your doctor immediately. (A fontanel that pulsates is normal.)

continued

CONDITION	DESCRIPTION	CAUSE	CARE ADVISE	CAUTIONS
Diaper rash	Angry red rash on buttocks or genital area.	Irritation of skin by urine or fecal matter—chafing can lead to bacterial or yeast infections.	Apply zinc oxide or other diaper-rash ointment to seal out moisture and soothe the skin. So air can keep the rash dry, try closing diapers more loosely, using a larger size, or letting the infant sleep without a diaper. Avoid plastic pants.	Call doctor if rash persists more than 3 days or if blisters or sores develop.
Cradle cap	Oily crusting on scalp (also other places sebaceous glands are present, including face, chest, and armpits). Sometimes thick and yellowish or reddish, or as slight-looking as dandruff. Appears at 3 to 4 weeks and usually disappears within 6 months.	Possibly due to maternal hormones from the womb.	If on scalp, wash hair daily with mild shampoo and brush away scales with a soft brush. The rash causes no discomfort to the baby.	Call doctor if skin oozes or appears red; medicated shampoo may be prescribed for severe cases.

continued

Eczema (*atopic dermatitis*)	Red, scaly, itchy rash on face and body marked by fluid-filled bumps that can open and crust over. Generally disappears by toddlerhood.	Often associated with asthma and allergies to food, pollen, and fabric; tends to be inherited.	Try to figure out the dietary triggers and avoid them. Use smooth-textured clothing, blankets, and sheets (100% cotton is best); avoid excessive bathing and extreme temperatures. Run a cool-air humidifier to keep air moist and cool. A doctor can recommend soothing ointments and medication.	One-third of infants with eczema later develop asthma or other allergies.
Heat rash (*prickly heat*)	Pink or white bumpy rash usually found in the skin creases of the neck, armpits, and diaper area.	Common in summer, it's caused by a temporary blockage of sweat glands—preventing sweat from reaching the skin's surface to evaporate, causing a rash.	Keep skin cool and dry; dress the baby loosely. Don't apply oil or cream, which further blocks pores.	Severe cases can become infected.

CONDITION	DESCRIPTION	CAUSE	CARE ADVISE	CAUTIONS
Thrush	Textured white patches on tongue, cheeks, lips, and roof of mouth; often mistaken for milk at first, but if rubbed off, the skin underneath will redden and bleed.	Yeast infection (*Candida albicans*), probably from exposure in birth canal.	Prescription liquid anti-fungicide.	A breastfeeding baby can pass thrush to mother, causing burning sensation in nipples; air-dry them after a feeding to prevent yeast's growth. Antifungal cream may be prescribed for infected breasts; the infant will also be treated.
Salmon patches (*neves simplex*)	Dull red to pink birthmarks, often at the back of the neck, hence the name *stork bites* (also called *angel's kisses* when on the forehead). Usually fade with time and disappear.	A cluster of large, visible blood vessels that disappears as the skin thickens and the blood vessels shrink.	No special care necessary.	None.
Strawberry marks (*hemangiomas*)	Raised, solid red bumps resembling the fruit for which they are named; size	Enlarged blood vessel.	No treatment necessary, though when located on a lip or eye,	None.

	can vary. Generally disappear over time, although they can get bigger for several months after the birth.		they can interfere with sucking or vision and may be removed surgically.	
Mongolian spots	Deep gray or bluish patches, usually on buttocks or lower back, most common on babies of African-American, Asian, Indian, or Mediterranean descent; sometimes mistaken for bruises. Disappear during early childhood.	Accumulations of pigment in a given area.	No special care necessary.	None.
Port wine stains (*nevus flammeus*)	First pink, then deep purple, these relatively uncommon marks usually occur on the face and neck or the limbs on one side of the body. They may fade over time but rarely disappear.	Cause unknown.	No special care necessary.	Some can be removed by laser when baby is older. They should be evaluated by a doctor.

Checklist: When to Call Your Pediatrician

Most new parents are constantly tempted to call their baby's doctor. When in doubt, do. Never hesitate to pick up the phone if you notice the following:

☐ Fever of more than 100.2 degrees F*
☐ Difficulty breathing
☐ Vomiting (not normal spitting up) more than once or forceful vomiting
☐ Repeated watery, foul-smelling stool (diarrhea)
☐ Blood in urine or stool
☐ Frequent, inconsolable crying or fussiness, or a high-pitched cry
☐ Persistent lethargy (sleeps for long periods and through feedings, or is hard to rouse)
☐ Yellowish or orange-hued skin and eyes (signs of worsening jaundice)
☐ Severe rash or blisters (signs of infected rash)
☐ White patches in mouth (signs of thrush)
☐ Greenish nasal discharge (sign of infection)
☐ Just doesn't seem "right" to you

*An axillary (armpit) thermometer reading is easiest with a baby. To take, use a regular oral thermometer or a rectal thermometer and hold it in the baby's armpit for 3 to 4 minutes.

Taking the temperature rectally provides the most accurate reading. First shake the thermo-meter down below 96 degrees; then lubricate the tip with petroleum jelly. Hold the baby belly-down on your lap or on a changing table as if you were changing a diaper; insert the thermometer bulb about 1 inch into the rectum with one hand. Hold the thermometer between your index and middle fingers while using the rest of that hand to cup your baby's bottom. Leave it in place for 2 minutes.

Tympanic (ear) thermometers, which are inserted in the ear for a few seconds, are the easiest to use but are not accurate for infants until about 12 months of age.

GOOD ADVICE: SOOTHING BABY'S CRIES

After you've checked to see that your baby's basic needs are being met—that he's not hungry, wet, or overtired—experiment with these tried-and-true soothers. Take care not to rush from one technique to the next in a frantic attempt to quell cries, however, which can cause the baby to get even more agitated.

• Carry the baby in a sling or soft carrier.
• Swaddle her (wrap her snugly) in a soft blanket.

- Rock and sing.
- Lay her on her tummy across your knees and rub her back, or lay her belly-down on a half-filled warm-water bottle covered by a cloth.
- Darken the room.
- Take her for a ride in a carriage or stroller.
- Encourage her to suck her fist or a pacifier.
- Give a soothing massage with warmed baby oil.
- Take a shower or bath together.
- Turn on the vacuum cleaner, a fan, or a radio between stations—steady "white noise" may lull her to sleep.
- Read to your baby in an even-toned voice. (Bonus: It can be a book *you* like—any book, not necessarily a children's story.)
- Place a strong-ticking clock near her bed.
- Hold her in front of a mirror.
- Try a wind-up or battery-operated swing (many models feature carriages or adjustable seats for newborns who can't sit up yet).
- Give a warm bath or shampoo (if she normally likes them).
- Play a recording of soft music or of soothing sounds such as a rainstorm or the ocean.
- Take a quick ride in the car.
- Always check with your doctor before trying any type of homemade remedy (such as herbal teas).

Is It True...

That a fat baby will be a fat child? Birthweight isn't a good predictor of future weight. In fact, your baby's spot on the growth charts tends to fluctuate throughout the first year, so that a fleshy child in the 90th percentile for her weight at 4 weeks may fall to average by 4 months. Genetics and diet play a role in determining a baby's weight later in life, but not until after age 2 do you need to worry about obesity (20 to 30 percent over ideal bodyweight).

That if my baby has acne, he'll have acne as a teenager? There's no relationship. Infant pimples usually erupt between the third and fifth weeks of life and disappear on their own by 3 months. Called *milia*, these tiny whiteheads are caused by clogged pores, which are common to immature infant skin. They may be aggravated by maternal hormones that the newborn body is shedding.

That binding a quarter to a baby's belly will ensure a firm navel? Alas, this tradition only makes the baby uncomfortable. (Ditto using an old-fashioned belly-band or a Band-Aid.) Sometimes when the stump falls off, the surrounding abdominal muscles fail to come together tightly, resulting in a slight bulge or swell, called an *umbilical hernia*. This poses no danger, requires no medical treatment, and often disappears in a few years.

That switching to soy-based formula or giving Mylicon drops will cure colic? When faced with a persistently fussy baby, some doctors will suggest a switch from a formula based on cow's milk to a soy brand in an effort to see if the baby has a milk allergy. That may relieve cries if an allergy is indeed the problem, but there's no link between colic and what a baby consumes. Simethecone drops (such as Mylicon) are an over-the-counter medication given to treat gas—which may relieve a gassy baby but won't make any difference in one who has colic.

That colic stops exactly at 3 months? Very little about babies is exact. Some cases of colic persist into a baby's fourth or even sixth month, but the overwhelming majority do indeed vanish around the 3-month mark.

That flashbulbs can hurt my baby's eyes? They certainly can be annoying, though probably not damaging. If natural light isn't sufficient for photos, try bouncing the flash off a nearby surface or standing several feet back. But an occasional close-up with a flash is okay.

What If ...

My baby smiles—can it really be "just gas"? Even a day-old infant can flash a grin during the REM (rapid-eye movement) stage of active sleep. But the genuine article—which usually appears before sleep or in response to a high-pitched voice or a face—doesn't show up until 4 to 6 weeks.

I feel compelled to check my baby's breathing all the time? That would make you normal, not neurotic. Some parents even find themselves jostling the child or laying a hand on their baby's chest to be sure it's rising and falling all right. Consider your vigilance a reflection of how seriously you're taking parent-hood. Remember, too, that babies have varying stages of slumber—sometimes active, sometimes deep and still, sometimes noisy and snuffly. Your comfort level will grow with experience, but don't be surprised if you're still creeping in to check on your sleeping child well into the elementary years!

Resources: Newborn Care

- SIDS Alliance, 800-221-SIDS. Ask for the free pamphlet, "What Every New Parent Should Know: Facts about Sudden Infant Death Syndrome and Reducing the Risk for SIDS."
- March of Dimes, 1275 Mamaroneck Ave., White Plains, NY 10605; 888-663-4637 or http://www.modimes.org. A toll-free resource center answers questions about newborn care, and you can request educational brochures or referrals to major medical centers in your area.
- American Academy of Pediatrics, P.O. Box 927, Elk Grove Village, IL 60009; 847-228-5005 or http://www.aap.org. Provides educational brochures and fact sheets on children's health and psychosocial issues.

MOTHER TO MOTHER:
"Easing Early Jitters"

Shirley Kathryn Woods, 32
Virginia Beach, Virginia

Rebecca was a perfect newborn: a healthy 7 pounds, 4 ounces. But to her mother Shirley, the baby seemed tiny and fragile. "I never had much experience with a newborn," she says. "I was really nervous about leaving the hospital where I was surrounded by experts."

At home, Shirley's anxieties mounted. "I didn't know how long to let her cry, so I never let her cry during the first month. I worried about breaking her fingers when I dressed her, and whether she had enough clothing on. I was nervous taking care of her belly button, too—it amazed me that it had once joined us together, and I didn't want it to get infected." Then there were the strange grunting noises Rebecca made, the scabby stuff on her head, and the red marks around her nose and eyes. "I wondered if everything was normal," she says. (It all was.) When they went out, Shirley found herself a much more cautious driver. "When I wasn't driving carefully, I was always fiddling with her car seat so she'd be safe."

It helped that Shirley's mother and sister stayed with her for a week. "My husband kept me positive, too, by saying things like, 'Hey, you're a good mom,' or 'You're doing the right thing,' " she recalls. Their support gave her permission to feel exhausted and overwhelmed. Encouragement also helped her stop making unhelpful comparisons to how she imagined other mothers might better handle various situations.

Another confidence booster was keeping her baby close. Shirley used a baby carriage as a crib during the first months, wheeling it from room to room so she could keep an eye on Rebecca. She'd also sit in a cozy spot reading aloud from her favorite mystery writer while breastfeeding. "I now keep a picture next to my computer of me reading to my daughter during those first 48 hours and it warms me every day to look at it," she says.

Shirley's tips for getting comfortable with newborn care:

• *Follow your instincts.* "My mom kept telling me to put the baby down, but holding her was my way to get to know her and feel more confident about caring for her."

• *Pump yourself up.* "I'd say positive, reassuring things to myself, like how happy and healthy my baby was."

• *Tune out unhelpful advice.* "Be confident and try not to overreact. Ignore what others say to you, especially out in public."

• *Talk to other mothers.* "I wish I'd done that more. It would have helped me to realize my concerns were common ones."

• *Enjoy!* "Revel in these weeks—falling in love with your newborn is incredible."

ILLUSTRATION CREDITS (by page number)

CHAPTER 1
4   Joyce Tenneson
5   Narda Lebo
6   Narda Lebo, Steve Rahn
7   Narda Lebo
10 Gabrielle S. Revere
41 Lori Eanes
52 David Roth
58 RJ Erwin, Photo Researchers (pasta)
    Nick Dolding, Tony Stone (milk)
    Gentl & Hyers, Photonica (chocolate cake)
    Seth Joel/Science Photo Library (potatoes)
60 David Roth
65 Joe Polillio/Liaison International (walking)
    Lyn Hughes/Liaison International
    (swimming)
67 Lori Adamski Peek/Tony Stone
72 David Roth
73 David Roth
79 Narda Lebo
83 Narda Lebo

CHAPTER 2
98   Joyce Tenneson
100 Lennart Nillson, *A Child Is Born*,
     Dell Publishing Co.
101 Narda Lebo
105 David Roth
107 David Roth
108 Gabrielle S. Revere
110 Narda Lebo
115 Narda Lebo
119 Narda Lebo
130 David Roth
132 David Roth
134 David Roth
135 David Roth
136 David Roth
138 Narda Lebo
139 Narda Lebo
144 Narda Lebo
152 Joseph Nettis/Photo Researchers, Inc.
154 Narda Lebo

CHAPTER 3
158 Joyce Tenneson

160 Narda Lebo
161 Narda Lebo
162 Narda Lebo
163 Narda Lebo
173 David Roth
186 David Roth
192 Narda Lebo
202 Narda Lebo
207 Gabrielle S. Revere
208 Gabrielle S. Revere
209 Gabrielle S. Revere

CHAPTER 4
214 Joyce Tenneson
216 Stella Johnson
231 Narda Lebo
233 David Roth
235 Narda Lebo
236 Narda Lebo
241 Narda Lebo
242 Narda Lebo
243 Narda Lebo
256 Narda Lebo
258 Narda Lebo
268 Narda Lebo
270 Stella Johnson
276 Stella Johnson

CHAPTER 5
286 Cristiana Ceppas
304 Patricia Arian
305 Patricia Arian
306 Steve Rahn
311 Leanne Schmidt/Swanstock
314 Gabrielle S. Revere
315 Patricia Arian
321 Rick Rickman
331 David Roth
332 David Roth
333 David Roth
343 K.L. Knief/Photonica
346 Lise Alexander
350 Patricia Arian
351 Gabrielle S. Revere

Thanks to the following companies for contributing products for use in the photos:

Avent America, Inc.
Babies Best, Inc.
Braun
Century
Evenflo Company, Inc.
Hoohobbers International, Inc.

House of Hatten, Inc.
Infantino
Kapoochi
Lamby Nursery Collection
Munchkin
Primo

Regal Lager, Inc.
Remond for Babies
Safety 1st, Inc.
The Company Store

INDEX

Illustrations in the text are indicated by an italicized "i" next to the page number.

Abortion, 48, 145
Abortion, spontaneous, 18, 81–83
Acetaminophen
 for fever, 18, 25
 for migraines, 85
 postpartum, 279, 289, 292, 310
 for prenatal pain, 17, 22, 25
Acupressure, 15, 177, 254
Acupuncture, 254, 263
Afterbirth, 239
Age, maternal
 forty plus, 10, 44, 78, 84
 thirty plus, 78, 84, 114
 thirty-five plus
  caregivers for, 36, 44
  increased risks for, 78
  prenatal tests for, 47, 48, 115
AIDS (acquired immune deficiency syndrome), and AZT, 40
Air embolism, 23, 142
Albumin, 39
Alcohol
 avoidance of, 2–3, 20–21, 180
 and breastfeeding, 318
 in cough medicine, 25
 effects of on fetus, 20
Allergies, maternal, 85
Alpha-fetoprotein (AFP) test
 anxiety about, 117–18
 choice about, 43, 48, 118
 purpose of, 113–14, 115, 117
 reliability of, 47, 87, 114
American Academy of Pediatrics, 200, 202, 213, 318, 361
American Cancer Society, 28
American College of Nurse-Midwives, 48
American College of Obstetricians and Gynecologists,
48, 52, 118, 193
American Council of Nanny Schools, 149
American Diabetes Association, 85
American Lung Association, 28
American Physical Therapy Association, 263
American Society for Psychoprophylaxis in Obstetrics (ASPO/Lamaze), 152, 154
Amniocentesis, 100, 115i
 choice about, 43–44, 46, 48, 117
 and fetal gender, 115, 173
 insurance payment for, 92
 purpose of, 42, 114, 115–16
 and Rh factor, 39–40
Amniotic fluid
 amount of, 41, 67, 143, 176
 inhaled by fetus, 100, 160
 weight of, 51, 53, 110i
Amniotic sac, rupture of, 222–24
 alerting doctor to, 164, 229, 230
 amniotomy for, 223, 240
 premature (PROM), 144, 223, 240
Analgesics, 177, 251, 255–57
Anemia
 causes of, 16, 40, 78, 127
 and fetal distress, 240
 postpartum, 291
Anesthetics
 for circumcision, 202
 for dental care, 107
Anesthetics, in childbirth
 minimization of, 36
 natural, 237, 241
 and pushing stage, 242, 251
 types of, 256–58
 See also Epidural block
Antacids, 18, 24, 103
Antibiotics, 10, 25, 107, 175, 308
Antihistamines, 17, 24, 25
Anxiety, 169–72

and breastfeeding, 309
and miscarriage, 29–30, 33–34, 96
myth regarding, 113
performance, 170–71, 295–96
and prenatal tests, 111, 117–18
Apgar scores, 275, 281
Appearance
 and body image, 109–11, 111–12
 and partner, 139, 140–41
 and peer support, 63
 postpartum, 296
 third trimester, 187–89
Arthritis, 77, 85, 86
Arthritis Foundation, 86
Artificial sweeteners, 23
Aspirin, 17, 18, 22, 77
Asthma, 85, 200, 355
Aversions, 9, 13–14, 49, 102

Baby blues ("milk fever"), 296, 297
 See also Depression, postpartum
Baby shower, 159, 161, 207, 210–11
Back labor, 254, 266–67
Backache
 causes of, 52, 63, 164
 as danger signal, 143
 in labor, 224, 254
 minimization of, 63, 104–5
Bedrest, 144–47
 for cervical incompetence, 145
 for hepatitis B carriers, 114
 for hypertension, 77
 and miscarriage, 81
 for preeclampsia, 191
 for preterm labor, 34, 144
 support network for, 85
Bilirubin, 318–19, 352
Biofeedback, 254, 263
Biophysical profile, 176
Birth announcements, 205–6

Birth canal, 161, 179, 222, 226, 234, 237, 268
Birth certificate, 277
Birth control
  choices of, 337–40
  counseling on, 36, 302
  and lactation amenorrhea, 341
  pills, 3, 9, 11, 187, 337–38
  stopping, 2, 11, 139
Birth defects
  diagnosing, 41–44, 46–47, 113–17
  in family, 37, 44, 115–16
  preterm labor with, 143
  risk factors for
    age over forty, 78
    diabetes, 2, 77
    maternal infections, 2, 18–19
    medications, 22, 43, 78
    overheating, 18, 21
    rubella, 2, 18–19, 40
    toxic substances, 3, 20–24, 49
    vitamin overdose, 23
    X-rays, 21
Birth plan, 177–79
  and caregivers, 176, 204
  and situational control, 219
  written, 160, 204
Birthing centers, 220, 254
  and natural birth, 153
  physician backup for, 35, 37
  resource for, 48
Birthing chairs/tubs, 225
Birthmarks, 113, 185, 356–57
Blastocyst, 5i, 6, 8
Bleeding
  after falling, 187
  first trimester, 80–81
    diagnosis for, 42
    with ectopic pregnancy, 83
    with exercise, 66, 68
    and miscarriage, 33–34, 81–82
  hemorrhage, 21, 84
  implantation, 7, 8, 80
  postpartum
    as danger sign, 293, 330

  See also Lochia
  and Rh factor, 39
  second trimester, 143, 144–45
  with sexual activity, 76
  third trimester, 167, 191–92, 229
Bloating, 17–18, 51, 127
Blood pressure
  baseline, 38, 77
  and dizziness, 16–17
  and fetal distress, 240
  high. See Hypertension
  monitoring, 113, 144, 175, 184
Blood tests
  and anemia, 10, 40
  for genetic disorders, 40–41
  infant, 277, 284, 352
  multiple marker, 100, 114, 115
  pregnancy verification, 10
  for Rh factor, 39–40
  routine, 48
  for rubella, 18–19, 40
  for STDs, 40
Blood type, 39–40, 275
Bloody show. See Mucus plug
Bonding with baby, 171
  delayed, 280, 281–82, 294
  prenatal, 109
Bottle feeding, 200, 313–16
  and breast care, 291
  supplemental, 319
  supplies for, 201, 314i
  of water, 179, 277, 319
Bradley Method, 53, 152, 154, 264
Brain defects, 21, 114
Brazelton neonatal scale, 277
Breast changes, 110i
  engorgement, 290–91, 305, 310
  first trimester, 8–9, 69, 75–76
  milk ducts, 70, 308
  third trimester, 69, 166
Breast implants/reduction, 317
Breast milk
  expressing, 291, 305, 312, 316, 320

  leakage of, 201, 307, 308, 317
  production of, 290–91, 306–7, 309
  storage of, 312
Breast pumps, 310–12, 311i, 321
Breastfeeding, 303–13, 306i
  advantages of, 200–201
  away from home, 321–22
  at birth, 275–76, 280
    advantages of, 238–39, 309
    with C-section, 269
  choices for, 179
  and infections, 308–9, 356
  learning about
    classes for, 153, 201
    and lactation consultants, 201, 303, 320, 322
  and midwives, 36
  and medications, 308, 310
  myths regarding, 317–19, 334
  painful, 308–9, 320–21
  positions for, 304i, 305i–6
  questions about, 317–19, 328–39
  resources for, 213, 321
  and rooming in, 277
  supplies for, 201
Breathing techniques
  for anxiety, 170
  choice about, 177
  cleansing, 238, 253, 263
  for contractions, 232, 234, 235, 250, 252–53, 289
  learning, 152–53
  for migraines, 85
  practicing, 160, 329
Breech position, 163i, 195, 268
Bromocryptine (Parlodel), 291

Caffeine, 50–51
  avoidance of, 15, 17, 57, 180
Calcium
  in antacids, 18
  deficiency in, 105, 191
  loss of, 50
  need for, 57, 59, 323, 324
  sources of, 23, 59, 127–28, 180

Carbon monoxide, 21, 24
Carcinogens, 20, 24
Caregivers
    at delivery, 237, 239
    insurance payment for, 92,
        200
    questions for, 38, 44–46
    relationship with, 48
        after pregnancy, 302–3
        and anxiety, 111, 170
        and birth plan, 2, 176–77
        and labor support, 219
    selection of, 35–37, 48
    when to alert, 164, 167–68,
        229
        in early labor, 176, 222,
            232
Cat litter, 3, 26–27
Centers for Disease Control, 26
Cephalopelvic disproportion,
    268
Certified nurse-midwives (CNM)
    and continuity of care, 45,
        225
    functions of, 36–37
    and physicians, 35–36, 37,
        46
    popularity of, 220
    resources for, 48, 272
    See also Caregivers
Cervical cerclage, 144i–45
Cervix
    effacement of, 143–44, 164,
        226, 230
    first trimester, 10, 16, 38
    incompetent, 16, 68, 144–45
    inflammation of, 80–81, 144
    ripening of, 175
    See also Dilatation
Cesarean delivery, 268–71, 270i
    anesthetic for, 257, 258, 268
    choices for, 178
    conditions for
        abnormal labor, 240, 268
        diabetes, 142, 268
        fetal distress, 240–41
        fetal position, 162–63,
            195–96, 268, 273
        herpes simplex, 19, 268
        placenta problems, 192,
            268

postterm pregnancy, 193
preeclampsia, 268
prolapsed cord, 224, 243
emergency, 37, 46
frequency of, 36, 45, 200,
    220, 270–71
myth regarding, 179
recovery from, 63, 279,
    291–92, 302, 334
resource for, 272
and weight gain, 52
Checkups. See Exams
Cheese Frittata, 56–57
Chemical products, 22, 24,
    70–71
Chicken pox (varicella), 19
Child Care Aware, 149
A Child Is Born (Nilsson), 31
Childbirth classes, 269, 298
    and birth plan, 177
    and C-sections, 269
    fathers and, 199, 247
    and informed birth, 170,
        219
    and pain management, 252
    selection of, 101, 109,
        151–54, 152i
    as support group, 34, 298
Childcare, 147–49, 198
Chloasma, 187
Chorionic villus sampling (CVS)
    choice about, 46
    and fetal blood type, 40
    in first trimester, 8, 47
    procedure for, 42, 47
Chromosomes, 26
    abnormalities in, 47, 82,
        115–16
    analysis of, 173
Circumcision, 201–2i
    care for, 349, 350
    choice about, 179
    resource for, 213
Civil Rights Act of 1991, 150
Cleft palate, 23, 50, 59, 275
Clothing, 71–74
    and attractiveness, 111
    for hospital, 211–12, 224
    lingerie, 67, 70, 73–74, 201
    maternity, 133–38, 135i, 136i
    need for, 71–73, 72i, 100

for nursing, 136, 137, 318,
    322
postpartum, 330
shoes, 74, 105, 189
variety in, 189
Coach, childbirth
    availability of, 229
    and Bradley Method, 152–53,
        174–75
    and C-section, 45, 178, 268
    items needed by, 212, 260
    as labor support, 225, 234,
        244, 248, 260–63
    selection of, 34, 178,
        199–200
    See also Fathers; Support,
        labor
Colostrum, 166, 290, 291
Constipation, 17, 60, 103, 180,
    290
Contractions, 167
    Braxton-Hicks, 143, 162,
        168, 224, 228, 230
    in labor, 222, 227, 230–38,
        250
    and oxytocin, 239, 240
    postpartum, 278, 288–89
    preterm, 143–44, 165,
        180
Cooley's anemia, 44
Coombs test, 275
Corn Chowder, 181–82
Cough medicines, 24, 25
Couvade syndrome, 174
Cradle cap, 354
Cramping
    as danger signal, 25, 66,
        80–82, 83, 143
    leg cramps, 105–6
    mild, 9
    near due date, 164
    postpartum, 278, 289
Cravings, 118, 125–26
Crowning, 216i
    and delivery, 225, 226,
        234–35i
    and episiotomy, 237, 241i
C-section. See Cesarean delivery
Cystic fibrosis, 44
Cystitis, 16
Cytomegalovirus (CMV), 19

Decongestants, 24, 25
Dehydration
  causes of
    exercise, 67
    overheating, 22
    pregnancy sickness, 14,
      15, 127
    vomiting/diarrhea, 25,
      61
  infant, 307, 316, 319, 353
  and thirstiness, 16, 60
Delivery, 216i, 235i
  anesthetics for, 242, 243,
    251, 257
  and birth plan, 160, 176,
    177–79
  positions for, 178, 236i, 238
  pushing stage, 230, 234–38,
    262–63
  recovery from, 287–94
Dental care, 2, 21, 107
Depression
  medications for, 10, 85
  and miscarriage, 82
  postpartum, 283, 291,
    296–97, 300–301, 302
Depression After Delivery, 299
Diabetes
  and birth defects, 2, 77
  detection of, 39
  development of, 78
  family history of, 114–15
  and miscarriage, 2, 77
  resource for, 85
Diabetes, gestational
  detection of, 101, 114–15,
    142–43
  exercise for, 54, 142
  and maternal age, 114
  monitoring for, 225
  and overweight, 3, 52, 54,
    114
Diabetics
  C-section for, 142, 268
  exercise for, 68, 77
  induced labor for, 239
  monitoring of, 36, 68, 77
Diaper rash, 354
Diarrhea
  infant, 200
  maternal, 25, 61, 224

Diet
  first trimester, 48–51, 57–59
    and digestion, 17
    and fetal growth, 48–49,
      53
    with nausea, 13–14, 49,
      90
  food substitutions for, 125
  foods to avoid in, 23, 27, 50,
    58, 103
  myths regarding, 57, 185
  with overweight, 53–54
  second trimester, 103,
    118–21,125–27
  third trimester, 180
  vegetarian, 3, 61–62, 329
  See also Nutrition
Dilatation and curettage
  (D & C), 82
Dilatation, cervical
  in labor, 164, 222, 226,
    230–35, 231i
  and miscarriage, 82
  premature, 16, 143–44
  rate of, 221, 230
Diuretics, 50, 77
Dizziness, 16–17, 66, 119, 278
Doppler, 8, 10, 41, 42, 226
Douching, 16, 23, 288
Doulas
  as labor support, 178, 200,
    225, 252
  postpartum, 206, 292
  resources for, 213, 299
Doulas of North America, 213
Down's syndrome, 44, 47, 114,
  117
Dreams, 171–72
Drugs, illegal, 2–3, 21
Due date
  calculation of, 11–12
  as estimate, 38, 161, 193,
    221
  myths regarding, 179, 185
  and ultrasound, 42, 100, 115,
    117
Dystocia, 268

Ectopic pregnancy, 42, 83i
  diagnosing, 42
  and pregnancy tests, 10

resource for, 86
  and Rh factor, 39
Edema. See Swelling
Effacement, cervical, 143–44,
  164, 226, 230
Embryo, 6i–7i, 13–14, 79, 81, 84
Embryoscopy, 43
Emotional changes
  first trimester, 28–31
  postpartum, 279–80, 294–96
  second trimester, 109–11
  third trimester, 168–73
  See also Anxiety
Employer
  and leave time, 32, 87–89,
    91–92, 196
  obligations of, 91
  and task modification, 150
  See also Workplace
Endometriosis, 84
Endorphins, 63, 254
Endoscope, 43
Enemas, 45, 220, 227
Engagement. See Lightening
Epidural block, 256i–57
  attitudes toward, 45
  availability of, 37
  choice about, 177, 259, 267
  complications of, 259
  IV with, 225, 256, 259
  monitoring with, 227
  vs. natural birth, 153, 220
  patient-controlled, 257
  for prolonged labor, 259,
    265–66
  and pushing stage, 243, 257
  when to request, 234, 267
Epilepsy, 44, 78
Episiotomies
  anesthetic for, 257–58
  choice about, 176, 178, 242
  and crowning, 237, 241i–42
  and epidurals, 259
  frequency of, 36, 45
  and midwives, 36
  recovery from, 249, 289, 302,
    334, 336
  repair of, 239, 241
Equal Employment Opportunity
  Commission (EEOC), 150
Estriol, 100, 114

Estrogen, after birth, 296, 336
Estrogen, effects of
  migraines, 17
  mood swings, 28
  on sexual desire, 75, 336
  on sleep quality, 15
  pregnancy sickness, 13
  skin changes, 70, 188
Exams, infant
  newborn, 275, 277
  for problems, 358
  well-baby, 93, 202–3, 309, 352
Exams, maternal, 11
  first trimester, 7, 18, 37–38,
    44–46
  internal, 38, 113, 224, 226,
    302
  postpartum, 279, 302
  pre-pregnancy, 2
  scheduling, 90
  second trimester, 113–18
  third trimester, 161, 175, 222
  See also Caregivers
Exercise, 63–69
  with bedrest, 145
  and diabetes, 77
  first trimester, 15, 17, 103
  with multiple fetuses, 79
  myths regarding, 69, 187,
    334
  postpartum, 296, 302,
    329–34
  pre-pregnancy, 3
  second trimester, 103,
    128–32
  and smoking cessation, 28
  third trimester, 164, 165,
    184,186
  and varicose veins, 104
  walking as, 15, 17, 65, 68,
    69, 103, 186, 329, 330
  and weight, 54, 66, 68
Exercise classes
  postnatal, 298, 330, 334
  prenatal, 67i, 69, 112
  selection of, 68
  as support group, 34, 298
Exercises, 129–33, 130i, 132i
  Kegels, 132–33
  pelvic tilts, 105, 132, 145,
    164

  postpartum, 329, 331i–33i
  yoga, 264, 265, 330
  See also Breathing techniques

Fallopian tubes, 38
  and conception, 5i, 6
  and ectopic pregnancy,
    83i–84
False labor, 167–68, 228
Families and Work Institute, 199
Family history
  of birth defects, 37, 44,
    115–16
  and diabetes, 114–15
Family Medical Leave Act, 88, 91
Family practitioner (FP), 36
Fathers
  and hazardous substances, 3
  for labor, 199, 247–48, 252
  postpartum, 248, 342
  prenatal, 174–75
  and sexual activity, 140–41
  as support, 220
Fatigue
  first trimester, 7, 8–9, 15–16,
    29
  postpartum, 291, 296–97,
    308–10
  second trimester, 102
  third trimester, 164
Fertility, 2, 3, 21
Fertility drugs, 10, 78, 84, 113
Fetal alcohol syndrome (FAS), 20
Fetal death, 21, 86, 191
Fetal distress
  causes of, 193–94, 240–41
  monitoring for, 227, 238
  symptoms of, 223, 240–41
Fetal fibronectin (fFN) test, 116
Fetal kick test, 162
Fetal monitoring
  and biophysical profile, 176
  and Cesarean delivery, 227
  during labor, 226–27, 240,
    256
  with epidural, 225, 256, 259
  for postterm pregnancy, 193
  preferences for, 177, 227
  and preterm labor, 144
  routine, 45, 151
Fetoscopy, 43, 102

Fetus
  age of, 11, 41
  first trimester, 6i–8, 7i
  in utero learning by, 157
  position of, 161i–62i,
    175–76, 195, 268
  second trimester, 99–102,
    101i
  third trimester, 159–61i, 160i
Fetus, gender of
  and amniocentesis, 47, 115,
    173
  and chorionic villus sampling
    (CVS), 47, 173
  myths regarding, 26, 74, 137,
    166, 173
  and name selection, 95,
    150–51
  and ultrasound, 8, 41, 100,
    101i, 151, 173–74
Fever, maternal
  as danger signal, 16, 25, 80,
    294
  in first trimester, 18, 25–26
  postpartum, 294, 308, 309
Fibroids, 78, 143
Finances, 34–35, 89
Flu shots, 25–26, 90
Fluid intake, 180
  and amniotic fluid, 67
  and digestive system, 103,
    165
  in early labor, 223, 232
  and exercise, 67
  postpartum, 290, 307, 313,
    324
  and preterm labor, 144, 165
  requirements for, 60
Folate
  as B vitamin, 59
  importance of, 3, 7, 50
  pre-pregnancy, 78
  requirement for, 3, 57, 59
Fontanels, 275, 353
Food pyramid, 49, 50, 118–19i
Forceps-assisted delivery, 242i,
  251, 257, 258, 259
Formula. See Bottle feeding
Friends
  advice from, 94, 112–13
  pregnant peers as, 31, 34

Friends (cont.)
   present at birth, 178, 204–5
   when to tell, 32, 87–88,
      96–97
Fruity Spritzer, 55
Gassiness, 17–18, 51, 292
Gastric reflux, 165, 180
Genetic counseling, 18, 44, 170
Genetic-defect disorders
   detection of, 40–41, 47,
      115–16
   risk factors for, 44
German measles. See Rubella
Gingivitis, pregnancy, 107
Glucose screen
   and gestational diabetes, 101,
      114–15, 142–43
   reliability of, 87

Hair, and dyes/perms, 24, 70–71
Headaches
   and anxiety, 113
   as danger signal, 25, 191
   medication for, 17, 22
   migraine, 17, 85
Healthy Tuna Pockets, 122
Hearing defects, 19, 20, 175
Heart defects, 18
Heartbeat, fetal
   first trimester, 8, 10, 41, 42
   See also Fetal monitoring
Heartburn, 17, 102–3, 109, 180
Hemophilia, 44
Hemorrhage, 21, 84
Hemorrhoids, 46, 103, 290
Heparin lock, 226
Hepatitis B virus (HBV), 114, 352
Hepatitis C virus, 39
Herbs
   in medicines, 14
   in teas, 46, 57, 103, 359
Herpes simplex, 19, 40, 76, 268
Herpes zoster, 19
High-risk pregnancy, 76–80
   caregivers for, 36, 37
   insurance coverage for, 93
   and maternal deaths, 218
   monitoring of, 38, 222, 225
   and obesity, 52
   resources for, 85
   and sexual abstinence, 76

HIV (human immunodeficiency
      virus), and RhoGAM, 39
Home births, 246–47
   in history, 220
   medical backup for, 37
   resource for, 272
Hospital bag
   contents of, 204, 211–12
   readiness of, 161, 168, 204,
      232
Hospitals, 35
   birthing rooms in, 37, 225
   labor procedures in, 225–28
   routine, 45, 151, 153,
      217
   length of stay in, 179,
      280–81, 283
   newborn security in, 282–83
   preregistration at, 160, 204,
      224
   tours of, 153, 170
Hot tubs/hot baths, 2, 21, 166
Household help, 206, 281, 292
Human chorionic gonadotrophin
      (hCG)
   blood tests for, 9–10, 33–34,
      81, 100, 114
   and metabolism, 67
   and pregnancy sickness, 13
   and urinalysis, 39
Humidifiers, 17, 25, 208
Hyperactivity, 20
Hyperemesis gravidarum, 15
Hypertension
   and calcium, 59
   and exercise, 68
   indications of, 17, 25, 38
   and induced labor, 239
   monitoring of, 77
   and placenta abruptio, 192
   risk factors for, 52, 78
   and sodium, 120, 191
   See also Preeclampsia
Hypnosis, 178, 254

Ibuprofen, 17, 22, 278, 289, 310
Immunizations, 2, 18–19, 25–26,
      90
In utero treatment, 44
In vitro fertilization, 26
Incontinence, 132, 165, 290

Indigestion
   acid. See Heartburn
   causes of, 17, 103, 113
   remedies for, 17–18, 103
Induced labor, 45
   for diabetics, 239
   for postterm pregnancy, 193
   and ruptured membrane,
      223, 240
Infant car seat, 204, 212
Infant phobia, 171
Infections, maternal
   and breastfeeding, 308–9
   cervical, 81
   detection of, 116
   first trimester, 18–19, 25–26
   hepatitis B, 114
   postpartum, 294, 308–9
   streptococcus, 161, 175
   of tooth, 107
   toxoplasmosis, 19, 23, 26,
      26–27, 116
Inherited disorders, 2, 44, 277
   See also Genetic-defect
      disorders
Insomnia, 113, 164, 297
Insurance
   and caregivers, 92, 200
   disability, 150
   employer obligation for, 91
   and hospital stay, 280–81
   learning about, 88, 92
   managed care plans, 92,
      115
   and pediatric care, 93, 203
   and prenatal tests, 42, 46,
      92,115
International Childbirth Educa-
      tion Association (ICEA),
      153, 154
Intrauterine growth retardation,
      53
Intravenous lines, 225–26
   with epidurals, 259
   for fluids, 15, 144, 177, 249
   for medications, 240, 255,
      268
   routine, 45, 177
Inverted nipples, 201, 309
Involution, 278, 279, 288–89
Iodine, 3

Iron
absorption of, 127, 180
deficiency in, 16, 40
function of, 50, 59
in infant formula, 314
need for, 57, 59, 60
sources of, 59, 120, 180

Jaundice, 358
and bilirubin, 318–19, 352
and cytomegalovirus, 19
and Rh factor, 39

Kegel, Arnold, 132
Kegel exercise, 132–33
and bedrest, 145
for incontinence, 165, 290
instructions for, 132
near due date, 186, 242
postpartum, 290, 329, 340
Ketonuria, 53

La Leche League, 201, 213, 303, 322
Labor, 231i, 248–49
abnormal, 268
back, 166–67, 254
and birth plan, 160, 176, 177–79, 219
early symptoms of, 221–24, 228–29, 230–31i, 250
fear of, 170, 217–18
hospital procedures for, 45, 151, 153, 225–28
length of, 221, 230, 240, 244–46
positions for, 178, 233i–34, 240
relaxation techniques for, 226, 232
stage one. See Dilatation
stage two. See Delivery
See also Induced labor;
Preterm labor; Transition
Lactation amenorrhea, 341
Lactation Consultant Association, International, 322
Lactose intolerance, 127
Lamaze method, 85, 152, 154, 254
Lanugo, 100, 101, 161

Le Boyer birth method, 237
Lead-based paint, 22, 90, 156, 157
Learning difficulties, 19, 258
Learning disabilities, 20
Legal issues
birth certificate, 277
hospital stay, 283
infant car seat, 212
medical leave, 91
pregnancy discrimination, 32, 94, 150
will, 96
Leukorrhea, 16
Lightening, 163–64, 169, 222
Linea negra, 187
Lochia
with C-section, 279
danger signs for, 293–94, 330
description of, 278, 288
and sexual activity, 341
Low birthweight, factors in
blood pressure, 77
infections, 27
nutrition, 53
prematurity, 79
smoking, 20

Magnesium, 105
Mammograms, 2, 21
Managed care plans, 92, 115
March of Dimes, 28, 361
Marijuana, 21
Massage, 152, 177, 253–54, 263
Mastitis, 308–9
Maternity centers. See Birthing centers
Meconium
description of, 161
and fetal stress, 223, 241
inhalation of, 193, 275
and newborn, 316, 348
Medications
for acne, 3, 22, 70
for allergies, 85
antidepressant, 85, 297
antiepileptic, 78
anti-inflammatory (NSAIDS), 22
anti-nausea, 14–15
and breastfeeding, 310

evaluation of, 7, 10, 24, 46
as hazards, 3, 17
for headache, 17, 22
for migraines, 85
over the counter, 22, 24, 50, 103
prescription, 24, 69–70, 85
Mediterranean Couscous Casserole, 121
Melanocyte-stimulating hormone, 187
Membranes. See Amniotic sac
Menstrual cycle
and breastfeeding, 319
and conception, 6, 8, 10
and due date, 11, 12
postpartum, 200
Mental development, 20
Mental retardation, 20, 175
Microwaves, 26, 312, 315
Midwives. See Certified nurse-midwives
Migraines, 17, 85
Minestrone Soup, 124–25
Miscarriage, 8
anxiety about, 29–30, 33–34, 96
multiple, 44, 68, 78
resources for, 86
Miscarriage, risk factors for
diabetes, 2, 77
high fever, 18
prenatal tests, 42–43, 47
previous miscarriage, 42
Rh factor, 39, 40
toxic substances, 3, 20, 24, 49
Miscarriage
and sexual activity, 76
spontaneous, 81–83, 144–45
symptoms of, 25, 80, 82
telling others of, 32, 82, 96–97
and video display terminals, 93
Montgomery's tubercles, 69
Mood swings. See Emotional changes
Morning sickness. See Pregnancy sickness
Mothers of Supertwins, 86

Movements, fetal
decline in, 167, 176, 229
and fetal kick test, 162
hiccups, 101
monitoring, 243
second trimester, 100, 101,
106–7, 109
third trimester, 160, 162
and ultrasound, 41
Mucus plug, 144, 164, 222
Multiple births
epidural for, 255, 272
monitoring of, 225
resources for, 86
Multiple fetuses, 79i, 86–87
caregivers for, 36
detection of, 11, 41, 42, 78, 115
exercise with, 68
factors favoring, 84
fraternal vs. identical, 79–80
and maternal age, 78, 84
risks with, 78–79, 88
sexual activity with, 76
weight change with, 52, 53
Muscular dystrophy, 44

Name selection, 94–95, 150–51,
277
Narcotics, 177, 251, 255–57
Nasal congestion, 17, 25
National Association for the
Education of Young Chil-
dren, 149
National Association of
Childbearing Centers, 48
National Center for Health
Statistics, 221
National Institute for Occupa-
tional Safety and Health,
89
National Organization for Single
Mothers, 35
National Organization of
Circumcision Information
Resource Centers, 213
National Organization of Mothers
of Twins Clubs, 86
Natural childbirth
at birthing centers, 37
Bradley Method for, 152–53,
264

as choice, 220
and fetal monitoring, 227
home births, 37, 246–47, 272
intravenous line for, 225–26
and Lamaze, 152
and pain management,
250–51
Nausea
during labor, 234, 248–49
from prenatal vitamins, 60
as symptom, 18, 294, 308
See also Pregnancy sickness
Nervous system, fetal, 7, 21, 27,
41
Neural tube defects
causes of, 2, 21, 50
diagnosis of, 47, 114
and folic acid, 3, 59
New Ways to Work, 199
Newborn
common concerns with,
353–57
fear of, 171
immediate access to, 176,
178, 238, 269, 275
insurance coverage for, 93,
203
myths regarding, 281–82,
359–60
and rooming in, 179, 283
skin problems of, 354–58,
359
weight of, 110, 161, 179,
316, 359
See also Bonding with baby
Newborn care, 283–84, 361–62
away from home, 351
bathing, 208, 349–51, 350i
burping, 315i
crying and colic, 328,
344–45, 358–60
diapering, 210, 348, 354
dressing, 210, 347–48
learning about, 153
resources for, 361
sleeping habits, 342–44, 360
swaddling, 345–46i, 345–46,
358
See also Exams, infant
Nicotine. See Smoking
Nilsson, Lennart, 31

Nosebleeds, 17
Nurse-practitioners, 35
Nursery
furnishings for, 155–57,
207–10
necessities for, 169, 206,
207–10
preparation of, 109, 150,
169, 224
Nurses, labor and delivery
dissatisfaction with, 229–30
as labor support, 36, 225
thanking, 239
Nutrition, fetal, 14, 48–49, 53,
54,180
Nutrition, infant
and breastfeeding, 200
criteria for, 309, 316
Nutrition, maternal
and food pyramid, 49, 50,
118–19i
postpartum, 296, 310,
323–24
pre-pregnancy, 3
See also Diet
Nutritionists, 53, 54, 181

Obstetrician-gynecologist, 35–36
in group practice, 116
in labor and delivery, 225
and pre-pregnancy exam, 2
resource for, 48
See also Caregivers
Orange and Ginger Rice Pudding,
327– 28
Organs, fetal
development of, 7–8, 15,
48–49, 101, 180
risks to, 18, 89–90
Oriental-Style Brown Rice Salad,
326–27
Osteoporosis, 200
Ovaries, 5i, 6, 15, 38
Overheating, 18, 21–22, 66, 67
Ovulation, 6, 8, 11, 84, 200
Oxygen supply, fetal, 21, 66,
240–41
and prolapsed cord, 224, 243
Oxytocin
and contractions, 239, 240
pitocin, 176, 240, 251, 269

release of, 176, 190, 278, 289
and sexual activity, 139

Pacifiers, 179, 202, 277, 319
Pain management, 45
choice in, 176, 177–78, 220, 267
medical, 255–59, 256i, 258i
nonmedical, 251–55, 264–65
resources for, 154, 263
See also Childbirth classes
Pap smears, 36, 39
Parasites, 19, 23, 27
Parenting, learning about, 298
Pediatrician
and newborn care, 44, 275–76, 277
selection of, 160, 202–4
when to call, 358
Pelvic inflammatory disease, 84
Percutaneous umbilical blood sampling (PUBS), 116
Perineum
postpartum, 278, 289–90
stretching of, 178, 237, 241–42
See also Episiotomies
Pesticides, 3, 22
Phenylketonuria (PKU), 23, 277
Physicians, 35–37
in group practice, 116
and pre-pregnancy exam, 2
See also Caregivers
Pitocin, 176, 240, 251, 269
Placenta, 41
delivery of, 230, 235, 239, 293
and fetal distress, 240
first trimester, 6–7, 15
hormone production by, 9, 114
location of, 115
second trimester, 100
third trimester, 191–92, 193
weight of, 51, 53, 110i
Placenta abruptio, 21, 78–79, 81, 191, 192, 268
Placenta previa, 76, 81, 191–92i, 268
Placental tears, 81

Postpartum Assistance for Mothers, 299
Postpartum Support International, 299
Postterm pregnancy, 161, 176, 193, 194–95
Posture, 128, 164, 185–86
Potassium, 61, 291
Preeclampsia, 190–91
Cesarean delivery for, 268
and exercise, 68
indications of, 191, 193
blood pressure, 38, 77
edema, 166, 184
urinalysis, 39
Pregnancy and Infant Loss Center, 86
Pregnancy Discrimination Act, 91
Pregnancy journal, 31
Pregnancy sickness
first trimester, 9, 13–16, 29, 49, 60–61, 70
myths regarding, 26
second trimester, 102, 127, 139
Pregnancy tests
at doctor's office, 10, 38, 82
home test, 7, 9–10i, 38, 81
Premature birth, 193–94
and blood pressure, 77
and folic acid, 59
frequency of, 193
and hazardous substances, 20, 21
and infections, 27, 39
of multiple fetuses, 79
and respiratory problems, 161, 194
and severe stress, 93
Preservatives, food, 23
Preterm labor, 222
detection of, 116, 143–44
folate to prevent, 59
history of
and exercise, 68
and sexual activity, 76
risk factors for, 143
dehydration, 60
excess weight gain, 52
multiple fetuses, 79
severe stress, 93

treatment for, 34, 144
Progesterone
after delivery, 296
effects of
on digestion, 17
heartburn, 103
on ligaments, 104
mood swings, 28
sedative, 15
on sexual desire, 75
skin changes, 70
and pregnancy sickness, 13
Prolactin, 106
Prostaglandin, 240
Pubic shaves, 45, 220, 227
Pubococcygeus (PC) muscle, 132–33

Quesadillas, 326
Quick Apple Crumble, 184
Quickening, 100, 106
See also Movements, fetal

Recipes, 55–57, 121–25, 181–84, 325–28
Relatives
advice from, 30
present at birth, 178, 204–5
when to tell, 32
Relaxation, 173, 298–99
Relaxation techniques, 173
in childbirth classes, 152
during labor, 226, 232, 234, 251
imagery, 128–29, 152
meditation, 85, 129, 178
practicing, 160, 170
progressive, 128–29
touch/massage, 128–29, 152, 253, 261
visualization, 152–53, 238, 253
Relaxin, 66, 104, 128
Respiratory problems, 161, 194
Rh factor, 39–40, 116, 275, 278
Rh immunoglobulin (RhIg), 102
brand names for, 39–40, 278
Rooming in, 179, 277, 283
Round ligament pain, 166
Rubella, 2, 18–19, 40

Salmon Cakes, 182–83
Salmonella, 23
Salt, 120, 125, 128, 191
Sexual activity, 74–76
 abstinence from, 76
 cervical abrasion from, 80–81
 and episiotomy, 249
 and Kegel exercise, 133
 myths regarding, 76, 142,
  190
 positions for, 138i, 139i
 postpartum, 302, 335–36,
  340–42
 second trimester, 138–42
 third trimester, 190
Sexually transmitted diseases
 (STDs), 19, 39, 40, 76
Shingles, 19
Shortness of breath, 166
Siblings, 171
 adjustment of to baby, 32–33
 classes for, 154
 as gradual process, 301–2
 during Mom's pregnancy
  activities with, 15
  anxieties about, 171
  lifting of, 108, 186i
 present at birth, 178, 205
 temporary care for, 205
Sickle-cell anemia, 41, 44, 277
Sidelines National Support Net-
 work, 85
SIDS Alliance, 361
Single mothers, 34–35
Sitz baths, 278, 389–90
Skin changes, 70, 187–88
Sleep, quality of, 15, 29, 102,
 164, 171–72
Sleep deprivation, 291, 301, 336
 and insomnia, 113, 164, 297
Sleeping positions, 107–8
Smoke, passive, 3
Smoking, 103
 as risk factor, 20–21, 50,
  143
 stopping, 2–3, 27–28
Social Security number, 277
Sonogram. See Ultrasound
Sperm, 3, 5–6
Spider veins, 187
Spina bifida, 3, 44, 114

Spinach and Ricotta Lasagna,
 325–26
Spinal cord defects, 50
Station, minus or plus, 226
Steroids, 22, 77
Stillbirth
 resource for, 86
 risk factors for
  diabetes, 77
  previous stillbirth, 44
  Rh factor, 40
  toxoplasmosis, 27
  unexpected, 243–44
Stirrups, 225, 228
Strawberry marks, 185, 356
Streptococcus, Group B, 161,
 175
Stress, emotional
 avoidance of, 78
 and miscarriage, 93
 and ovulation, 8
 and pregnancy sickness, 13
 See also Anxiety
Stretch marks, 188, 189
Sudden infant death syndrome
 (SIDS), 20, 343
Sugar
 in diet, 15, 126
 in urine, 39
Supplements, dietary
 calcium, 105, 127
 folic acid, 3
 hazards in, 3, 23, 121, 127
 iron, 16, 40, 60
 magnesium, 105
 with multiple fetuses, 79
 prenatal vitamins, 18, 40,
  60, 127, 180, 329
Support, labor, 200, 219, 225
 See also Caregivers; Coach
Support network
 postpartum, 206, 248, 298,
  361–62
  for depression, 296, 297
  online, 194, 300
 prenatal, 87, 171
  national, 85
  online, 31, 34, 146, 195
  resources for, 299
 See also Household help
Sweet-Potato Chips, 56

Swelling
 as danger signal, 17, 25, 184,
  191
 and fluid retention, 120, 166,
  184

Tanning booths, 22
Tay-Sachs disease, 41, 44
Teas, 50, 58, 128
Teas, herbal, 46, 57, 103, 359
Testing, prenatal, 8
 first trimester, 38–44, 46–47,
  48
 reliability of, 11, 118
 risks in, 42–43, 47, 48,
  116
 second trimester, 100, 101,
  111, 113–18
 third trimester, 161, 175–76
 See also Blood tests
Thalassemia, 44
Thirstiness, 16, 60, 166, 223
Thrush, 308, 356
Thyroid defects, 3, 277
Tocolytics, 144
Toxemia. See Preeclampsia
Toxoplasmosis, 19, 23, 26–27,
 116
Transcutaneous electrical nerve
 stimulation (TENS), 254
Transition, 234–38
 coaching for, 262
 pain relief for
  medical, 255, 257, 259
  nonmedical, 252–55
 vomiting during, 248
Transverse position, 163i, 268
Traveling, 94, 109, 154
The Triplet Connection, 86
Twin Services, 86
Twins. See Multiple fetuses

Ultrasound
 as alternative to X-rays, 21
 and biophysical profile, 176
 and due date, 11, 100, 115,
  117
 and fetal gender, 8, 41, 100,
  101i, 151, 173, 173–74
 first trimester, 41i–43
 and fetal heartbeat, 10

and miscarriage, 34, 81, 82
insurance payment for, 92
limitations of, 117, 151, 174
and multiple fetuses, 78
for preterm labor, 144
second trimester, 100
diagnostic, 114, 115
and fetal movement, 109
third trimester, 193
diagnostic, 191–92
and fetal position, 162,
175
vaginal, 41–42
See also Doppler
Umbilical cord
around neck, 237, 240, 275
blood tests from, 116, 275
blood transfusion to, 40
cutting, 178, 216i, 237
first trimester, 7
myth regarding, 108
prolapsed, 224, 243
second trimester, 100
Umbilical cord blood, 196
Umbilical hernia, 360
Umbilical stump, 348–49, 350
U.S. Department of Agriculture
(USDA), 50, 118
U.S. Department of Labor, 197
U.S. Environmental Protection
Agency (EPA), 20
U.S. Food and Drug Administration (FDA), 26, 59, 291
Unplanned pregnancy, 29, 34–35
Urinalysis, 39, 48, 113
Urinary tract infection (UTI)
and breastfeeding, 200
diagnosis of, 39
and pregnancy tests, 10
symptoms of, 16
Urination
frequent
first trimester, 7, 8–9, 16,
60
postpartum, 290
painful, 16, 19, 80, 294
third trimester, 164, 165,
171–72

Uterus, 41
first trimester, 5i, 6–8, 16, 38,
83i
growth of, 11, 84, 161
postpartum, 200, 278,
279, 288, 302
prolapsed, 132
second trimester, 102, 103,
104, 113
weight of, 51, 53, 110i, 165
See also Contractions

Vacuum extraction, 242–43i,
257, 258, 259
Vaginal birth after Cesarean
(VBAC), 220, 221, 227,
271–72, 274
Vaginal discharge, 16, 143
mucus plug as, 144, 164,
222
See also Bleeding; Lochia
Vaginal infection, 16, 39
Varicose veins, 52, 104, 187
Vegetarianism, 3, 61–62, 329
Vernix, 100, 161, 237, 275
Vertex position, 162i
Video display terminals (VDTs),
93
Videotaping birth, 249
Vision, maternal, changes in, 25,
106, 191
Vision defects, 20, 175
Vitamins
vitamin B complex, 180
vitamin C, 23, 59, 180, 323,
324
vitamin E, 189
See also Supplements
Vomiting
as danger signal, 25, 294
during transition, 248
See also Pregnancy sickness

Water
contaminated, 24, 314–15
laboring in, 178, 225, 231,
254
and lead-lined pipes, 22

well, 314–15
See also Fluid intake
Water breaking. *See* Amniotic sac
Weekly highlights
first trimester, 6–8
second trimester, 99–102
third trimester, 159–61
Weight, baseline, 38
and exercise, 68
food journal for, 54
and gestational diabetes, 3,
52, 54, 114
overweight, 62–63
underweight, 3, 52, 68
Weight change, 51–54, 66
as danger signal, 191
first trimester, 14, 15, 52, 102
with multiple fetuses, 52, 79
myth regarding, 137
postpartum, 53, 302,
322–21, 334–35
second trimester, 102,
109–11, 117
third trimester
distribution of, 110i
peak of, 161, 175
rate of, 160, 180, 184–85
White Beans Provençal, 182
Whole Wheat Pizza, 123–24
Women's Bureau, U.S. Department of Commerce, 94,
199
Workplace, 87–91, 196–98
alternatives for, 197–98
discrimination in, 32, 94,
150
resources for, 94, 199
stress level in, 93
survival kit for, 149
See also Employer; Friends

X-rays, 2, 20, 90, 107

Yoga, 264, 265, 330
Yogurt Fruit Smoothie, 55

Zinc, 57, 59
Zygote, 6

ABOUT THE AUTHOR

PAULA SPENCER is a contributing editor of PARENTING Magazine. She writes about women's health, children, and family issues for many national magazines. A graduate of the University of Iowa, she worked as a magazine editor in New York City and as an editorial director of Whittle Communications before becoming a freelance writer. She lives in Knoxville, Tennessee, with her husband, George, and their three children.